Contemporary Feminisms in Social Work Practice

T0262859

Contemporary Feminisms in Social Work Practice explores feminism as core to social work knowledge, practice and ethics. It demonstrates how gender-neutral perspectives and practices obscure gender discourses and power relations. It also shows feminist social work practice can transform areas of social work not specifically concerned with gender, through its emphasis on relationships and power.

Within and outside feminism, there is a growing assumption that equality has been won and is readily available to all women. However, women continue to dominate the ranks of the poor in developed and developing countries around the world; male perpetrated violence against women and children has not reduced; women outnumber men by up to three to one in the diagnosis of common mental health problems; and women continue to be severely underrepresented in every realm of power, decision making and wealth. This worrying context draws attention to the ways gender relations structure most of the problems faced by the women, men and children in the day-to-day worlds in which social work operates. Drawing together key contemporary thinking about feminism and its place in social work, this international collection looks both at core curriculum areas taught in social work programmes and at a wide range of practice fields that involve key challenges and opportunities for future feminist social work.

This book is suitable for all social work students and academics. It examines the nuanced nature of power relationships in the everyday and areas such as working with cross-cultural communities, mental health, interpersonal violence and abuse, homelessness, child protection, ageing, disability and sexuality.

Sarah Wendt is a Professor of Social Work at Flinders University, South Australia.

Nicole Moulding is a Senior Lecturer in social work at the University of South Australia.

Routledge Advances in Social Work

New titles

Analysing Social Work Communication
Discourse in practice
Edited by Christopher Hall, Kirsi Juhila, Maureen Matarese and Carolus van Nijnatten

Feminisms in Social Work Research
Promise and possibilities for justice-based knowledge
Edited by Stéphanie Wahab, Ben Anderson-Nathe and Christina Gringeri

Chronic Illness, Vulnerability and Social Work
Autoimmunity and the contemporary disease experience
Liz Walker and Elizabeth Price

Social Work in a Global Context
Issues and challenges
Edited by George Palattiyil, Dina Sidhva and Mono Chakrabarti

Contemporary Feminisms in Social Work Practice
Edited by Sarah Wendt and Nicole Moulding

Forthcoming titles

Domestic Violence Perpetrators
Evidence-informed responses
John Devaney, Anne Lazenbatt and Maurice Mahon

Transnational Social Work and Social Welfare
Challenges for the social work profession
Edited by Ursula Kämmerer-Rütten, Alexandra Schleyer-Lindemann, Beatrix Schwarzer and Yafang Wang

Responsibilization at the Margins of Welfare Services
Edited by Kirsi Juhila, Suvi Raitakari and Christopher Hall

Contemporary Feminisms in Social Work Practice

Edited by
Sarah Wendt and
Nicole Moulding

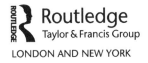
Routledge
Taylor & Francis Group

LONDON AND NEW YORK

First published 2016
by Routledge
2 Park Square, Milton Park, Abingdon, Oxon OX14 4RN

and by Routledge
711 Third Avenue, New York, NY 10017

First issued in paperback 2017

Routledge is an imprint of the Taylor & Francis Group, an informa business

British Library Cataloguing-in-Publication Data
A catalogue record for this book is available from the British Library

Library of Congress Cataloging in Publication Data
Contemporary feminisms in social work practice / edited by Sarah
Wendt and Nicole Moulding.
    p. ; cm.
    Includes bibliographical references and index.
    I. Wendt, Sarah, editor. II. Moulding, Nicole, editor.
    [DNLM: 1. Social Work–methods. 2. Feminism. 3. Interpersonal
    Relations. 4. Women's Rights. HV 41]
    HD6955
    306.3'6–dc23   2015031117

ISBN 13: 978-1-138-49453-4 (pbk)
ISBN 13: 978-1-138-02570-7 (hbk)

Typeset in Baskerville
by Wearset Ltd, Boldon, Tyne and Wear

Contents

Contributors

Margaret Alston is Head of Department of Social Work at Monash University where she has also established the Gender, Leadership and Social Sustainability (GLASS) research unit. Prior to commencing at Monash she was Professor of Social Work and Human Services and Director of the Centre for Rural Social Research at Charles Sturt University. She is a Foundation Fellow of the Australian College of Social Workers and is past-Chair of the Australian Council of Heads of Schools of Social Work. She has published widely in the field of rural gender and rural social issues. She has acted as a gender expert for UN–Habitat in Kenya, the Food and Agricultural Organisation in Rome, UNESCO in the Pacific and UNEP in Geneva. She received her Medal of the Order of Australia in 2010 for services to social work and the advancement of women, particularly in rural areas.

Lia Bryant is Associate Professor of Social Work and Sociology and Director, Centre for Social Change in the School of Psychology, Social Work and Social Policy, University of South Australia, Australia. She has published widely on research methodologies, gender and rural communities covering emotions, sexuality, suicide, embodiment, work and intersectionality. Her most recent books are L. Bryant and K. Jaworski, *Women Supervising and Writing Doctoral Theses, Walking on the Grass* (Lexington Books, 2015); and L. Bryant (ed.) *Critical and Creative Research Methodologies in Social Work* (Ashgate, 2015).

Fiona Buchanan is a Lecturer in the School of Psychology, Social Work and Social Policy at the University of South Australia. After working for many years as a social worker in community health and feminist non-government agencies in the UK and in Australia she completed her PhD at Flinders University: 'The effects of domestic violence on the relationships between women and their babies: beyond attachment theory'. Her research has focused on violence against women, mothering, child wellbeing and growing up with domestic violence. She applies a critical lens to the application of dominant discourses which operate across disciplines in health, welfare and child/family centred services.

Noël Busch-Armendariz is a Professor and the Associate Dean for Research at the School of Social Work, the University of Texas at Austin. She is also the director of the Institute on Domestic Violence and Sexual Assault (IDVSA), a collaboration of the Schools of Social Work, Nursing, and Law, and the Bureau for Business Research with more than 150 affiliate community organisations. Her areas of specialisation are human trafficking, domestic violence, sexual assault and campus sexual assault, refugees, asylees and international social work. She is regularly called as an expert witness in criminal (including the prosecution of human trafficking), civil and federal cases (including immigration and Hague cases) and directs statewide and national training on the topic. She serves as editor-in-chief of *AFFILIA: The Journal of Women and Social Work*. She is under contract with Sage, Inc. to author a textbook on human trafficking.

Jill Chonody is an Associate Professor of Social Work at Indiana University Northwest and adjunct research fellow at University of South Australia. She is a former social work practitioner in mental health and researches issues related to ageism, sexism, social work education issues, and creative techniques for research and practice. Her book, *Community Art: Creative Approaches to Practice* (Common Ground Publishing LLC, 2014), explores alternative ways to engage in social work practice.

Laurie Cook Heffron is a Harrington Fellow and doctoral candidate at the University of Texas at Austin and Associate Director for Research at UT-Austin's Institute on Domestic Violence and Sexual Assault (IDVSA). She has both direct social work practice and research experience related to domestic violence, sexual violence and human trafficking, and with a variety of communities, including refugees, asylum-seekers and other immigrant communities. She serves as a pro bono expert witness in immigration cases of immigrant women and children seeking T visas, U visas and asylum based on domestic violence. Her current research explores the experiences of, and relationships between, violence against women and migration, with a focus on migration from Central America to the United States.

Lena Dominelli holds a Chair in the School of Applied Social Sciences and is Co-Director at the Institute of Hazards, Risk and Resilience Research at Durham University, UK, where she Heads the Programme on Vulnerability and Resilience. She has recently completed major research projects for the Economic and Social Research Council. She has published widely in social work, social policy and sociology and several of her books have become classics and have been translated into many languages. She was elected President of the International Association of Schools of Social Work (IASSW) from 1996 to 2004, and is currently chairing the IASSW Committee on Disaster Interventions, Climate

Change and Sustainability. She has also been the recipient of various honours including a medal in 2002 for her contribution to social work given by the Social Affairs Committee of the French Senate, an honorary doctorate in 2008 from the University of KwaZulu-Natal in Durban, South Africa, and the Katherine A Kendall Memorial Award in 2012.

Lake Dziengel is an Assistant Professor in Social Work at the University of Minnesota Duluth, USA. He is a life long social work educator and practitioner, with primary research interests in sexual minorities and ageing, medical social work, grief and loss, anti-oppressive practice and social justice. He is the author of publications on resilience and ambiguous loss in older same sex couples, gender identity, Be/Coming Out, policy processes in securing civil protections for sexual minorities, and co-author on the resilience factors for older same sex couples in long term relationships.

Barbara Fawcett is Professor of Social Work (Adults and Communities) in the Department of Social Policy and Social Work at the University of Birmingham, UK. Previously she was Professor of Social Work and Policy Studies at the University of Sydney, Australia. She has authored and co-authored nine books and numerous journal articles. Her areas of research include postmodern feminism, mental health, 'disability' and research methodology.

Christine Fejo-King is an Aboriginal woman from Australia's Northern Territory and a senior Larrakia Elder. She has been a social worker for 34 years and worked in mental health, substance misuse, palliative care, child protection, juvenile justice, family and individual counselling, mentoring, course development, education, community development and reconciliation. She was very involved in the National Apology to Australia's Indigenous Peoples in 2008, as Co-Chair of the Stolen Generations Alliance. She is the current Chairperson of the National Coalition of Aboriginal and Torres Strait Islander Social Workers and continues to consult and publish widely on Indigenous social work.

Mel Gray is Professor of Social Work in the School of Humanities and Social Science at the University of Newcastle in New South Wales, Australia. Her wide-ranging research interests include social work, social policy and social development. Her most recent research focus, and contribution, has been in the complex areas of knowledge production, research use and evidence-based practice in social work and the human services. Theory and knowledge for practice, including culturally relevant knowledge along with the influence of global forces, such as neo-liberalism, on local welfare and development, are constant themes in her research.

Lynn Jamieson is a Professor of Sociology in the School of Social and Political Science at the University of Edinburgh, Scotland. She is also a researcher at the Centre for Research on Families and Relationships (CRFR). Her research has focused on intimacy, historical and cultural shifts in practices of intimacy, and globalisation and personal life. She has also researched sexuality, sexual offences and gender violence, and relationships and 'othering'. She has published numerous books on these topics.

Sue King is a Board Member of several not for profit organisations including the human service organisations Uniting Communities and Summerhill Aged Care Inc. She is an active member of the Australian Association of Social Workers and a member of the National Research Committee and the South Australian Social Justice Committee. As a member of the University of South Australia Centre for Social Change, her research interests are in the impact of social policy on the delivery of human services, the governance of human service organisations and the conceptualisation of workers.

Lesley Laing is Associate Professor in Social Work and Policy Studies at the University of Sydney, Australia, where her research and teaching focus on violence against women and children. Grounded in feminist theories and research methodologies, her research is collaborative and privileges the voices of those most vitally affected by public policy – the victim/survivors of violence and the practitioners who work with them. She was the founding Director of the Australian Domestic and Family Violence Clearinghouse and the NSW Health Education Centre against Violence. She is currently a member of the NSW Domestic Violence Death Review Team.

Nicole Moulding is a Senior Lecturer in social work at the University of South Australia, with research and teaching interests in gender and mental health, in particular gendered violence, abuse and mental health. She has worked as a researcher and educator in social work and public health for almost 20 years and, prior to this, was a professional social worker in women's health. Her published research includes a sole-authored book entitled *Gendered Violence, Mental Health and Recovery in Everyday Lives: Beyond Trauma* (Routledge, 2016), and a substantial body of journal articles about gender and mental health, including feminist social work approaches to practice in this area. Her most recent research explores the gendered dimensions of childhood emotional abuse and the implications for women's mental health.

Maura Nsonwu is an Associate Professor, Interim BSW Director and former Associate Chair in the Department of Sociology and Social Work at North Carolina Agricultural and Technical State University, USA. She has practised as a clinician, educator and researcher in the areas of refugee resettlement, human trafficking, health care, child welfare and social work education for 30 years. She has received external funding and produced numerous publications in this area of inquiry. She is a research fellow with the Center for New North Carolinians at the University of North Carolina at Greensboro serving refugee/immigrant communities as an advocate/scholar.

Bob Pease is Professor of Social Work at the University of Tasmania, Australia. His main research interests are in the fields of men's violence against women, cross-cultural and global perspectives on men and masculinities, the interrogation of privilege and critical social work practice. His most recent books are *Undoing Privilege: Unearned Advantage in a Divided World* (Zed, 2010), *Men and Masculinities Around the World: Transforming Men's Practices* (co-editor, Palgrave, 2011), *Men, Masculinities and Methodologies* (co-editor, Palgrave, 2013) and *The Politics of Recognition and Social Justice: Transforming Subjectivities and New Forms of Resistance* (co-editor, Routledge, 2014).

Annie Pullen Sansfaçon is Associate Professor at the University of Montreal's School of Social Work. After obtaining her PhD in ethics and social work, she continued working on the development of anti-oppressive theories, approaches and methodologies to promote ethical and emancipatory practice. Recent projects include research related the adaptation of migrant social workers and the barriers they navigate to practise in Canada, as well as the experience of parents of transgender children. She has co-authored the book *Ethical Foundations of Social Work* (Routledge, 2012) and *Supporting Transgender and Gender Creative Youth: Schools, Families and Communities in Action* (Peter Lang, 2014).

Margaret Rowntree was a Lecturer in the School of Psychology, Social Work and Social Policy at the University of South Australia between 2011 and 2015. She has published widely in national and international feminist and social work journals on gender, sexuality and sexual violence. Her PhD dissertation, entitled 'Trimillennium Feminine Sexualities: Representations, Lives and Daydreams', explores the intersections and interstices between the symbolic, material and imaginary realms of women's sexualities in the new millennium. She is also interested in the value of emotion in knowledge production.

Leanne Schubert is a private social work practitioner, who has worked with co-author Professor Mel Gray as a research associate for several years. She is currently team leader of Community Connect, a programme that takes an assets-based community development approach to inspiring members of low SES communities to learning and education being run by the Family Action Centre at the University of Newcastle, New South Wales, Australia. Her research interests include the relationship between social work and art, community practice, and domestic and family violence, and how these are influenced by the contemporary sociopolitical context.

Melanie Shepard is an Emeritus Professor of Social Work at the University of Minnesota Duluth, USA. She has published numerous articles primarily in the field of domestic violence, and co-edited the book, *Coordinating Community Responses to Domestic Violence: Lessons from Duluth and Beyond* (Sage, 1999). She has received federal grants from the Centers for Disease Control and Prevention and Health Resources and Services Administration. She was a practitioner in the fields of mental health, child welfare and domestic violence and taught for over 30 years. Currently she is a consulting editor for *AFFILIA: The Journal of Women and Social Work*.

Susanna Snyder is Research Fellow at Ripon College, Cuddesdon, and an Associate Member of the Faculty of Theology and Religion at the University of Oxford. Formerly an Assistant Professor at the University of Texas at Austin, her work focuses on the intersections between immigration, refugees, faith-based action and ethics. Her first book was *Asylum-Seeking, Migration and Church* (Ashgate, 2012), and she is widely published in journals and edited volumes. She co-chaired the Religion and Migration Group at the American Academy of Religion from 2012–2015, and is founding co-editor of the Palgrave book series on Religion and Global Migrations.

Barbra Teater is an Associate Professor at the College of Staten Island, City University of New York where she is Program Director of the Bachelor of Science in Social Work (BSSW) and the minor in Disability Studies. She teaches research methods to MSW students. Her research interests include social work education, research methods for social work, and the health and wellbeing of older adults, particularly the promotion of active ageing through preventative programmes. She has authored or co-authored over 35 articles, book chapters and books including the bestselling text, *An Introduction to Applying Social Work Theories and Methods* (Open University Press, 2010).

Deirdre Tedmanson is Program Director for social sciences in the School of Psychology, Social Work and Social Policy at the University of South Australia and a member of its Centre for Social Change. She lectures in the School in the areas of social analysis, community development and human service project management. Her research interests include Indigenous sovereignty and rights, social work in Indigenous contexts, social policy, post-colonial theory, critical management studies, sociocultural and gendered aspects of human service organisation, social enterprise and entrepreneurship, social justice and participatory action research methodologies.

Karin Wachter is a doctoral student in the School of Social Work at the University of Texas at Austin and a Project Director at the Institute on Domestic Violence and Sexual Assault. Previously, she worked for ten years with the International Rescue Committee as a humanitarian aid worker and senior technical adviser focused on violence against women in war-affected contexts, primarily in Africa. Her expertise includes intervention design, logic models, and programme monitoring and evaluation. Her current research interests include displaced women's experiences pre- and post-settlement in the United States, in order to inform policy and practice.

Sarah Wendt is Professor of Social Work at Flinders University, South Australia. She has published extensively on violence against women including most recently *Domestic Violence in Diverse Contexts: A Re-examination of Gender* (Routledge, 2015). Her current research projects explore the impact of domestic violence on women's citizenship, service provision for Aboriginal communities experiencing family violence and engaging men to address domestic violence. In particular, she has been researching rural women's experiences of domestic violence for over a decade in Australia. She is currently exploring rural women's help seeking decisions and coping with domestic violence.

Carole Zufferey is a Senior Lecturer at the School of Psychology, Social Work and Social Policy, University of South Australia, where she completed her PhD on social work and homelessness in 2008. Her research interests include social work, homelessness, intersectionality, social policy, social work education, social work responses to housing, home, homelessness, domestic violence and children.

Introduction

Nicole Moulding and Sarah Wendt

Feminism and social work share an imperative for social change. This goal has connected the feminist movement and the social work profession for more than a century, stretching back to their mutual beginnings in the late nineteenth century and the social upheavals of that period. This is not to suggest that the relationship between feminism and social work has been unproblematic: social work has often been, and continues to be, complicit in the state control of many women's lives (Bell, 2011). However, there has also been a natural alignment between feminism and much of social work throughout the past 100 years, with many social workers drawing on feminist insights into how gender frames women's lives in the course of their day-to-day work. This interconnection has been so enduring that feminist thought, ethics and practice might be now understood as mainstream to social work rather than as simply complementary to it. This book illuminates the interconnections between contemporary feminism and modern social work across diverse everyday practice worlds. It also considers some of the tensions borne of practising feminist social work in neo-liberal sociopolitical contexts that simultaneously 'ignore' gender and exploit and exacerbate relative female disadvantage. Importantly, the book is framed by the contemporary feminist insight that gender intersects with other dimensions of social disadvantage, such as those of race, class, disability and sexuality, which has critical implications for social work as a profession whose central concern lies with understanding and responding to hardship and oppression.

A re-evaluation of the relationship between feminism and social work is arguably timely. Within and outside feminism, the post-feminist school of thought suggests that equality is now readily available to all women. Within the academy and broader society, gender neutrality remains the prevailing stance, and aligning with a feminist position is often met with confusion and discomfort. However, women continue to dominate the ranks of the poor and the homeless in developed and developing countries around the world; male perpetrated violence against women and children has not reduced; women outnumber men by up to three to one in the diagnosis of common mental health problems; and women continue to be severely underrepresented in every realm of power and decision making across the globe. This paints a very different picture from more popular understandings, and draws attention to the ways gender relations continue to structure most of the problems faced by women, men and children in the day-to-day worlds in which social work operates. Gender also continues to structure the very profession itself. As Orme (2013) points out, social work is a profession mainly providing services for women by women.

While gender remains pivotal to many, if not all, of the social problems social workers encounter in their everyday work, the idea that equality has been 'won' often complicates an upfront engagement with feminist ideas. The veil of gender neutrality that has been drawn over women's (and men's) lives works to obscure gender oppression, and professional practices are often complicit in this by failing to attend explicitly to gender while continuing to draw on profoundly gendered assumptions about women and men. In this contemporary period, then, there is often a substantial disconnect between *explicit* discourses about gender and the *implicit* gendered social practices that women encounter in their everyday lives. Thus, while the idea of women's rights to equality has been widely accepted at an abstract level (Lamanna, 1999; Sharpe, 2001), in all countries across the world, everyday social practices (including professional practices) continue to be framed by unspoken, even unconscious, discourses about women, their rights and their responsibilities as qualitatively different from those of men. These implicit discourses and practices include the continuing treatment of women as sexualised body objects and the property of men, most graphically reflected in widespread rape, sexual abuse and domestic violence; continuing double-standards about female and male sexual behaviour; assumptions about women's place as primarily and more 'naturally' in the home and family, resulting in heavier burdens of care and double-shifts of paid and unpaid work; assumptions about women as more psychologically unstable, emotional and irrational than men, and therefore as less authoritative, competent and credible; and the laying of responsibility for men's behaviour, especially violence and rape, at women's feet. Thus, women continue to encounter diverse forms of gender oppression in their day-to-day lives based on implicit gender discourses and practices that are very often hidden from view, perhaps at least in part because of the success of the feminist movement in challenging more overt forms of sexism and discrimination.

In order to re-evaluate the place and value of feminism to social work in this contemporary moment, we bring together many of the foremost feminist social workers from around to world to examine and explore the theoretical, ethical and practical intersections between feminism and social work, and directions for the future. The aims of the book are to highlight in an illustrative way the centrality of feminism to contemporary social work; to show how gender-neutral perspectives and practices obscure gender and how feminism can challenge these practices; and, to

showcase the specific ways feminist social work practice can be transformative into the future through its emphasis on relationships and power.
The uniqueness of this book primarily lies in the fact that, in contrast to
other works that use more singular feminist approaches, our contributors
draw on a diversity of feminisms, including post-structuralist feminism,
radical feminism, liberal feminism, intersectional feminism, feminist
appropriations of critical race theory, structuralist feminism and materialist feminism. This enables multi-faceted insights into the complex
dynamics of gender relations and how they play out in the many 'problems of living' social work engages with.[1] As has been pointed out by
Freeman, in using diverse feminist perspectives to examine the status of
women in society,

> [e]ach interpretation yields a different interpretation of the social
> world and influences the assumptions, observations, and conclusions
> that are made regarding women's experiences in society, as well as the
> strategies that are used to change that status and those experiences.
>
> (1990, p. 75)

While some of the contributors to this book do not name a particular feminist theoretical tradition per se, what unites all the chapters is the feminist insight that systems of male privilege frame the lives of women, men
and children in myriad ways, and that fairer societies will not be achieved
without transformation of these social relations of advantage and disadvantage. All contributions, irrespective of specific theoretical orientation, are also united by an awareness that gender intersects with other
social relations of advantage and disadvantage. As such, it is universally
appreciated throughout the book that the concerns of all groups of
women must be considered, not just those of white, western, heterosexual,
'able-bodied', middle-class women. The book is also distinctive for its
global focus through its attention to feminist responses to global poverty
and refugees, and for the inclusion of diverse areas of feminist social work
practice such as sexualities in social work, body image and ageing, working
with Indigenous communities and working with men.

In order to maximise the relevance of the book for feminist social
workers, researchers, educators and students, we have divided the chapters
into two main parts. Part I engages with the core knowledge and curriculum areas taught in social work programmes, including theory, feminist
approaches to social policy, direct practice, management and leadership,
social work organisations and community development. In Chapter 1,
Sarah Wendt explores the influences of modernism and postmodernism
on both social work and feminism to argue the importance of theory for
the profession. She shows how feminism enables eclecticism within social
work. She argues that feminism and social work have both demonstrated a
level of reflexivity and development over time in terms of a capacity to

incorporate new theoretical insights, without losing the original impetus for social transformation. In Chapter 2, Melanie Shepard and Lake Dziengel consider the future of feminist social work practice into the twenty-first century. They argue that while social work practice and feminism have sprung from the same roots with similar values and goals for personal and social transformation, the impact of feminism on social work practice in the future is less clear. The authors explore the characteristics of feminist social work practice as shaped by the past, the influence of a changing social and practice environment, and their vision for feminist social work practice in the future. In Chapter 3, Annie Pullen Sansfaçon considers ethics in social work. She overviews the main ethical perspectives in this field, mapping some of the tensions and exploring the potential of feminist ethics of care, elaborating how this approach might be distinctive from other ethical positions in social work and its implications for future feminist-informed practice. In Chapter 4, Lesley Laing undertakes an analysis of feminism and social policy using the example of policies in family law as they are applied to 'shared parenting' arrangements. She shows how these supposedly gender-neutral policies obscure the gendered nature of parenting and the gendered assumptions that influence policy development and decision making. In Chapter 5, Sue King and Deirdre Tedmanson also explore feminist perspectives on social policy and its delivery, focusing on the gendered nature of social and economic disadvantage and the consequent social exclusion of women, in particular in their role as heads of sole parent families. This chapter also explores women's participation in the political and bureaucratic decision-making processes and looks at the impact of neo-liberalism on women's access to services.

Repositioning social work research is considered by Lia Bryant in Chapter 6. The chapter argues that it is timely to mainstream feminist approaches in social work because they have the potential to use critical and interpretive methodologies at the interstices between research and practice, thereby creating the potential for powerful social change. The chapter considers two key critical feminist approaches to research, Foucauldian archaeological discourse analyses and intersectionality, and introduces creative methods that may accompany these approaches. In Chapter 7, Margaret Alston focuses on rural community development in Australia and the Asia-Pacific region as sites of major restructuring, climate challenges and environmental degradation. She shows how rural spaces and policy responses take the masculine as the norm, with the consequence that women's efforts to sustain families and communities through their paid and unpaid work are marginalised and their interests and needs overlooked. The chapter draws out the importance of taking a feminist lens to rural issues and policy, and to community development strategies and actions, and argues that social workers have a significant role to play in challenging the dominant framing of rural life and advocating for policies and practices that advance gender equality and foster quality of life for women. In Chapter 8, Mel Gray and Leanne Schubert explore leadership in social work through a feminist lens, drawing out how feminist perspectives diverge from gender-neutral theoretical approaches. They critically examine the implications for feminist leadership in social work where women predominate in the social work workforce and also as service users, specifically contextualising feminist leadership within current managerialist models of service delivery and management, and exploring the scope of feminist social work leadership and mentoring to influence change. In Chapter 9, Lena Dominelli critically examines poverty alleviation strategies for their potential to increase the burden that women already carry for family wellbeing, especially that of children and older people. The chapter examines the Millennium Development Goals (MDGs), which allege to have women and children at their heart, and the more recent 'social protection floor', demonstrating their gender-neutral approach and failure to engage with the limitations of neo-liberal forms of social development. The chapter draws out the implications of this for research and teaching in social work.

Part II looks to the everyday practice worlds of social work, bringing to life the ways gender plays out in the social problems and relationships social workers encounter in practice through the authors' research and practice, and offering feminist approaches to practice. In Chapter 10, Deirdre Tedmanson and Christine Fejo-King consider some of the gendered dimensions of social work's contemporary engagement with Australian Aboriginal and Torres Strait Islander peoples and issues. The chapter draws on critical race theory to analyse how white privilege remains one of the most powerful, pervasive and under-discussed forms of contemporary racism. The chapter also identifyies the ways white privilege continues to adversely impact on Aboriginal and Torres Strait Islander women, and argues for strategies that dismantle 'whiteness' and build greater reflexivity in professional practice around the intersections of gender and race issues. In Chapter 11, Laurie Cook Heffron, Susanna Snyder, Karin Wachter, Maura Nsonwu and Noël Busch-Armendariz explore the weaving of feminist theories into social work practice with refugees. The chapter points out that women account for approximately one-half of those displaced in the world, with many facing a complex array of challenges, including trauma and gender-based violence. The chapter specifically discusses the gendered nature of resettlement experiences in the US, and explores the implications of four aspects of feminist theory for social work practice with refugees. In Chapter 12, Nicole Moulding critically examines the gendered dimensions of mental health and the potential of feminist-informed social work practice for challenging individualising and pathologising approaches. The chapter focuses specifically on mental health in contexts of gendered violence and abuse because much of the heavier burden of mental health problems experienced by women is traceable to these experiences. Drawing on the author's empirical research, the chapter argues for a feminist approach to practice that challenges the discursive construction of mental illness as individual pathology, situates mental health in the context of social relationships and engages with the material impact of unequal gender relations on women's mental health and wellbeing. In Chapter 13, Fiona Buchanan offers a radical feminist approach to working with women and children. The chapter examines how knowledge of childhood and attachments has been appropriated by experts who classify relationships between women and their children by means of observation and survey. By drawing on the author's own research, the chapter adds to feminist understandings of women's knowledge about protectiveness and argues that children's wellbeing is best promoted in a society that honours and supports women's mothering abilities. In Chapter 14, Sarah Wendt makes the case that domestic violence can only be properly understood and responded to by understanding gender. The chapter outlines the debates of gender to explain why men are predominantly perpetrators of domestic violence and women and children victims, exploring how feminism has been instrumental in exposing domestic violence as part of a range of tactics used by men to exercise power and control over women and children. The chapter concludes by examining how feminism has influenced practice and policy responses to domestic violence in social work.

In Chapter 15, Fiona Buchanan and Lynn Jamieson bring an intersectional feminist perspective to the issue of rape and sexual assault. Whether rape is committed against women, trans-gendered people or men, they argue that it is an attack on self-worth exercised as an act of control by the perpetrator. While outlining the contributions of earlier feminist analyses of rape, the chapter examines how an understanding of how rape and sexual assault intersect with other categories of social disadvantage such as race, class and disability. The authors offer a more nuanced perspective and explore the implications for social work practice. In Chapter 16, Carole Zufferey demonstrates how homelessness is a gendered and embodied experience, with gendered violence the main cause of women's homelessness. The chapter argues that intersectional feminism is an important lens through which to examine social work research, policy and practice responses to homelessness because it enables social workers to recognise and address the diverse and intersecting disadvantages that constitute the lived experiences of homelessness for women. Margaret Rowntree explores sexuality in social work as an emerging area of scholarship in Chapter 17. The chapter examines why knowledge about sexuality is important for social work practice and, by drawing on the author's research, it discusses how gender impacts on the experience, practice and portrayal of sexuality. The chapter concludes by offering a feminist perspective on the way in which knowledge about sexuality can be embedded into social work practice, theory, values and ethics. In Chapter 18, Jill Chonody and Barbra Teater explore the gendered dimensions of ageing with a particular focus on western societies' obsessions with beauty and youthful sexualities as symbols of social worth. They examine the gendered experience of growing older in western cultures, and show that youth-dominated cultures impact more negatively on women through drawing on contemporary examples and research. This chapter examines the implications for feminist social work approaches to working with older women. In Chapter 19, Barbara Fawcett demonstrates how the social model of disability has drawn from feminist perspectives in order to challenge and change disabling constructions. This chapter explores 'disability' by means of the various lenses that feminism has to offer, highlighting the opportunities and also the challenges posed by these perspectives and appraising how the various feminisms have influenced social work responses. In Chapter 20, Bob Pease explores some of the issues associated with engaging men in feminist social work. He points out that feminist social workers have emphasised the need for feminist thinking to inform work with men, but that few men in social work have taken up the feminist challenge. The chapter explores the personal, professional and practice implications for men of feminist principles in social work, arguing that it is possible for men to change their subjectivities and practices to constitute a profeminist men's standpoint by recognising their own gender privilege and the gender privilege of their male clients. The chapter also explores ways of encouraging men to reflect critically on the social construction of their own masculinities, and the consequences for women and for themselves of the male privilege that flows from their structural location. In the final chapter, we draw together the key ideas that have been showcased throughout the book, summarising the centrality of feminism to contemporary social work.

Note

1 British social worker Jerry Tew (2008) specifically reframes 'mental illnesses' as 'problems of living' to emphasise the social nature of mental health and illness rather than relying on pathologising and individualising medical discourses. We suggest that this term could be extended to describe more generally most, if not all, of the problems social work engages with.

References

Bell, S. (2011) Through a Foucauldian lens: a geneology of child abuse. *Journal of Family Violence*, 26, pp. 101–108.

Freeman, M. (1990) Beyond women's issues: feminism and social work. *AFFILIA: The Journal of Women and Social Work*, 5(2), pp. 72–89.

Lamanna, M. (1999) Living the postmodern dream: adolescent women's discourse on relationships, sexuality and reproduction. *Journal of Family Issues*, 20(2), pp. 181–217.

Orme, J. (2013) Feminist social work. In M. Gray & S. Webb (eds), *Social Work Theories and Methods*, 2nd edn. Sage, London, pp. 87–98.

Sharpe, S. (2001) Going for it: young women face the future. *Feminism and Psychology*, 11(2), pp. 177–181.

Tew, J. (2008) Social perspectives on mental distress. In T. Stickley & T. Basset (eds), *Learning about Mental Health Practice*. John Wiley & Sons Ltd, Chichester, pp. 235–252

Part I
Social work knowledge

1 Conversations about theory

Feminism and social work

Sarah Wendt

Introduction

This chapter is written from my reflections on teaching social work theory to undergraduate and masters students. I write this chapter imagining that I am having a conversation with a social work student. The person I am talking with believes feminism is not relevant to social work. In my course on social work theory, in the week we examine feminism, it is not uncommon for me to hear 'I am not a feminist', 'equality is won, we don't need feminism anymore' and 'feminism should lighten up'. Let me also say, though, that not all students agree. Many come to class either already identifying strongly with feminist politics or engage enthusiastically with the ideas introduced to them. So perhaps I also write this chapter for other reasons. These include that I want to showcase and show off the richness of feminism, I want feminism to remain an integral part of social work and I want future social work students to see its applicability, relevance and close relationship with the profession.

In this chapter, I show how feminism and social work have evolved over time in similar ways in response to complex debates and competing ways of knowing. This journey enables me to argue that feminism is core to social work knowledge and hence cannot be separated from the values and ideals of social work. Similar to Phillips and Cree (2014), I engage in a form of reflection as a feminist researcher, teacher and scholar in social work. These are my thoughts about why I believe in the continuing relevance of feminism in all its diversity, richness and contradictions, as a body of knowledge that must remain central to social work. I also argue that feminism enriches other theories and approaches used in social work.

Modernism and postmodernism: parallel journeys for feminism and social work

Modernism and postmodernism denote a range of theoretical orientations characterising particular periods of thought in the twentieth century. Modernism captures ideas and values that rest on strong notions of order, and the belief in unity, progress and rational scientific objectivity (Fawcett, 2013). Modernism is also often associated with the operation of grand narratives or 'big stories', which are viewed as having a universal application and principles, for example psychoanalysis, liberalism and Marxism (Fawcett, 2013, p. 148). On the other hand, postmodernism involves key ideas and values that reject the view that any one theory, system or belief can ever reveal the truth. Instead, postmodernism brings an emphasis on the plurality of truth and a critical appreciation of 'the will to truth' (Parton & O'Bryne, 2000; Parton, 2000). Postmodernism also embraces deconstruction, plurality and relativity, questioning taken-for-granted assumptions and emphasising that a wide range of understandings can be operating at any one time (Fawcett, 2013).

Both social work and feminism have been influenced by modernism and postmodernism and have grown in similar ways. Social work has become increasingly comfortable with discussing the implications of modernism and postmodernism. Many scholars have posed questions about the wide-ranging theoretical perspectives shaping social work (Morley & Macfarlane, 2012). It was recognised some time ago that social work has primarily arisen within a modernist tradition. As Howe (1994) has pointed out, social work is located in modernity because professional organisations have formed and social work departments have emerged. There has been considerable intellectual effort to analyse social work practice and write about its knowledge bases. As a profession, social work has synthesised various modernist theories and practices, which are evident in a range of contemporary textbooks today (see Payne 2014; Gray & Webb, 2013; Teater, 2010). For example, attachment and cognitive behaviour therapy often feature in textbooks, highlighting the importance of social workers understanding individuals and the psychological dimensions of their problems. Systems and empowerment theories are rarely missed in textbooks as they have a long history within social work, emphasising the importance of social workers understanding the interactions of the person within their environments. Critical theories include structural and radical social work, feminism, and anti-oppressive and anti-discriminatory practice, all of which take the view that many social problems are caused by the structures of society (Payne, 2014). A range of theories is included in social work education because they aim to improve both individuals and society.

Since the 1990s social work has considered postmodernism and what this body of thought means for the profession. Drawing on the influences of postmodernism, some have argued that social work needs to revisit its claims to 'cure and control' arising from modernist assumptions of progress, emancipation and perfection (Howe, 1994; Healy, 2005). Thus, there has been a questioning of the possibilities for human liberty and equality (Morley & Macfarlane, 2012). Instead, it can be argued that social work is more about interpreting. The focus of social work is therefore understanding local details, complexities and diverse experiences of people. Being self-reflexive, de-centred and deconstructive is what charac-terises social work influenced by postmodernism (Howe, 1994; Healy, 2005; Fawcett, 2013). For example, discourse, subjectivity and relations of power have been particularly picked up as tools for theorising and analysis (Healy, 2005). Similarly, implications for practice and hence approaches such as narrative therapy are now discussed in textbooks. In addition we see approaches showing engagement with and development from post-modern influences such as strengths approaches and solution-focused practice; these acknowledge how discourses construct clients as 'problem-atic' or 'deficit' (Payne, 2014). In summary, through consideration of post-modern ideas, social work as a profession has tried to shift away from 'problem solving' to a more forward-looking approach that contextualises the experiences of people. People are positioned as experts in their own lives and as active in developing their knowledge of the world; hence the social worker takes a stance of curiosity and a non-expert position (Teater, 2010; Payne, 2014).

Feminism too has become comfortable, discussing modernism and post-modernism and, like social work, has been shaped by these ideas. As Morley and MacFarlane (2012, p. 690) point out, feminism is also a modernist emancipatory project. It has a particular political agenda pertaining to a particular identity (i.e. woman). It has a grand narrative espousing a 'truth' about how patriarchy oppresses women. Feminism therefore seeks changes through structural reform, addressing social and political disadvantage by challenging inequitable social arrangements. As Gray and Boddy (2010) point out, feminism has achieved much under the influences of modern-ism. Feminism has challenged employment discrimination, advocated for voting and reproductive rights, and sought rights to property ownership and education. Feminism has raised awareness about and responded to male violence against women and children, including domestic violence, sexual assault and pornography. Under modernism feminism showcased various schools of thought with emancipatory ideals. For example, radical feminism focuses on practices of sexism in relationships between men and women. Marxist and socialist feminism highlight the need to differentiate between structures of production and reproduction to gain a fuller under-standing of the historical material basis of patriarchal oppression (Swigon-ski & Raheim, 2011). Liberal feminism focuses on reform through juridical means and hence lobbies for legal and civil reforms through affirmative action and anti-discrimination campaigns. Lesbian feminism highlights the dominance of heterosexuality in feminism and hence challenges the hege-mony of the white, middle-class, heterosexual woman. Black feminism highlights racism, domination and white privilege (Gray & Boddy, 2010). Like social work, there has been considerable intellectual effort within fem-inism to analyse the oppression of women and bodies of knowledge have emerged as a result along with academic journals devoted to feminist thought both in and outside social work.

Also similar to social work, feminism has questioned its emancipatory claims as a result of postmodernist challenges and insights. The power and authority of feminist claims about women's oppression have been widely questioned over the past 30 years. Some have argued that the third wave of feminism reflects the postmodern mood, as feminism has re-considered its social actions and theorisations of women as a homogeneous group. Feminism therefore embarked on a commitment to be more inclusive of race, class and sexual orientation. The third wave has been characterised as striving to be inclusive, non-judgemental, multifocal and multivocal, and focused on the complexity of identities and systems of oppression (Swigonski & Raheim, 2011, p. 18). In this era, we see feminism being self-critical, diverse and contradictory. For example, feminism has engaged with post-structuralist ideas to understand dominant discourses of gender. Feminism has embraced intersectionality to develop nuanced and inclusive understandings of gender, race and class. Feminism has been influenced by postcolonial thought which critiques western imperialism and its subordination of whole peoples, races and ethnic groups, hence drawing attention to the importance of Indigenous and local cultures (Gray & Boddy, 2010; Swigonski & Raheim, 2011). In summary, feminism has moved away from the notion that women are unified and uniform and instead embraced theorising about women's differences, diversity and the contextualised experiences of women. Like social work, feminism takes a position of curiosity, to embrace the ambiguity, contestations and richness of women's lives (McCann & Kim, 2013).

When one examines the journeys of both social work and feminism, it is clear they have similar emancipatory values and that during the 1990s in western societies they together entered a space of critical reflection prompted at least in part by the influence of postmodernism. To position feminism as no longer relevant to social work, as some contemporary social work professionals and students suggest, is a denial of the importance of feminist critical analysis and questioning over this period. In the remainder of this chapter, I show how feminism enables the development of sophisticated understandings and responses to the problems faced by women. First, I elaborate the contribution of feminism to more nuanced understandings of domestic violence, followed by critical feminist analysis of three key social work practice theories and their implications for working with women.

Feminism and social work: my example of the dual journey

I predominantly work in the practice field of domestic violence. In understanding domestic violence, feminism has argued historically that patriarchy and its associated economic and social processes are central. Power differences between men and women therefore contribute to domestic violence (Walby, 1990). With influences from postmodernism, explaining domestic violence as resulting from patriarchy has been seen as limiting because it assumes that gender roles are dichotomous or essential. The critique has pointed out that such explanations do not account for complex ways in which gender operates in social interactions between people (McHugh, 2005). As a social worker, I understood this debate and agreed with such insights; however, simultaneously, as a feminist working in the area of domestic violence, for me, gender needed to remain central because the statistics of violence against women and children by male partners remain alarmingly high (Phillips, 2008). For these reasons, as a feminist, I have turned to post-structuralist ideas to expose how violence plays out in gendered social contexts. Through examining complexities and nuances of gendered positioning, I argue that feminism can and should continue to centralise gender in understanding domestic violence (Wendt & Zannettino, 2015).

I have interviewed diverse groups of women and written about their experiences of domestic violence including mothers, religious women, rural women, Aboriginal women and women living with intellectual disabilities. As a social worker, both feminist and post-structuralist theories push me to be reflective, reflexive and open in writing about women's stories. My work could be considered an example of interpretation and understanding within social work influenced by the insights of postmodernism. In line with this, I focus on local details, complexities and the diverse experiences of women, arguing that change follows from questioning and challenging gendered discourses and subject positions.

Why feminist theory matters in social work

As the discussion above has shown, social workers have an ethical and professional responsibility to have knowledge of established social theories that are grounded in social work values. Or as Orme (2003, p. 132) argues, theoretical debates are relevant to social work because understanding how others come to experience, know and make sense of the world is core to social work practice. Theories help social workers explain phenomena and shape social work's purpose (Chenoweth & McAuliffe, 2008). Theory brings together a range of explanations that have a bearing on interpretations, decisions, assessment and interventions, and advocacy strategies (Cleak & Wilson, 2007). I argue that feminism exemplifies this for social work because feminism has a willingness to engage with debates, analyse and reflect, which can benefit social work. Social work is a profession that requires the integration of complex and evolving knowledge to inform practice.

Theory guides the focus, objectives and processes of social work practice. Through this guidance, theory provides accountability to service users, employers and funding bodies. In simple terms, theory enables social workers to be clear about what they are doing and why they are doing it. Theory pushes social workers to review their own assumptions and accepted ways of doing things as well as their own opinions and personal values; hence theory enables and demands critical engagement, thinking and reflection. Theory also creates a shared identity in social work (Healy, 2005; Osmond & O'Connor, 2006). I argue the continued growth and diversity of feminism is an example of what theory can do, and therefore enables a shared identity in social work. Developments within feminism can be used to guide processes and practices. Feminism is not static because feminist theorising over time continues to expand the tools and strategies that can be used in social work (Swigonski & Raheim, 2011). Feminism stimulates awareness and change, promotes reflection and opens up processes that can build egalitarian relationships. It emanates values of empowerment and these ways of working matter to social work (Payne, 2014). In summary, feminism particularly matters in social work because, as Swigonski and Raheim (2011, p. 11) eloquently point out, the actions and tasks of feminism and social work are often one and the same. Similarly, Barretti (2011, p. 264) points out that there are compatibilities and partnerships between social work and feminism because both come from a similar foundation of shared responsibility for social change and development.

Feminism: a lens for interacting with social work theories

Theory is essential in social work and so I do not argue in this chapter that feminism is and should be the only theory that social work requires. In teaching social work, I believe we have a responsibility to cover the breadth of theories that influence social work and it is ethical practice for social workers to acknowledge and use a range of established researched theories. As Phillips and Cree point out, it is important for social work to examine continually 'how it is best done and how it best responds to the complexity of the lives of the people that it aims to serve' (2014, p. 941). In the remaining part of the chapter, I therefore also want to show how feminism provides me with a social work identity that comes from critical social work, which questions taken-for-granted ideas and arguments. I want to understand and change 'harmful divisions, unequal power relations, injustices and disadvantage' (Morley, Macfarlane & Ablett, 2014, p. 2). Feminism provides me with a lens to engage with other social work theories, enabling me to practise eclecticism and draw on the rich bodies of thought that social work has embraced across time. I therefore present three social work theories that are being used in contemporary Australian social work. I draw out the strengths and limitations of such theories for working with women by examining these theories through my feminist lens. By engaging with feminism I am able to enact critical thinking, which is an important part of social work. Feminism helps social workers question existing assumptions and taken-for-granted ways of being and knowing, and aids one to remain open minded to take account of different perspectives (Payne, 2014, p. 87).

Systems theory

Social work has a long history with systems theory (Besthorn, 2013) and has distinguished itself from other helping professions through its dual focus on the person and the environment (Norton, 2012). The purpose of engaging with systems theory is to help the social worker customise their intervention to the person, the environment and the interaction between the two. The aim of practice is to facilitate the restoration of an adaptive balance between the person and environment by reducing stress, improving coping and therefore establishing stability (O'Donoghue & Maidment, 2005). Systems theory has enabled social workers to understand the developing person in the context of family, social network, community and wider society (the environment) (Scott, Arney & Vimpani, 2010). For example, human development is seen to be based in a concentric arrangement of systems (micro, meso, exo and macro) and analysing each systems level provides different insights (Ambrosino et al., 2008; Scott et al., 2010).

As Besthorn (2013, p. 179) points out, systems theory has relevance to social work because it provides a comprehensive, multidisciplinary and holistic framework within which the complex and interrelational elements of people's lives can be connected and understood. However, systems theory has been criticised for being conservative and justifying the status quo (Hanson, 2001). Furthermore, some argue that systems theory has no organised methodology and therefore its complexity of concepts and assertions act as a barrier to clear prescriptions for action (Payne, 2014). Systems theory has also been criticised for its lack of critical perspective and, despite its claims to focus on both person and environment, many argue that the adaption perspective within systems prevails and in most cases individuals and their adaption is the focus, not changing environments (Besthorn, 2013).

In responding to some of these critiques, feminism offers additional important insights. For example, Stephens (2012) introduces feminist systems theory (FST) as an emerging theory grounded in cultural ecofeminism and critical systems theory; hence, it brings to social work a set of principles that contain implications for community development, social research and intervention practice. Specifically, FST adopts a gender-sensitive approach that is missing from systems theory and thereby centralises what is distinctive about women's experiences. One could also argue that FST has been influenced by postmodernism because it promotes practice that is contextualised, where change happens when it is locally embedded. Similarly, Norton (2012) argues that for social work to respond to the critiques of systems theory it could look to feminist psychology and ecofeminism. Specifically, she argues that social work needs to redefine its central 'person-in-environment' mantra to embrace the natural world more fully. She introduces concepts of empathy and empowerment from relational cultural theory as important ideas to integrate into systems theory in order to promote deeper awareness of the parallels between the oppression of women and domination of nature.

Feminism can offer systems theory the critical edge it needs. As Swigonski and Raheim (2011, pp. 10–11) point out, feminism brings with it a range of tools and strategies that have been developed across modernism and postmodernism. These include, for example, tools and strategies for deconstructing systems of oppression and dominant ideologies that impact on and influence women's lives. The conceptualisations of gender, care, power, difference and diversity that have emerged from feminism enable further theorising about the person in their environment, through the micro-, mezzo- and macro-level human interactions that affect the well-being of women and, therefore, their families and communities.

Cognitive behavioural therapy (CBT)

As Teater (2010) points out, CBT is a well-researched psychological approach that is based on theories of learning and has been highly influential in social work. CBT is generally used in social work to understand clients' behaviours, thoughts and feelings and how these are contributing to the source of their problems (Payne, 2014). CBT provides social workers with interventions that can assist clients in altering thoughts or behaviours to produce more positive and acceptable outcomes (Teater, 2010). Theories of CBT are primarily a western model of practice that emphasises psychological change within individuals, rather than more broad social change. CBT has been particularly used in specialised settings with particular client groups such as those experiencing phobias, anxiety and depression (Payne, 2014).

Some argue that CBT promotes particular social work values and ways of working. For example, CBT is a brief intervention that provides clients with tools for the future. CBT teaches clients new skills, and new ways of thinking and feeling that can be transferred to other situations or future problems. Furthermore, some argue CBT enables the social worker to engage the client in a collaborative relationship in which goals and activities are designed together (Teater, 2010; Garland & Thyer, 2013).

On the other hand, CBT has also been criticised because the individual is the focus of the work; hence social and political factors contributing to the problem are ignored. For example, discrimination, racism, sexism, poverty and/or cultural expectations that may be contributing to the problem are not addressed. The focus of CBT shifts attention away from oppressive systems to individual defects (Teater, 2010). Furthermore, some view the claim of collaboration with a level of caution because CBT requires the social worker to be directive and, without high levels of interpersonal skills, CBT therefore risks becoming a disempowering experience for clients (Teater, 2010).

Feminism can offer CBT tools of empowerment and space to be political. For example, Dietz (2000) argues that individual practice is a critical component of feminist practice because challenging oppression requires social workers to support individuals in naming their experiences of oppression and its effects. Feminism brings with it practice that recognises that the personal is political. By supporting women in naming their experiences of oppression, examining the effects of oppression and challenging oppression both personally and politically, CBT can acknowledge critical examination of individuals' experiences in the context of larger societal systems of oppression and domination. Feminism brings the empowerment tradition in social work to CBT (Dietz, 2000, p. 371). Without feminism, CBT risks individualising and pathologising public issues (such as domestic violence and sexual assault), or risks denying gender role socialisation and inequality as central to many women's experiences (Morley & Macfarlane, 2012). Without feminism, emphasis is placed on personal change or women are expected to work on themselves; hence the structural analysis of women's lives is missed and social problems individualised, pathologised and depoliticised (McDonald, 2005).

Attachment theory

Attachment theory has been taken up in social work because if offers a life-course perspective. It helps practitioners understand how adverse conditions such as poverty, parental stress, maltreatment, rejection and abandonment impact on the development and wellbeing of children (Howe, 2013). Attachment theory generally posits that children who develop secure patterns of attachments (not avoidant, ambivalent or disorganised) through positive caregiving are more likely to experience lower levels of stress and other associated benefits. In turn, they are more able to contribute positively to society and care for future generations. Attachment theory also has a sound foundation of empirical support (Connors, 2011) and has found that ways 'parents regulate their children's arousal, or respond to the joy, has profound implications for children's neurological, physiological and psychosocial development' (Howe, 2013, p. 78).

Attachment theory helps social workers make sense of children's development and behaviour in conditions of adversity and it can guide and help workers plan assessments and interventions (Howe, 2013). However, attachment theorists have mainly focused their research on mothers and children and hence have been critiqued for attributing blame and causality to mothers. This concern has particularly come from feminist researchers and practitioners working in the areas of child sexual abuse and family and domestic violence (Bolen, 2000). Feminism does not refute that attachment theory makes a valuable contribution in recognising the important role of mothering and caring for babies and children. The concern for feminism is the indiscriminate application of the concept of attachment without due attention to, or acknowledgement of, the contexts in which women form relationships with their babies. In short, feminism points out that, within attachment theorising and practices, the environment can often be excluded from scrutiny and the lived context of women's lives can remain invisible (Buchanan, Power & Verity, 2013; Buchanan, 2008, 2013). Without attention to societal issues and gender analysis, feminism points out that attachment can prescribe narrow, unrealistic and conservative roles for women as mothers. Furthermore, it creates societal pressures by holding women solely responsible for the human condition, which can compound women's feelings of inadequacy and exacerbate feelings of low self-esteem (Franzblau, 1999a, 1999b).

Feminism offers attachment theory a lens to regard both micro and macro contexts of women's lives (Buchanan, 2013). It brings with it a continuum of politics and research that exposes historical, exploitative and oppressive conditions under which women may have children and mother (Franzblau, 1999a, 1999b). This is particularly important for understanding contexts of domestic violence and child sexual abuse, where fear and coercive control are present (Buchanan et al., 2013).

Feminisms: conclusions and implications for social work

Using feminism as a lens does two things in social work. First, feminism assists social workers to merge theory with practice by engaging with gender oppression and inequality in women's lives rather than applying theory in a gender-blind way. Feminism enables frameworks for practice by using gender analysis, reflection and dialogue. Second, because theories can become polarised and competitive with each other (Featherstone & Fawcett, 1995), feminism offers eclecticism.

As Orme (2013, p. 87) clearly states, there are multiple feminisms and feminist theorising is developmental in an iterative and reflective way. Feminism raises questions about the nature of theory in social work and its relationship to practice. It brings a lens to social work that enables reflections on theories and a questioning of the implications of how they construct women and/or address the conditions of women. Feminist theory and practice is anti-oppressive in nature and can be used in conjunction with other theories and methods. It has a commitment to empowerment, social change, challenging inequalities and ending oppression (Teater, 2010). The breadth of feminist theory encompasses individual, social, political and cultural considerations of women's lives for social work. Feminism's complexity and maturity therefore have important implications for social work.

In casting my mind back to conversations with social work students and colleagues, I have written this chapter in answer to their questions about the relevance of feminism, showing the wide-ranging contributions of feminist thought and practice to the social work profession. Feminism is not about being in 'opposition to', or of having 'power over' or 'hating men': it is a rich continuum of thought that gives attention to analysis of gender relations for both women and men, and provides tools of reflection for social work (Orme, 2013). As Featherstone and Fawcett (1995) point out, because of feminism we have a rich appreciation of masculinity and femininity as constituting each other rather than occupying distinct oppositional locations. If we rely on, or fail to challenge, simplistic assumptions about feminism and what it is, this strips feminism of its complexity and hinders creative and productive dialogue and critical engagement. My main aim for this chapter was that it open up space for dialogue and conversation about the place of feminism in contemporary social work. Feminism and social work have grown together through the influences of modernism and postmodernism, and hence have created conditions for ongoing dialogue and interpretation (Morley & Macfarlane, 2012). Embracing this journey is important for continuous growth within feminism and in the profession of social work.

Further reading

Gray, M. & Webb, S. (eds) (2013) *Social Work Theories and Methods*, 2nd edn. Sage, London.

Morley, C. & Macfarlane, S. (2012) The nexus between feminism and postmodernism: still a central concern for critical social work. *British Journal of Social Work*, 42(4), pp. 687–705.

Swigonski, M. & Raheim, S. (2011) Feminist contributions to understanding women's lives and the social environment. *AFFILIA: The Journal of Women and Social Work*, 26(1), pp. 10–21.

References

Ambrosino, R., Heffernan, J., Shuttlesworth, G. & Ambrosino, R. (2008) *Social Work and Social Welfare: An Introduction*, 6th edn. Thomson/Brooks Coles, Belmont, CA.

Barretti, M. (2011) Women, feminism, and social work journals 10 years later. *AFFILIA: The Journal of Women and Social Work*, 26(3), pp. 264–277.

Besthorn, F. (2013) Ecological approach. In M. Gray & S. Webb (eds), *Social Work Theories and Methods*, 2nd edn. Sage, London, pp. 173–182.

Bolen, R. (2000) Validity of attachment theory. *Trauma, Violence and Abuse*, 1(2), pp. 128–153.

Buchanan, F. (2008) *Mother and Infant Attachment Theory and Domestic Violence: Crossing the Divide*. Stakeholder Paper No. 5. Sydney: Australian Domestic & Family Violence Clearinghouse.

Buchanan, F. (2013) A critical analysis of the use of attachment theory in cases of domestic violence. *Critical Social Work*, 14(2). www1.uwindsor.ca/criticalsocial work/critical_analysis_attachment_theory (accessed 15 July 2015).

Buchanan, F., Power, C. & Verity, F. (2013) Domestic violence and the place of fear in mother/baby relationships: 'What was I afraid of? Of making it worse'. *Journal of Interpersonal Violence*, 28(9), pp. 1817–1838.

Chenoweth, L. & McAuliffe, D. (2008) *The Road to Social Work and Human Service Practice*, 2nd edn. Cengage Learning, South Melbourne.

Cleak, H. & Wilson, J. (2007) *Making the Most of Field Placement*, 2nd edn. Thomson, South Melbourne.

Connors, M. (2011) Attachment theory: a 'secure base' for psychotherapy integration. *Journal of Psychotherapy Integration*, 21(3), pp. 348–362.

Dietz, C. (2000) Responding to oppression and abuse: a feminist challenge to clinical social work. *AFFILIA: The Journal of Women and Social Work*, 15(3), pp. 369–389.

Fawcett, B. (2013) Postmodernism. In M. Gray & S. Webb (eds), *Social Work Theories and Methods*, 2nd edn. Sage, London, pp. 147–156.

Featherstone, B. & Fawcett, B. (1995) Oh no! Not more isms: feminism, postmodernism, poststructuralism and social work education. *Social Work Education: The International Journal*, 14(3), pp. 25–43.

Franzblau, S.H. (1999a) Attachment theory. *Feminism and Psychology*, 9(1), pp. 5–9.

Franzblau, S.H. (1999b) Historicizing attachment theory: binding the ties that bind. *Feminism and Psychology*, 9(1), pp. 22–31.

Garland, E. & Thyer, B. (2013) Cognitive-behavioural approach. In M. Gray & S. Webb (eds), *Social Work Theories and Methods*, 2nd edn. Sage, London, pp. 159–172.

Gray, M. & Boddy, J. (2010) Making sense of the waves: wipeout or still riding high? *AFFILIA: The Journal of Women and Social Work*, 25(4), pp. 368–389.

Gray, M. & Webb, S. (eds) (2013) *Social Work Theories and Methods*, 2nd edn. Sage, London.

Hanson, B. (2001) Systems theory and the spirit of feminism: grounds for a connection. *Systems Research and Behavioural Science*, 18, pp. 545–556.

Healy, K. (2005) *Social Work Theories in Context: Creating Frameworks for Practice*. Palgrave Macmillan, Houndsmill, UK.

Howe, D. (1994) Modernity, post modernity and social work. *British Journal of Social Work*, 24, pp. 513–532.

Howe, D. (2013) Attachment theory. In M. Gray & S. Webb (eds), *Social Work Theories and Methods*, 2nd edn. Sage, London, pp. 75–86.

McCann, C. & Kim, S. (eds) (2013) *Feminist Theory Reader: Local and Global Perspectives*, 3rd edn. Routledge, New York.

McDonald, J. (2005) Neo-liberalism and the pathologising of public issues: the displacement of feminist service models in domestic violence support services. *Australian Social Work*, 58(3), pp. 275–284.

McHugh, M. (2005) Understanding gender and intimate partner violence. *Sex Roles*, 52(11/12), pp. 717–724.

Morley, C. & Macfarlane, S. (2012) The nexus between feminism and postmodernism: still a central concern for critical social work. *British Journal of Social Work*, 42(4), pp. 687–705.

Morley, C., Macfarlane, S. & Ablett, P. (2014) *Engaging with Social Work: A Critical Introduction*. Cambridge University Press, Cambridge.

Norton, C.L. (2012) Social work and the environment: an ecosocial approach. *International Journal of Social Welfare*, 21, pp. 299–308.

O'Donoghue, K. & Maidment, J. (2005) The ecological systems metaphor in Australasia. In M. Nash, R. Munford & K. O'Donoghue (eds), *Social Work Theories in Action.* Jessica Kingsley Publishers, London, pp. 32–49.

Orme, J. (2003) 'It's feminist because I say so!' Feminism, social work and critical practice in the UK. *Qualitative Social Work*, 2(2), pp. 131–153.

Orme, J. (2013) Feminist social work. In M. Gray & S. Webb (eds), *Social Work Theories and Methods*, 2nd edn. Sage, London, pp. 87–98.

Osmond, J. & O'Connor, I. (2006) Use of theory and research in social work practice: implications for knowledge-based practice. *Australian Social Work*, 59(1), pp. 5–19.

Parton, N. (2000) Some thoughts on the relationship between theory and practice in and for social work. *British Journal of Social Work*, 30(4), pp. 449–463.

Parton, N. & O'Bryne, P. (2000) What do we mean by constructive social work? *Critical Social Work*, 1(2). www1.uwindsor.ca/criticalsocialwork/what-do-we-mean-by-constructive-social-work (accessed 15 July 2015).

Payne, M. (2014) *Modern Social Work Theory*, 4th edn. Palgrave Macmillan, Basingstoke, UK.

Phillips, R. (2008) Feminism, policy and women's safety during Australia's 'war on terror'. *Feminist Review*, 89, pp. 57–72.

Phillips, R. & Cree, V. (2014) What does the 'fourth wave' mean for teaching feminism in twenty-first century social work? *Social Work Education: The International Journal*, 33(7), pp. 930–943.

Scott, D., Arney, F. & Vimpani, G. (2010) Think child, think family, think community. In F. Arney & D. Scott (eds), *Working with Vulnerable Families: A Partnership Approach.* Cambridge University Press, Melbourne, pp. 7–28.

Stephens, A. (2012) Feminist systems theory: learning by praxis. *Systemic Practice and Action Research*, 25, pp. 1–14.

Swigonski, M. & Raheim, S. (2011) Feminist contributions to understanding women's lives and the social environment. *AFFILIA: The Journal of Women and Social Work*, 26(1), pp. 10–21.

Teater, B. (2010) *An Introduction to Applying Social Work Theories and Methods.* McGraw Hill and Open University Press, Maidenhead, UK.

Walby, S. (1990) *Theorising Patriarchy.* Blackwell, Oxford.

Wendt, S. & Zannettino, L. (2015) *Domestic Violence in Diverse Contexts: A Reexamination of Gender.* Routledge, London.

2 Feminist social work practice

Implications for the twenty-first century

Melanie Shepard and Lake Dziengel

Feminist social work practice: a review of the past

In the United States, the emergence of the social work profession largely coincided with the progressive era in the early twentieth century, a time of major social reform led in part by women who were the predecessors of the profession and who were also active in the movement for women's suffrage. The second wave of the feminist movement beginning in the 1960s influenced feminist social work educators and practitioners to advocate for the inclusion of feminist perspectives in social work practice and to articulate feminist social work practice methods. In 1975 the National Association of Social Workers (NASW) formed a National Committee on Women Issues. The work of this committee led to the Feminist Practice Project, designed to 'describe and disseminate information on feminist theory and models and to evolve new models of practice grounded in theory and practice' (Bricker-Jenkins & Hooyman, 1983, p. 3). At a 1983 NASW Institute on Feminist Practice there was an extensive examination of what it meant to be a feminist social worker. Based upon a pilot study conducted earlier that year at a Council on Social Work Education (CSWE) Conference, a broad definition of feminist practice emerged and characteristics of feminist practice were identified.

According to Bricker-Jenkins and Hooyman (1983), feminist social work practitioners approach social issues with 'a view to identifying their implications for women' and are concerned with problems created by institutionalised sexism that limit the full potential of 'individuals and groups'. They 'tend to view social work practice as "political" in working toward an egalitarian society' (pp. 26–27). Subsequent feminist social workers have further conceptualised feminist social work practice. Table 2.1 lists characteristics identified across three decades: by the 1983 NASW institute, more recent conceptualisations of clinical feminist practice (Van Den Bergh, 1995) and feminist generalist direct practice (Saulnier, 2008).

While the language and emphasis has varied, key themes are consistent across the three decades: empowerment, relationship building, contextual analysis and social change. These aspects of feminism have strongly

Table 2.1 Characteristics of feminist social work practice across three decades

Bricker-Jenkins and Hooyman (1983)	Van Den Bergh (1995)	Saulnier (2008)
• Use of consciousness raising • Emphasis on process • Use of networking, support and self-help groups • Valuing of diversity • Emphasis on women's experiences • Multidimensional thinking and analysis • Emphasis on empowerment • Orientation to social, political or economic change • Political–normative–ideological orientation • Emphasis on basic needs and objective conditions • Preference for consensus democratic decision-making • Orientation to 'praxis' (theory/practice) • Preference for 'collectivism'	• Validating the social context • Revaluing the positions of women (e.g. placing greater value on caregiving and other traditional feminine attributes) • Recognising differences in male and female experience of psychological development • Rebalancing perceptions of normality and deviance • Inclusive stance; valuing diversity • Attention to power dynamics in the therapeutic relationship • Recognising how the personal is political • Adopting a deconstructive stance (breaking down and re-examining language and experiences) • Partnering stance with clients • Challenging traditional gender roles • Empowerment practice • Rejecting the myth of value-free psychotherapy	• Engagement phase focuses on empowerment and minimising power differentials • Data collection and assessment examines contextual factors at both the micro and macro levels • Planning and contracting with the 'service user' or 'community member' to set goals that focus on addressing individual needs and/or promoting social justice • Evaluate by use of ongoing 'service user' feedback • Focus on changing systems of oppression, particularly sex-based oppression

influenced key components of what is known as 'generalist' social work practice, which is at the core of social work education in the United States today. Students are provided a practice foundation in the ecological-systems perspective, which emphasises assessing contextual factors, the problem-solving method, empowerment and multilevel intervention (Coady & Lehmann, 2008). However, these practice methods are often taught to students without acknowledging the influence of feminism. Social workers have frequently been criticised by feminist activists in the domestic violence movement for failing to take into account contextual factors that trap women in abusive relationships and for implementing gender-neutral interventions that obscure social realities. Social workers, particularly those working in child welfare bureaucracies, are often seen more as adversaries than allies by feminist activists. We believe that this disconnect between social work practice and feminism is partly due to the failure to recognise common ground, as well as organisational constraints placed on social workers in the field.

The Council on Social Work Education in the United States also took action during the second wave of the women's movement by establishing the Commission on the Role and Status of Women in 1974 after several years of member advocacy for more attention to women's issues. Of significance was the addition in 1977 of a 'required focus on women to the accreditation standards, which already specified race, ethnicity, and cultural diversity' (Alvarez et al., 2008, p. 72). Accreditation sites teams actively explored issues around the status of women faculty and the integration of women's issues into the curriculum.

Social work educators approached this mandate from different orientations, depending upon the degree to which they embraced and integrated feminism in their work. Hooyman (1994) distinguishes between a women's issues approach, a non-sexist perspective and a feminist perspective. The women's issues or 'add women and stir' approach addresses bias and the need to gain greater equity for women, but also focuses on how women can be more successful in a male-dominated society without emphasising the need for structural change. A non-sexist approach recognises the need to challenge institutional sexism and sexist stereotypes, but integrates content on gender with only minor revisions to the traditional curriculum. A feminist perspective seeks fundamental changes in institutional norms and challenges 'a worldview based on male experiences or on helping women to acquire male privileges' (Hooyman, 1994, p. 325). It seeks to create institutional structures and norms that are empowering for all. Integrating a feminist perspective into the social work curriculum rarely occurs at this level. Despite efforts to promote change, there have been ongoing concerns that the integration of content on women is inadequate and does not reflect women's lived experiences (Nichols-Casebolt, Figueria-McDonough & Netting, 2000). Tice has called for a 'gender inclusive curriculum' that does not 'collapse the multiplicity of women's expressions, preoccupations and experiences into the universal women' (1990, p. 136).

While gaining a stronghold in the 1970s, feminist theory in social work as a focal point has lost considerable ground in the present day. Very little has been written about feminist perspectives in the social work literature in recent years. Barretti (2011) found a substantial reduction in journal articles containing women's content when comparing 1988–1997 with 1998–2007 and an even greater decline in articles written from a feminist perspective. A study conducted in the late 1980s of Masters of Social Work students at a major US university found that they had 'little awareness of feminist issues and did not identify themselves as feminists' (Lincoln & Koeske, 1987, p. 50). Current social work students are likely to be even less influenced by feminism. Third wave feminists of the 1990s into the present have been criticised for being more concerned with self-actualisation, lifestyle choices and consumer culture than with structural injustices (Valentich, 2011). In the following section we will explore whether feminist social work practice is still relevant in the twenty-first century. Can it continue to be influential in a multicultural practice milieu that has moved increasingly towards an individualistic focus and which embraces empiricism?

Current challenges to feminist social work practice

There is no doubt that social work practice settings have experienced significant changes in response to new technologies, a changing social environment, and the demand for accountability and demonstrated outcomes. Four areas that we will explore in relation to feminism are addressing diversity, the impact of evidence-based practice, the growing dominance of clinical social work practice over macro practice and binary perceptions of gender.

Addressing diversity

There has been a strong push in social work education to prepare students for twenty-first century practice that embraces diversity and culturally competent practice. It can be argued that this drive has resulted in less importance being placed specifically on addressing the needs and concerns of women. For example, in 2004 the Council on Social Work created, amidst some controversy, a Commission for Diversity and Social Economic Justice, which subsumed a re-designated women's commission to the status of a council (along with other special population groups). The word 'women' no longer appears in the current Educational Policy and Accreditation Standards established in 2008. However, there is a standard that addresses engaging diversity and difference in practice. According to this standard, 'dimensions of diversity are understood as the intersectionality of multiple factors including age, class, color, culture, disability, ethnicity, gender,

gender identity and expression, immigration status, political ideology, race, religion, sex, and sexual orientation' (CSWE, 2008, p. 5). This standard reflects an intersectionality framework first advanced by feminist women of colour to understand better the complex nature of oppression and human experiences (Murphy et al., 2009). According to Lockhart and Danis, 'a women's lived experiences, [therefore] reflect the complex, irreducible realities that result when multiple social, political, cultural and experiential axes of differentiation interact in shaping our lived experiences' (2010, p. 18).

Against the backdrop of mandatory infusion of content on multiple populations, the content on the exploitation, discrimination and oppression of women can sometimes be diluted. Feminist principles are often at odds with religious beliefs or cultural/ethnic traditions. Intersectional feminism can help students and practitioners to conceptualise the intersection of multiple identities and their impact on client's lives, while recognising the need to challenge oppression for all. Social workers must consider whether or not methods are anti-oppressive in nature with respect to diverse groups, while assessing for cultural sensitivity and appropriateness of practice methods. According to Lum (2011, p. 153) social workers can engage in steps to promote interpersonal and systemic change through ethnoconsciousness, ethnic sensitivity and empowerment, all of which appreciate the role of 'critical consciousness', and change can occur through individual and social transformation.

Yet to say that social work in the US is a radical profession that works to end oppression and promote feminist principles would be a misstep. The contribution of feminist theory in shaping social work theory and practice continues to be largely unrecognised. The current social, political and economic environment has shaped contemporary social work practice to focus on clinical practice and demonstrated outcomes, with less emphasis being given to social change and advocacy (Reisch & Andrews, 2002). What is most current in US social work practice is the emphasis on knowledge and skills to engage in evidence-based practice.

Evidence-based practice

Evidence-based practice (EBP) and its emphasis on effectiveness dominate social work practice today. It requires the use of practice methods that have clearly designed protocols and research-based intervention strategies that demonstrate positive outcomes for clients. The medical community moved to a standard of care with what became known as evidence-based medicine (EBM) in the 1970s (Drisko, 2014; Gilgun, 2005; Rosenthal, 2006). EBM launched the criteria for guiding the decision-making processes that inform treatment intervention. These include the client's circumstances, the best research evidence, the client's choice and the expertise of the provider (Drisko, 2014). EBP as a standard of care was accepted slowly in the social work profession due to the broad scope of service provision, modalities, client systems and the lack of training and resources, as well as professional reticence and scepticism (Roberts, Yeager & Regehr, 2006).

Social work practice has historically been focused on the client relationship, and has relied on the expertise and ethics of the profession in the provision of services. Practice models traditionally were not well grounded in empirical study (Fortune, 2012). Reid and Epstein introduced the task-centred model in the 1980s and began a movement within the social work profession towards the EBP standard that exists today. The Campbell Collaboration, a clearinghouse for EBP research, was founded in 2000, and in 2008 the Council on Social Work Education required that schools of social work incorporate evidence-based interventions into their curriculum (Fortune, 2012), yet did not provide a clear definition of EBP.

Despite the lack of clarity, EBP influences how social work is currently taught in higher education and practised in agency settings. The rise of EBP also created somewhat dichotomous thinking and confusion as to what it really means (Mitchell, 2010) or its intentions. Some practitioners remain sceptical of whether or not the applicability of EBP can be generalised, while others cite the lack of administrative and organisational supports for practitioner training to learn EBP methods accurately (McCracken et al., 2012). Mullen and Streiner (2006) argue that EBP must recognise that randomised controlled trials (RCT) are not the only source of 'evidence': that good research and practice can guide the design for EBP. Drisko (2014) further notes that workers must continue to be competent and attend to the process of relationship building as it remains a key factor in influencing client outcomes, and that researchers still need to consider using qualitative methods and exploratory research to understand the implications of practice interventions. According to McCracken et al. (2012), there is limited data to support the use of EBP in terms of better outcomes or more effective and timely service provision, yet agencies and funding sources have an expectation that EBP should guide interventions. Thus, while social workers are now expected to use EBP, there remains limited demonstration of improved service. Yet others would argue that the focus on EBP has advanced a measure of accountability and critical thinking within the profession.

Feminist social workers today are challenged to maintain their focus on feminist practice principles in settings that emphasise EBP. Feminist research emphasises qualitative methods that examine contextual factors over the quantitative approaches that have been the hallmark of EBP. There are times when the implementation of an EBP in one setting developed from an RCT in another setting presents distinct challenges. McCallion and Ferretii (2010) note potential problems such as conflict with the agency culture, the client's values or inability to engage in all aspects of the intervention modality due to restricted resources. These factors are in direct conflict with empowerment-oriented feminist social work practice.

Additionally, EBP may not always appreciate the implications of how a problem is viewed or whether it is the result of larger, more systemic and oppressive structures. The model of implementing EBP research and interventions holds that the provider or researcher must first understand the client problem and situation, whether it is a micro or macro problem (Drisko, 2014) and design an answerable question (Thyer, 2006; Yeager & Roberts, 2006). This supposes that the researcher will identify key words or terms that can be objectively measured to collect data or 'evidence' based upon predetermined descriptors of the data. These types of measures become finite and do not usually allow for much variance between or within groups, or the impact of societal structures and factors such as systemic oppression. Thyer (2007) wrote that EBP includes an objective reality, and that we can deduce an understanding of psychosocial events in the context of that objective reality through scientific inquiry and measurement of phenomena. Thyer further stated that

> realism need not imply that the only reality is that which is objective and material, just that there is such a reality … to claim … that the world is a social construction is certainly acceptable, as long as the position is that social constructivism may be a part of the universe, not the whole thing.
>
> (2007, p. 8)

This position is somewhat at odds with the theory of social constructionism, which questions the notion of reality and the role of hegemony. Whether or not the 'truth' can be reduced to objectively determined evidence that leads to EBP is a question that critiques the researcher's role and the subtle subjective interpretations that can result when personal values go unrecognised. Social constructionism questions the generalisability and validity of 'evidence' that does not acknowledge the role of power and language in social norms, mores and structures, particularly when viewed through the feminist lens of intersectionality.

While the foundation of EBP is to include the client in decision-making processes (Drisko, 2014), congruent with feminist practice principles, the implementation of EBP in agency settings can fail to fulfil this mandate. For example, EBP research has sometimes 'screened out' clients, or has been completed with a limited client group and has not sought consumer input (McCallion & Ferretii, 2010). Feminist social work practice focuses on the relationship, fosters client collaboration and seeks to reach a common understanding of problems and solutions. This is vitally important given that the client–worker relationship has been documented as accounting for 30–40 per cent of variance in treatment outcomes (Mitchell, 2010). EBP interventions informed by feminist principles must promote the integration of critical thinking and reflection on the part of the practitioner, as well as partnerships with clients built upon mutual trust and appropriate self-disclosure to diminish power differentials.

Clinical focus

Social work students today increasingly pursue careers in clinical practice, which are considered to be more lucrative and prestigious, but provide limited opportunities for the social change mission of the social work profession. While we believe that there are opportunities to embrace feminist principles within clinical practice, there are also many barriers. Insurance reimbursement requires a focus on pathology, prescribes treatment length, and often type, and diminishes opportunities to engage clients in partnerships. Increasingly, the social work clinical curriculum is being dictated by state and licensure requirements. These requirements understandably focus on mental health diagnoses and treatment methods that have been shown to be evidence based. However, these standards are silent about many important issues that are critical for helping individuals recover from mental illness: coping with stigma, marginalisation and discrimination. Feminist tenets of empowerment practice, such as attention to diversity and social context, are often ignored in favour of the 'medicalisation' of mental health, an imperfect science that has resulted in many individuals with mental illness living on the margins of our society.

The structure and culture of agency settings are also significant barriers to implementing feminist social work direct practice with clients. White refers to 'the defining features of social work as a state mediated profession charged with implementing statutory duties' (2006, p. 38), which limits the ability of social workers to engage in egalitarian relationships with their clients and practice autonomously. While it can be argued that feminist social work practice can take place within these constraints, bureaucratic structures and processes can be experienced as oppressive by social workers and clients alike. Working in these organisations can lead feminist social workers to lose their ability to promote empowerment in both their clients and themselves. For example, one clinical modality that is compatible with the tenets of feminism is dialectical behavioural therapy, which was designed specifically for use with women to support and affirm personal growth. However, agencies and funding sources do not always support the resources needed to implement the model fully, particularly that of practitioner availability to the client whenever needed.

Lack of awareness and insight about feminist theory has contributed to many clinically focused (and other) social workers engaging in 'gender neutrality' in their practice. Just as it was once common to deny seeing 'race' and overlook the cultural context, social workers often view it as more egalitarian to ignore gender. For example, in the field of domestic violence 'battered women' became 'spouse abuse'. According to Dominelli, 'feminist social workers have challenged the gender neutrality regarding this social division usually upheld in traditional professional social work theories and practice' (2002, p. 8). Social workers must seek to understand the context in which women are abused and use violence themselves (Shepard, 2008). The use of violence by men and women in their intimate partner relationships differs in terms of motivation and consequence and is shaped by social and economic factors. However, many states have policies that require standard programme models for both genders as if they can be effectively treated using the same approaches (Tower, 2007). Social workers who do not have an understanding of the historical oppression of women will miss how it subtlety plays out in the lives of their clients. Feminist social workers find themselves continually pushing at the margins of mainstream social work practice to sustain the progress that has been made in addressing oppressive practices in regard to gender.

Redefining gender as fluid

We must examine the gender binary and our understandings of gender, expression and roles typically assigned as feminine and masculine. Ferree 'defines gender as a social relation characterized by power inequalities that hierarchically produce, organize, and evaluate masculinities and femininities through the contested but controlling practices of individuals, organizations and societies' (2010, p. 424). Thus, we must ask: does promoting feminist theory, research and practice reinforce this binary view of gender and indirectly undermine its own goals?

The social construction of gender as either male or female influenced social work practice and perhaps limited the vision, understanding and application of feminist theory as it relates to gender. Focused efforts to address women's needs may have inadvertently fostered oppression and stereotyping, conflicting with core feminist principles. Nagoshi and Brzuzy (2010) write that a positive and affirming view of gender needs to allow for fluidity in the individual experience and interaction with larger social structures, and empowering people who may live outside the gender binary. They note that we often unconsciously assign people a 'gender' without thinking, which potentially reinforces the heteronormative binary of being gendered into either this or that. This circumvents feminism's view of intersectionality and seeing differences within groups.

Rubin and Tanenbaum (2011) asked lesbian and bisexual breast cancer patients about their perceptions of medical staff regarding breast reconstruction. Most participants described feeling pressured to choose reconstruction, talked about 'feminist body politics' (p. 410) and felt urged to conform to a female appearance. Rubin and Tanenbaum strike a telling chord when they note that what should certainly be considered a medical crisis becomes recast as a 'cosmetic crisis' (p. 408). Gendered norms of appearance, identity and context reinforce these social structures of what it means to be a woman. This is a mechanism of oppression that impacts on those who are gender nonconforming and a factor frequently overlooked in social work practice. Feminism must participate in this dialogue about feminine identity, gender and unconscious bias regarding appearance, personal beliefs and gender. This conversation is ever evolving. We address gender and gender identity as social constructions and implications for feminist practice further in the next section.

Future directions for feminist social work practice

Feminist social work practice can play a vital role in addressing the practice challenges of the twenty-first century by promoting an understanding of intersectionality, encouraging critical thinking and enhancing practice approaches that promote client empowerment (see Figure 2.1). In our rapidly changing practice environment, future practitioners must integrate critical thinking, reflect on personal skills and decision-making processes, and address personal biases and limitations. We must consider the ways that the feminist movement can move forward to challenge the power and structural norms that remain so deeply embedded in society. We revisit the key contemporary challenges of diversity, EBP, clinical practice and gender, and propose that these four areas should be a focus in fostering the future of feminist social work practice in the twenty-first century.

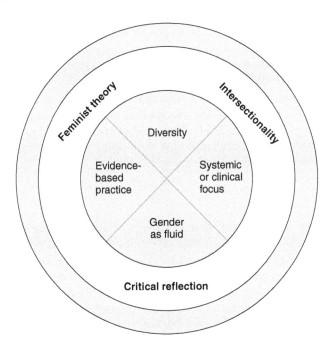

Figure 2.1 Future challenges for feminist theory.

Addressing diversity

We must continue to identify and challenge systemic oppression, particularly in the areas of race, class, sexuality and gender. Intersectionality provides a structural framework to assess power dynamics in relationships, as well as mechanisms that reinforce oppression. Engaging others in critical reflection at multiple levels (micro, mezzo and macro) can foster change in viewpoints and behaviour (Mattsson, 2014). Social workers must internalise feminist perspectives in order to promote social change and empower clients, while simultaneously respecting the uniqueness of individuals and their cultural beliefs and context. We must find ways to support and empower all groups that experience marginalisation and commit ourselves to gender equity on a global scale. Integration of feminist principles into conversations about topics of race, ethnicity or religious beliefs can be done using a proactive and respectful stance that promotes social justice and focuses on empowerment.

Evidence-based practice

Feminist theory offers a critical lens for examining the complex variables that will shape effective social work practice in the future. Qualitative research that focuses on lived experiences and the multiple contextual variables that impact client lives must be considered as valuable as studies using EBP that measure outcomes (Furman, 2009). Feminist research examines the multiple systems and multilayered impacts of oppression, and can be used to analyse how some populations are affected by inequalities within systemic structures. Using intersectionality as a conceptual framework requires the researcher to consider factors such as identity development, power structures and the categorisation of aspects of people into finite parameters (Mattsson, 2014). This kind of critical thinking must be utilised when designing research aimed at developing effective practice interventions in an increasingly complex world.

Clinical focus

Social work practice in the twenty-first century is at risk of being dominated by a focus on clinical practice that has become disengaged from the systemic nature of the problems we address. This is further fuelled by the push for EBP, which 'privileges micro-level approaches that focus on problems that fit more neatly into a biological or mechanistic model' (Furman, 2009, p. 83), and maintains a focus on knowledge rather than the core values of the profession. Feminist social work practice can help keep the need for systematic change and client empowerment at the forefront of social work practice.

Valentich (2011) calls for social work educators to demonstrate a commitment to feminist principles and ideals in the classroom, and to promote the social change mission of the profession. Mentoring, assignments focused on advocacy and creating supportive classroom environments that assist students to develop their own identity can give them the confidence to challenge patriarchal systems. Organisational and societal change, and social justice require that practitioners revisit the roots of social work and their ethical commitment to advocacy and anti-oppressive practice. Continuing education, leadership and mentoring, political work and advocacy, and community engagement are all vehicles for social workers to demonstrate feminist practice at macro levels in supporting and empowering oppressed groups. Clinical social workers who have been rooted in feminist theory will be better able to empower clients from diverse backgrounds in their practice.

Gender as fluid: identity and roles

Future conceptualisations of feminism incorporating critical reflection will require us to consider power and structural norms so deeply engrained in society that we 'cannot see the forest for the trees'. In an effort to support and empower people grounded in feminist principles, we may unintentionally reinforce gender stereotypes. Gilbert (2009) notes that breaking down gendered thinking about roles and identity could result in the transformation of other 'isms', including sexism, which is a goal of feminism. The earlier discussion of women's health needs, particularly around surgery and gendered appearance, remains an area of research inadequately addressed from a feminist perspective. Another practice area that remains largely gender defined involves the role of women as mother. Birthing frequently focuses on the mother–child context, with supports provided in 'mother-baby centres'. Reinforcing gendered mothering roles could result in disempowering other women who do not have children, whether by choice or circumstance.

Additionally, construction of gender and gender identity must be part of the ongoing development of feminist theory. Research on lesbian and gay parenting too often focuses on the notion that children are experiencing 'normal' gender development (Hicks, 2013, p. 159). We must reconsider 'normal' gender identity and expression, and assess our personal biases as to what we perceive as gender-normative identifiers or gender roles. Social expectations of conformity challenge feminist theory to deconstruct gendered hierarchies and ideals, which are often couched in moral beliefs. This is no small task, and yet cannot be ignored. Similar to the incorporation of voices of women of colour and sexual minorities, challenging the gender binary must become part of feminism's future. We must act in ways that reduce the limitations and barriers set by social norms and mores regarding gender as binary and transform our perceptions of gender (Dziengel, 2014). We can recognise the social pre-scriptions of roles, respect the differences within, and address the isms and barriers that support a gendered stance in agency, and political and social structures. Again, an intersectionality framework provides a useful mech-anism to examine and deconstruct gender. More research from a feminist paradigm can advance this perspective.

Conclusion

It was noted by bell hooks that the 'new' feminist movement has to change: 'our emphasis must be on cultural transformation: destroying dualism, eradicating systems of domination' (2000, p. 165). Social work educators and practitioners must engage in this transformation by putting their feminist principles into action at the micro and macro levels of practice. Evidence-based practices should be evaluated based upon the extent to which they incorporate interventions that support the feminist ideals of empowerment, shared power and equity. Feminist principles are deeply aligned with social work's core values of the importance of relationship, social justice, integrity, and dignity and worth of the person. Social work educators can reaffirm feminist per-spectives in the classroom by drawing connections with the core of social work practice and highlighting the role of patriarchal systems as the root of oppression for all groups. This discussion must also include an expanded view of gender to reduce the tendency to see gender as binary and to eliminate stereotypical thinking about gender. Reclaiming a fem-inist identity can advance the social work profession in the twenty-first century as we work towards a more just society.

Further reading

Baum, N., Yedidya, T., Schwartz, C. & Ofra, A. (2014) Women pursuing higher education in ultra-Orthodox society. *Journal of Social Work Education*, 50(1), pp. 164–175.

Giflus, M.E., O'Brien, P., Trabold, N. & Fleck-Henderson, A. (2010) Gender and intimate partner violence: evaluating the evidence. *Journal of Social Work Educa-tion*, 46(2), pp. 245–263.

Lockhart, L. & Danis, F. (2010) *Domestic Violence: Intersectionality and Culturally Com-petent Practice*. Columbia University Press, New York.

Mattsson, T. (2014) Intersectionality as a useful tool: anti-oppressive social work and critical reflection. *Afflia: Journal of Women and Social Work*, 29, pp. 8–17.

References

Alvarez, A.R., Collins, K.S., Graber, H.V. & Lazzari, M.M. (2008) 'What about women?' Historical perspectives on the CSWE Council on the Role and Status of Women in Social Work Education (Women's Council). *Journal of Social Work Education*, 44, pp. 63–83.

Barretti, M.A. (2011) Women, feminism, and social work journals 10 years later: 1998–2007. *AFFILIA: The Journal of Women and Social Work*, 26, pp. 264–276.

Bricker-Jenkins, M. & Hooyman, N.R. (eds) (1983) *Not for Women Only: Social Work Practice for a Feminist Future.* National Association of Social Workers, Silver Springs, MD.

Coady, N. & Lehmann, P. (eds) (2008) *Theoretical Perspectives for Direct Social Work Practice: A Generalist-Eclectic Approach.* Springer, New York.

Council on Social Work Education (2008) *Educational Policy and Accreditation Standards.* Council on Social Work Education, Alexandria, VA.

Dominelli, L. (2002) *Feminist Social Work Theory and Practice.* Palgrave, New York.

Drisko, J. (2014) Research evidence and social work practice: the place of evidence-based practice. *Journal of Clinical Social Work*, 42(2), pp. 123–133.

Dziengel, L. (2014) Renaming, reclaiming, renewing the self: intersections of gender, identity and health care. *AFFILIA: The Journal of Women and Social Work*, 29(1), pp. 105–110.

Ferree, M.M. (2010) Filling the glass: gender perspectives on families. *Journal of Marriage and Family*, 72, pp. 420–439.

Fortune, A.E. (2012) Development of the task-centered model. In T.L Rzepnicki, S.G. McCracken & H.E. Briggs (eds), *From Task-Centered Social Work to Evidence-Based and Integrative Practice: Reflections on History and Implementation.* Lyceum Books, Chicago, IL, pp. 15–39.

Furman, R. (2009) Ethical considerations of evidence-based practice. *Social Work*, 54(1), pp. 82–84.

Gilbert, M.A. (2009) Defeating bigenderism: changing gender assumptions in the twenty-first century. *Hypatia*, 24(3), pp. 94–112.

Gilgun, J.F. (2005) The four cornerstones of evidence-based practice in social work. *Research on Social Work Practice*, 15(1), pp. 52–61.

Hicks, S. (2013) Lesbian, gay, bisexual and transgender parents and the question of gender. In A.E. Goldberg & K.R. Allen (eds), *LGBT Parent Families: Innovations in Research and Implications for Practice.* Spring Science+Business Media, New York, pp. 149–162.

hooks, b. (2000) *Feminist Theory: From Margin to Center.* South End Press, Cambridge, MA.

Hooyman, N.R. (1994) Diversity and populations at risk: women. In F. Reamer (ed.), *The Foundations of Social Work Knowledge.* Columbia University Press, New York, pp. 309–345.

Lincoln, R. & Koeske, R.D. (1987) Feminism among social work students. *AFFILIA: The Journal of Women and Social Work*, 2, pp. 50–56.

Lockhart, L.L. & Danis, F.S. (2010) *Domestic Violence and Culturally Competent Practice.* Columbia University Press, New York.

Lum, D. (2011) *Culturally Competent Practice: A Framework for Understanding Diverse Groups and Justice Issues*, 4th edn. Brooks Cole, Belmont, CA.

McCallion, P. & Ferretii, L. (2010) Social work and aging: the challenges for evidence-based practice. *Generations: Journal of the American Society on Aging*, 34(1), pp. 66–71.

McCracken, S.G., Kinnel, E., Steffen, F., Vimont, M. & Mallon, C. (2012) Implementing and sustaining evidence-based practice: case example of leadership, organization, infrastructure and consultation. In T.L Rzepnicki, S.G. McCracken & H.E. Briggs (eds), *From Task-Centered Social Work to Evidence-Based and Integrative*

Practice: Reflections on History and Implementation. Lyceum Books, Chicago, IL, pp. 111–135.

Mattsson, T. (2014) Intersectionality as a useful tool: anti-oppressive social work and critical reflection. *AFFILIA: The Journal of Women and Social Work,* 29(1), pp. 8–17.

Mitchell, P. (2010) Evidence-based practice in real-world services for young people with complex needs: new opportunities suggested by recent implementation science. *Children and Youth Services Review,* 33, pp. 207–216.

Mullen, E.J. & Streiner, D.L. (2006) The evidence for and against evidence-based practice. In A.R. Roberts & K.R. Yeager (eds), *Foundations of Evidence-Based Social Work Practice.* Oxford University Press, Oxford, pp. 21–34.

Murphy, Y., Hunt, V., Zajicek, A., Norris, A. & Hamilton, L. (2009) *Incorporating Intersectionality in Social Work Practice, Research, Policy and Education.* National Association of Social Workers, Washington, DC.

Nagoshi, J.L. & Brzuzy, S. (2010) Transgender theory: embodying research and practice. *AFFILIA: The Journal of Women and Social Work,* 25(4), pp. 431–443.

Nichols-Casebolt, A., Figueria-McDonough, J. & Netting, F.E. (2000) Change strategies for integrating women's knowledge into social work curricula. *Journal of Social Work Education,* 36, pp. 65–78.

Reisch, M. & Andrews, J. (2002) *The Road not Taken: A History of Radical Social Work in the United States.* Routledge, New York.

Roberts, A.R., Yeager, K. & Regehr, C. (2006) Bridging evidence-based health care and social work: how to search for, develop and use evidence-based studies. In A.R. Roberts & K.R. Yeager (eds), *Foundations of Evidence-Based Social Work Practice.* Oxford University Press, Oxford, pp. 3–20.

Rosenthal, R.N. (2006) Overview of evidence-based practices. In A.R. Roberts & K.R. Yeager (eds), *Foundations of Evidence-Based Social Work Practice.* Oxford University Press, Oxford, pp. 67–80.

Rubin, L.R. & Tanenbaum, M. (2011) 'Does it make me a woman?': breast cancer, mastectomy, and breast reconstruction decisions among sexual minority women. *Psychology of Women Quarterly,* 35(3), pp. 401–414.

Saulnier, C.F. (2008) Feminist theories. In N. Coady & P. Lehmann (eds), *Theoretical Perspectives for Direct Social Work Practice: A Generalist-Eclectic Approach.* Springer, New York, pp. 343–366.

Shepard, M. (2008) Battered women who use force: implications for practice. In J. Keeling & T. Mason (eds), *Domestic Violence: Recognition, Reaction, Involvement and Outcome.* McGraw Hill, Maidenhead, UK, pp. 99–105.

Thyer, B. (2006) What is evidence-based practice? In A.R. Roberts & K.R. Yeager (eds), *Foundations of Evidence-Based Social Work Practice.* Oxford University Press, Oxford, pp. 35–46.

Thyer, B. (2007) Evidence-based social work: an overview. In B.A. Thyer & J.S. Wodarski (eds), *Social Work in Mental Health: An Evidence-Based Approach.* Wiley & Sons, New York, pp. 1–28.

Tice, K. (1990) Gender and social work education: directions for the 1990s. *Journal of Social Work Education,* 26, pp. 134–144.

Tower, L. (2007) Group work with a new population: women in domestic violence relationships responding to violence. *Women in Therapy,* 30(1/2), pp. 35–60.

Valentich, M. (2011) On being and calling oneself a feminist social worker. *AFFILIA: The Journal of Women and Social Work,* 26(1), pp. 22–31.

Van Den Bergh, N. (1995) *Feminist Practice in the 21st Century.* NASW Press, Washington, DC.

White, V. (2006) *The State of Feminist Social Work.* Routledge, New York.

Yeager K.R. & Roberts, A.R. (2006) A practical approach to formulating evidence-based questions in social work. In A.R. Roberts & K.R. Yeager (eds), *Foundations of Evidence-Based Social Work Practice.* Oxford University Press, Oxford, pp. 47–58.

3   Ethics and feminist social work

Annie Pullen Sansfaçon

Publications about ethics in social work have increased steadily since the 1990s, and have proliferated over the past ten years. In addition to exploring the different ways of understanding ethics, a number of these publications have discussed how best to manage ethical problems and dilemmas in everyday situations or, more broadly, ethical issues in professional practice. Authors have also described and analysed various ethical and moral perspectives as a way to manage ethical practice, and some have argued for the use of one perspective over another in specific contexts of social work practice. However, only a few publications in social work have seriously considered ethics from a feminist perspective. Where does feminist social work fit within these analyses? What theoretical foundations can be used by feminist social workers?

In this chapter, I will explore various ethical theories used in social work and their criticisms from a feminist perspective. To do so, I will briefly explore standpoint feminism as my starting epistemological position. Next, I will describe two broad ethical perspectives, namely principle-based approaches, which include utilitarian and Kantian ethics, and relationship and character-based approaches, which comprise ethics of care as well as virtue ethics. I will provide detailed discussions of character- and relationship-based perspectives and their potential fit within a feminist social work perspective. I will conclude this chapter with a discussion of the possibilities offered by a feminist perspective as applied to virtue ethics in social work, highlighting its strengths and weaknesses for practice.

Epistemological roots: a standpoint feminist perspective

While I have long been involved in various social struggles and scholarly debates about ethics, resistance and oppression, it took me a few years to identify as a *feminist*. As a scholar inspired by the ideas expressed by Foucault, Freire and MacIntyre, I strongly believe that oppressed groups, regardless of their gender, are tangled, though differently, in webs of power relationships, and that the emancipation of these groups is possible

through consciousness raising, dialogue, development of personal dispositions and collective action. While these ideas are mainly inspired by male-
identified scholars, I nevertheless feel that they transfer well to various
analyses I engage with.

Why write from this specific perspective now? Over the past few years I
have been increasingly involved in various social movements, particularly
those that relate to trans rights for children and young people, in Canada.
As the mother of a transgender child, my experience and analysis of power
have been strongly influenced by the following experience: that of a
middle-class cisgender female, a heterosexual parent and a fierce advocate
for the rights of my trans child, and an active member of a growing community fighting for the rights and equality of trans youth. This experience
has put gender at the forefront of my analysis and has led me to identify
specifically with standpoint feminism. A feminist standpoint is a perspective grounded in the experience of women 'who are reflexively
engaged in a struggle and knowledge arises from this intellectual and
political engagement' (Letherby, 2003, p. 45). In this sense, a standpoint
requires the person to be engaged as opposed to simply having an interest
in a particular matter (Hartsock, 2003). Given my scholarly focus on collective action and ethics, not to mention my experience as a member of a
growing community that engages in dialogue about gender norms and the
impact on trans youth, I am writing this chapter with this specific feminist
perspective in mind.

Ethics in social work

Social work ethics tend to gravitate around two main perspectives:
principle-based ethics and character- or relationship-based ethics. While it
is possible to find other ethical perspectives in social work literature (see
for example Houston, 2008; Wilks, 2005), these two ways of thinking seem
to dominate the debates in social work and, more broadly, society in
general. Banks (2006) explains that principle-based ethics relate to ethical
theories that draw on principles or rules used to determine the right
action, while character- and relationship-based ethics focus on the person
or moral agent that is making the decision. I shall now briefly explore the
main differences between these broad ethical perspectives and discuss
their suitability for feminist social work, drawing from specific moral
theories.

Principle-based ethics

Principle-based ethics concern a person's ability to live according to
certain moral principles, which are to be applied in everyday situations.
Examples of principle-based ethics include Kantian and utilitarian ethics,
which both articulate principles to follow in order to live an ethical life.

For example, in Kantian ethics, principles such as 'the intention behind the action should always be good', or 'the decision must always be based on respect for the person' should be applied consistently, among other Kantian principles, to form the moral basis of ethical decision making (Pullen Sansfaçon & Cowden, 2012). The utilitarian approach is another example of principle-based ethics. Utilitarianism usually promotes that the principle of 'greatest happiness for the greatest number', when applied to situations, will lead to ethical actions (Burn, 2005).

Despite different principles being promoted by different perspectives, such as Kantian and utilitarian, principle-based ethics generally require the decision maker to apply a set of abstract principles to the problem situation or, more broadly, to one's life. This may be one of the strengths of principle-based ethics: they provide relatively clear guidance on how an ethical dilemma should be managed and offer a sense of objectivity with regards to the decision-making process. Indeed, applying principles regardless of who is applying them should ensure a certain level of detachment and impartiality. However, principle-based ethics are exposed to significant criticism, which is specifically evident from a feminist perspective. First, because they are meant to be applicable to all situations, they neglect to take into consideration the singular characteristics of the person making the decision, or the context in which the decision is taken. In a way, principle-based ethics treat decision makers as though they are all the same, whether it is a mother faced with making a life-altering decision about her child's medical care, or a probation officer making a decision about a young offender in his caseload. The contextual element of the decision being made and the person who is making the decision could, however, have some impact on such a decision. As Gray (2010) asserts, principle-based ethics fail to take into account gender differences in decision making, as well as account for the relationship that may be established between those involved in the situation, the emotions one may feel or the responsibility one may have for another. Furthermore, although principle-based ethics may look as though they protect against subjective decisions, values and principles are always open to interpretation, and therefore even well-crafted principles could be applied differently depending on the person making the decision. Additionally, as described above, different ethical theories, for example Kantian and utilitarian ethics, propose different principles. It then becomes legitimate to ask what principle-based theory most deserves to be followed. In fact, one can rarely promote the greatest happiness for the greatest number while at the same time respecting the worth and dignity of each individual. Also, principles such as the greatest happiness for the greatest number are likely to overlook the most vulnerable segments of the population, including women and minorities, trans youth and gender non-conforming children. Principle-based ethics therefore fail to take into consideration and read-dress the complex power relationships present in society.

A feminist standpoint perspective requires that the actor questions the ideas and ideologies that disadvantage women, in order to achieve a less biased understanding of the various realities, as opposed to taking for granted ideas that are only constructed and validated by dominant groups (Bowell, 2011). Simply applying principles for ethical conduct without deconstructing them, taking into consideration the context, the person or the privilege that may come with applying such and such principles, therefore, does not offer a satisfactory basis for feminist ethics in social work.

Relationship- and character-based ethics

Relationship- and character-based ethics are broadly understood not as an ethical perspective that requires adherence to a set of principles, but rather as a way of looking at the moral agent, that is, the type of person making the decision, and the context in which the dilemma takes place. Ethics of care (EC) and virtue ethics (VE) are two ethical perspectives discussed under this broad umbrella.

Developed as a critique of Kolberg's work, which asserts that all people go through universal stages of moral development, Gilligan (1982) posits that instead women and men are not the same. In EC, it is believed that women are not naturally drawn to principles, and therefore alternative ethical perspectives are needed to truly give a role to women in morality. As Noddings says, 'it is well known that many women – perhaps most women – do not approach moral problems as problems of principle, reasoning, and judgment' (2003, p. 28).

EC therefore offers an alternative in ethics by positioning the person at the forefront of the decision. It also sees the concept of care as central to a type of ethics that takes into account womanhood 'not as practices under male domination, but as it should be practiced in post patriarchal society, of which we do not yet have traditions of wide experience' (Held, 2006, p. 19). In the tradition of EC, 'caring' (not as an unpaid task under male authority, but instead as central to ensuring the survival of humankind) is therefore perceived as central to most human activities.

In the EC, the notion of 'relationships' between people is also fundamental. By forging relationships, individuals always engage in giving or needing 'care' at some point in their lives, and it is a human responsibility to care for others (Held, 2006). Furthermore, while people are considered autonomous, the status of the relationships in which they are engaged can never be abstracted from their decision making. Thus, by being contextually relevant, EC also considers the role of emotions, an aspect that is often dismissed by principle-based approaches. According to the EC, not only is it reasonable to account for emotions that emerge from a situation; it is essential. The concept of impartiality is therefore refuted (Held, 2006). Furthermore, since context is so important in the decision-making process, EC is aware of the role played by the structures around the agent, and therefore always attempts to connect the private and public spheres (Held, 2006) so 'the personal is political'.

Despite the enormous contribution made by Gilligan, Noddings and Held to develop a type of ethics that focuses more on the feminine traits of decision making, EC is also criticised. For example, it is sometimes perceived as relying too much on a binary understanding of gender. While I do not refute that there may be several ways to engage in ethical reasoning and that perhaps the reasoning of some males may differ from their female counterparts, it may not always be so clear-cut. As Dworkin explains, 'dangerous and static associations between women and femininity and men and masculinity are often assumed, eroding much of the diversity that exists within and among these categories' (2005, quoted in Johnson & Repta, 2012, p. 18). From a feminist standpoint perspective, these gender differences, highlighted by the EC, 'may not fully reflect the multiple realities that women may experience, since both sex and gender are socially constructed and therefore subject to change over time' (Johnson & Repta, 2012, p. 20). Hence, there may be some issues with categorising women as caring and nurturing and men as otherwise. Not only can it contribute to reinforcing traditional gender roles for women (Gray, 2010), but it can also contribute to maintaining an understanding of 'womanhood' based on a set of dispositions that are inherent to their anatomical or birth sex. To classify male and female as having a specific set of traits therefore falls short of the ever-growing evidence about gender diversity. For example, some gender non-conforming children who were assigned 'male' at birth may display more feminine traits than some children who were assigned as 'female'. Furthermore, some intersex children may have genitals that are differently determined from a rigid binary perspective and develop a gender identity of their own. In this regard, EC, or at least some of its versions, may contribute to the development of a 'moral trap' because of the link between women and care, which may in turn lead to situations 'in which they will become even more subordinate to men than they are now' (Tong, 1998, p. 148). Finally, EC can be criticised for focusing too much on 'a private, relational or moral matter' and to neglect, in the end, the political aspects of how care is shaped in a patriarchal society (Gray, 2010, p. 1802). On the basis of the above criticism, a feminist standpoint-oriented perspective on ethics that is inclusive of gender diversity should instead present *a range of character traits that promote greater gender equity and gender justice as opposed to traits that are only related to women.* Maintaining the concept of relationships and moral agency at the centre of the discussion, I shall now turn to virtue ethics.

Virtue ethics (VE) originated with Aristotle, but was furthered by contemporary scholars such as Philippa Foot (2001) and Alasdair MacIntyre (1999). Today, different versions of VE exist, and the ethics of care is often considered a form of VE (see for example Meyers, 2001; Halwani, 2003; Pullen Sansfaçon & Cowden, 2012). VE can be summarised as a moral philosophy that focuses on the person, or moral agent, through the development of character traits or personal dispositions, also called virtues. These virtues should promote what is referred to as *eudemonia*, or human flourishing, not only of self, but also of others. In other words, from a VE perspective, the personality traits developed by the person will not only help them to flourish and be happy, but will also help others to do so. Examples of virtues include compassion, self-control, humility, courage, trustworthiness and patience (Pullen Sansfaçon & Cowden, 2012, p. 169). Care is also considered a virtue by some (Meyers, 2001). In fact, many other character qualities or traits can be considered virtues, as long as the disposition is stable, strikes a balance between vice and excess, and promotes human flourishing. A personality trait such as self-denial would not be considered a virtue because, while it may promote the flourishing of a person close to the moral agent, it will certainly not promote self-flourishing. By definition, self-denial is foregoing one's needs to help others. To be considered a virtue, a personal disposition must also be developed through habituation, and draw from the ability of practical reasoning. Once developed, the virtue needs to be practised in order to become part of one's life as opposed to a one-off act of heroism (Lynch & Lynch, 2006). The notion of relationships between people is also central, as it constitutes the grounds for practical reasoning and the development of virtues through a community of practice.

VE, like other moral perspectives, has been subjected to a number of critiques. First, VE is often perceived as being very 'masculine'. In fact, many point out that the traditional version of VE does not even refer to virtues such as 'care', 'benevolence' and 'compassion', character traits that tend to be labelled as being on the feminine end of the spectrum (Tong, 1998). Also, VE is often described as a moral philosophy that neglects the role that emotions play when managing an ethical dilemma. As MacIntyre explains, a virtue is an acquired human quality (1985, p. 191) rather than a feeling about rightness or wrongness. From a feminist point of view, this moral perspective can therefore be problematic in so far that it neglects to consider the criticism that Gilligan raised in her early work to move away from principle-based ethics to a more feminine version of ethics.

That said, VE also has some important strengths that should not be neglected, especially when seeking a feminist social work ethics perspective. Its main strength probably lies in the fact that VE is a powerful platform from which to address power struggles. For example, Foucault, in his later work, described ways of resisting power that were inspired by VE. Just as he began to recognise that the subject can be 'self-determining, capable of challenging and resisting the structures of domination in modern society' (McNay, 1992, p. 4, quoted in Besley, 2005, p. 79), an idea he coined as the *Technologies of the Self*, so some commentators have exposed a close link between increasing resistance through the *Technologies of the Self* and the integration of 'virtue ethics' into Foucault's work. As Levy explains,

Foucault's virtue ethics thus focuses, not on the subject, but on the character of the individual. While a subject is something given in advance, character is the set of dispositions and motivations to act into which we are acculturated and which we may then choose to cultivate or reject. According to this picture, if the self has depths, it is only because it has created them. Here too, though, Foucault is not a lone voice, but working in an area that has also been cultivated by at least some virtue ethicists.

(2004, p. 30)

Therefore, VE has great potential to facilitate the rejection of subjugating structures and relationships of power, including gender inequalities which feminist social work aims to challenge, by cultivating personal dispositions or virtues that can increase resistance to those power relationships in society. Thus, I believe it is not only possible, but also necessary, to read-dress the critiques of virtue ethics and make it move towards a more feminist social work ethics. This will be possible by integrating a standpoint perspective into it.

The contribution of standpoint perspectives to virtue ethics to inform the development of ethically based feminist social work practice

Furthering the theory of VE by drawing from a feminist standpoint perspective in social work means that the approach needs to include the values and objectives of feminism, as well as to draw on the specificity of social work practice. In the final section of this chapter I therefore explore how virtue theory can build from a feminist standpoint and further the debates around feminist ethics in social work. I will also illustrate, drawing from my own experience whenever possible, how VE can assist a community of parents fighting for their trans children's rights.

A brief review of the literature shows that a small number of scholars have already defended the idea of a feminist VE perspective (see for example Tong, 1998; Gray, 2010; Daukas, 2011). Specifically in social work, Gray asserts that feminist VE is possible by distancing itself from '"difference" feminism, which gave rise to the Ethics of Care, by seeing the virtues as distinctly human capacities' (2010, p. 1798). One can in fact ask whether the feminine characteristics identified by ethics of care scholars are really specific to a single gender or if, instead, a feminist ethics perspective should rather be influenced by the specific goal pursued in achieving good. On this point, Vanderberg (1996) makes a useful distinction between *feminist* and *feminine* ethics. He explains that a 'feminine ethics eschews the language and thought of "male ethics" when formulating a putative female perspective on how to promote the good' (p. 253), while feminist ethics uses ethical language regardless of the gender of its origin to promote justice, equity and the liberation of women. Virtue ethics can definitely achieve the goals of *feminist ethics*.

Some ethics of care scholars have strongly criticised VE for being too individual in its nature (Held, 2006), but the concept of *telos* (or purpose in human life) in VE theory is anything but individualistic. In fact, most versions of VE theory stress the importance of a person developing virtues *within a community* so that *telos* and *eudemonia* are defined together through practical reasoning activities. As such, through the development of, or engagement within, a community participants can be exposed to discussion and reflection or, as MacIntyre calls it, practical reasoning. This enables the participants to draw from the force of numbers, directly readdress power relationships and resist through collective action.

Therefore, drawing on VE and carefully integrating a concept of community, it becomes possible to begin rejecting subjugating structures and relationships of power through cultivating personal dispositions or virtues that increase resistance to power relationships in society (Levy, 2004). The central point of my argument is therefore that cultivating personal dispositions or virtues in the context of a strong community (MacIntyre, 1999) can be a powerful ground from which to begin to increase opportunities to resist power and challenge gender inequalities.

From my personal involvement with other parents of transgender kids, it is evident that having a forum to discuss in depth the situation faced by our children, and ourselves as parents and as families, allowed us to realise that the problems identified laid deep in the structure of society (i.e. one that only caters for people who fit within the binary). From forming a community of gender-creative kids' families, we not only had the opportunity to enquire about each other's experience, but also to understand the underlying commonalities, and thus to begin to identify the chief enemy, that is, the oppressive structures that forbid our trans children to exist as such.

In this sense, a feminist version of VE not only highlights the importance of developing virtues at an individual level but also focuses on achieving a collective definition and understanding of the nature of human flourishing and *telos*, based on a specific feminist orientation. As MacIntyre points out, practical reasoning as a collective activity is central to the development of virtues:

> Rational enquiry about my practical beliefs, relationships, and commitments is therefore not something that I undertake by attempting to separate myself from the whole set of my beliefs, relationships and commitments and to view them from some external standpoint. It is something that we undertake from within our shared mode of practice by asking, when we have good reason to do so, what the strongest and soundest objections are to this or that particular belief or concept

that we have up to this point taken for granted. Such rational enquiry extends and amplifies our everyday practical reasoning.

(1999, p. 157)

Practical reasoning within a community of feminist social workers may therefore draw from feminist values, not only by pursuing the general aim of social work, but also by aiming specifically at the liberation of women, and genders more broadly (and I see the term 'women' here in its broad sense, not only as an assigned sex birth), from oppression. Whether from a feminist standpoint or any other epistemological basis, the development of virtues in the tradition of virtue ethics theory should be socially located and should fully draw on relationships and community. By focusing on practical reasoning as a collective activity (see Pullen Sansfaçon, 2010 for further discussion), and sharing the process to identify the virtues needed to achieve the *telos* of the community, feminist values and orientations can be integrated so that that social workers who belong to this community can directly reflect feminist values, as well as the collective and subjective experience of the group's diverse reality, within a professional context through the development of personal dispositions.

To illustrate this point from my involvement with the Gender Creative Kids community, I have been involved in a monthly social action and support group with other parents that need reassurance and encouragement to better support their children, but also to take action to challenge the oppressive structures that are at the root of many of their concerns. Using critical pedagogies approaches, we have begun to unpack the many difficulties we face as parents and articulate strategies to achieve a more just society (*telos*). Personally, I have submitted a complaint to the Canadian Human Rights Commission with the aim of challenging the current law that forbids a person under the age of 18 years to request a change of sex marker on official birth certificate documents. If this law is changed, it will allow trans youth to be recognised legally, and will allow our children to live their life without having to make 'coming outs' every time they have to provide an ID, whether on the bus, at the health clinic or at the airport. To go through this difficult process of challenging the law, I had to draw on some personal qualities: *courage* to assert myself and identify publicly as a parent of a trans youth, but also *critical analysis* to choose the right forum to do so; *perseverance* to continue with the human rights challenges despite the many barriers that have come our way but *patience* to understand that these changes take time to happen; *empathy* to understand that not everyone is experiencing it the same way, and *care* to continue supporting those who are not yet affirming of their children's gender identity. Many of those goals are related to achieving a society that is inclusive of all, regardless of sex or gender.

Practical reasoning as a collective activity fits well within a feminist standpoint perspective by allowing for the emergence of a specific political analysis. MacIntyre explains that practical reasoning is an 'enquiry that provides us with grounds for the critique, revision or even rejection of many of our judgments, our standards of judgment, our relationships and our institutions' (1999, p. 157). Thus, practical reasoning, according to VE theory, allows us to integrate the feminist standpoint by engaging in a critique where 'conceptual frameworks emanating from patriarchal systems fail to provide the cognitive tools that enable women and others who are marginalized to make sense of their experiences in and of the world' (Bowell, 2011). As such, ethical practice in the tradition of feminist VE will focus on working towards a *telos* aimed specifically at challenging the social norms and institutions that contribute to maintaining gender inequality, in order to achieve the flourishing of self and others.

So what virtues would be needed in feminist virtue ethics? To identify relevant virtues for a specific community of practice, the values of the group may be a good starting point. For a feminist social work community, values associated with social work and feminism should therefore be considered. In the case of feminist social work, the values may be spelled out as being related to the liberation of women from oppression and the attainment of a more just society though social change, critical thinking and empowerment. Gender rights, equal opportunity and self-determination would also be important values to uphold. As such, a community of practice made of feminist social workers, if they are inspired by both feminist and social work values, should include diverse conceptions of womanhood so the empowerment of one does not contribute to the oppression of another. This would allow the multitude of experience to be included. The feminist standpoint perspective constantly questions what is considered reality so that it is possible to uncover the power relationships that contribute to building and maintaining the dominant ideology (Bowell, 2011). The dominant group here should not only be identified as 'male', that is, the bearer of the medico-legal category 'M' on birth certificates, but rather the dominant and static gender roles and performances that contribute to maintaining the oppression of one gender over another through the culture and structure of society.

From a standpoint perspective, I have found, from my experience of getting involved in the Gender Creative Kids movement in Quebec and beyond, that the development of a community of practice has allowed the necessary values to be integrated in our work towards achieving a more just society for all young people, regardless of their gender expression or their gender identity. This involvement has helped deconstruct knowledge that, according to a standpoint perspective, 'is socially located and arises in social positions that are structured by power relations' (O'Brien Hallstein, 1999, p. 35). As a result of this process, the moral agent will draw from virtues such as critical thinking to deconstruct, within their own community of practice, the concept of gender and work towards the development of a concept of womanhood that is inclusive and equally respected in society. The community members will also probably want to develop virtues of care and compassion to intervene on a day-to-day basis with groups oppressed by gender norms. Courage and justice will also be important to organise actions in order to challenge, at a more structural level, systems that are in place to maintain and reinforce oppressive structures identified through practical reasoning.

Using feminist VE, any social workers, regardless of their social location (gender, sex, sexual orientation, race, class, disability, etc.), may contribute to a society that is more just for all, as long as the practical reasoning activities are happening within a community of practice that shares feminist social work values and *telos*. Once the virtues or traits of character are developed and nurtured, feminist social workers should be in a position to practise ethically in a multitude of contexts or types of relationship. As Gardiner explains,

> as there are no rigid rules to be obeyed, it allows any choices to be adapted to the particulars of a situation and the people involved. Two people might both behave well when resolving the same situation in different ways.
>
> (2003, p. 301)

By allowing for the development of virtues that are contextually relevant and coherent with feminist social work, virtue ethics theory can allow for the repositioning of the actors, whomever they may be, to achieve ethical practice that is both inclusive and anti-oppressive, as Gray rightly points out:

> By attributing morality to human nature, rather than to differences between men and women, Virtue Ethics enables feminists to focus on fundamental human interests and needs. This fits well with social work's view of itself as a profession, which helps people achieve their full potential by actualizing their innate capacities.
>
> (2010, p. 1799)

Combining virtue ethics with a feminist standpoint perspective offers opportunities for the development of a community of practice that will work towards identifying what dispositions are necessary and what knowledge is needed to achieve a more equal society with regard to gender. Integration of feminist and social work values within a community of practice will also serve as the basis for questioning and challenging dominant ideologies through practice and the development of virtues. The community of practice will also serve as group mobilisation towards challenging unequal power relationships. Thus, it is possible to achieve a feminist virtue ethics perspective that is socially located, cognisant of the systems of domination that contribute to liberation from gender oppression, by allowing for the development of personal disposition, not on the basis of feminine or masculine traits of character, but, instead, on the basis of agreeing on a *telos* and conception of *eudemonia* that focuses on liberating 'gender' from oppression.

Conclusion

Undertaking practical reasoning within a community of practice that works towards a specific *telos* of gender liberation through the development of personal dispositions can facilitate ethical practice according to a feminist standpoint social work perspective. The work undertaken with families of transgender children in Canada can serve as an illustration for this point. While the growing community of parents and allies has been rather diverse, not only in terms of gender and gender identity, but also in terms of class, ethnicity and sexuality, they have nevertheless managed to come together around the same goal: that of working towards a society that is inclusive of gender diversity for people of all ages through directly confronting gender oppression. Through a process of critical reflection and defining the issues collectively, we have started to achieve social change (see Pullen Sansfaçon, Dumais-Michaud & Robichaud, 2014). Despite the challenge faced, the group has continued to highlight the importance of *critical analysis* and *justice* through identifying structural causes in the search for a solution, and *compassion* and *trustworthiness* in providing support to other parents and carers who may be struggling to accept their children's gender identity. Those characters traits, which will vary from one person to another, are all put forward so that a common goal, that of liberating children and young people from gender oppression so they can begin living according to their true gender self, can become possible. Examples such as this highlight the possibility of drawing from a feminist standpoint and a VE perspective, which combined offer early promises for a range of ethical feminist social work practice that can contribute to promoting 'social change and development, social cohesion, and the empowerment and liberation of people' (IFSW, 2014).

Further reading

Banks, S. & Gallagher, A. (2009) *Ethics in Professional Life: Virtues for Health and Social Care.* Palgrave Macmillan, Basingstoke.

Berges, S. (2015) *A Feminist Perspective on Virtue Ethics.* Palgrave Macmillan, Basingstoke.

Gray, M. (2010) Moral sources and emergent ethical theories in social work. *British Journal of Social Work,* 40, pp. 1794–1811.

References

Banks, S. (2006) *Values and Ethics in Social Work.* Palgrave-Macmillan, Basingstoke.

Besley, T. (2005) Foucault, truth telling and technologies of the self in schools. *Journal of Educational Enquiry,* 6(1), pp. 76–89.

Bowell, T. (2011) Feminist standpoint theory. In C.M. Bellon (ed.), *The Internet Encyclopedia of Philosophy.* www.iep.utm.edu/fem-stan/ (accessed 6 May 2014).

Burn, J.H. (2005) Happiness and utility: Jeremy Bentham's equation. *Utilitas,* 17(1), pp. 46–61.

Daukas, N. (2011) Altogether now: a virtue-theoretic approach to pluralism in feminist epistemology. In H.E. Grasswick (ed.), *Feminist Epistemology and Philosophy of Sciences: Power in Knowledge*. Springer, Dordrecht, pp. 45–67.

Foot, P. (2001) *Natural Goodness*. Clarendon Press, Oxford.

Gardiner, P. (2003) A virtue ethics approach to moral dilemmas in medicine. *Journal of Medical Ethics*, 29, pp. 297–302.

Gilligan, C. (1982) *In a Different Voice: Psychological Theory and Women's Development*. Harvard University Press, Cambridge, MA.

Gray, M. (2010) Moral sources and emergent ethical theories in social work. *British Journal of Social Work*, 40, pp. 1794–1811.

Halwani, R. (2003) Care ethics and virtue ethics. *Hypatia*, 18(3), pp. 161–192.

Hartsock, N.C.M. (2003) The feminist standpoint: developing the ground for a specifically feminist historical materialism. In S. Harding & M.B. Hintikka (eds), *Discovering Reality: Feminist Perspectives on Epistemology, Metaphysics, Methodology and Philosophy of Sciences*. Kluwer Academic Publishers, Dordrecht, pp. 283–310.

Held, V. (2006) *The Ethics of Care: Personal, Political and Global*. Oxford University Press, New York.

Houston, S. (2008) Communication, recognition and social work: aligning the ethical theories of Habermas and Honneth. *British Journal of Social Work*, 39(7), pp. 1274–1290.

IFSW (2014) *Update on the Review of the Global Definition of Social Work*. International Federation of Social Workers. http://ifsw.org/news/update-on-the-review-of-the-global-definition-of-social-work/ (accessed 8 May 2014).

Johnson, J.L. & Repta, R. (2012) Sex and gender: beyond binaries. In L.F. Oliffe & L. Greaves (eds), *Designing and Conducting Gender, Sex, and Health Research*. Sage, London, pp. 17–37.

Letherby, G. (2003) *Feminist Research in Theory and Practice*. Open University Press, Buckingham.

Levy, N. (2004) Foucault as virtue ethicist. *Foucault Studies*, 1, pp. 20–31.

Lynch, D.T. & Lynch, C.E (2006) Aristotle, MacIntyre and virtue ethics. *Public Administration and Public Policy*, 116, pp. 55–74.

MacIntyre, A. (1985) *After Virtue*, 2nd edn, Duckworth, London.

MacIntyre, A. (1999) *Dependent Rational Animals*. Duckworth, London.

Meyers, D.T. (2001) Social groups and individual identities: individuality, agency and theory. In P. Desautels & J. Vaugh (eds), *Feminist Doing Ethics*. Rowman & Littlefield, Oxford, pp. 35–44.

Noddings, N. (2003) *Caring: A Feminine Approach to Ethics and Moral Education*, 2nd edn. University of California Press, Berkeley, CA.

O'Brien Hallstein, D.L. (1999) A postmodern caring: feminist standpoint theories, revisioned caring, and communication ethics. *Western Journal of Communication*, 63(1), pp. 32–56.

Pullen Sansfaçon, A. (2010) Virtue ethics for social work: toward a new pedagogy for practical reasoning. *Social Work Education: The International Journal*, 29(4), pp. 402–415.

Pullen Sansfaçon, A. & Cowden, S. (2012) *The Ethical Foundations of Social Work*. Routledge, London.

Pullen Sansfaçon, A., Dumais-Michaud, A.A. & Robichaud, M.J. (2014) Transforming challenges into action: researching the experience of parents of gender-creative children through social action and self-directed groupwork. In E.J.

Meyer & A. Pullen Sansfaçon (eds), *Supporting Transgender and Gender Creative Youth: Schools, Families and Communities in Action.* Peter Lang, New York, pp. 159–173.

Tong, R. (1998) The ethics of care: a feminist virtue ethics of care for healthcare practitioners. *Journal of Medicine and Philosophy*, 23(2), pp. 131–152.

Vanderberg, D. (1996) Caring: feminine ethics or maternalistic misandry? A hermeneutical critique of Nel Noddings' phenomenology of the moral subject and education. *Journal of Philosophy of Education*, 30(2), pp. 253–269.

Wilks, T. (2005) Social work and narrative ethics. *British Journal of Social Work*, 35, pp. 1249–1264.

4 Feminism and social policy

Lesley Laing

Introduction

In this chapter I argue that engagement with the social policy process is integral to social work and that the application of a feminist lens can assist in critical analysis of social policies and inform actions that are consistent with social work's commitment to promoting human rights and social justice. Following a brief discussion of the social policy process, I provide examples of the ways in which the application of a critical feminist lens can strengthen social work's contribution to this process.

Feminist policy analysis is commonly associated with policies that are readily identified as vitally concerned with women's equality and well-being, such as domestic violence, equal pay and child care. In addition, the broader application of a feminist lens can also uncover hidden gender bias and inequality in broader policy areas which may not be as readily identified as topics for feminist analysis. Policies that claim gender neutrality, for example addressing 'parents' and 'families', can be interrogated to identify the ways in which they obscure gender inequality. I explore this through the example of changes to Australian family law regarding decision making about post-separation parenting arrangements.

Social policy processes

I adopt the definition of social policy as 'systematic public interventions relating to social needs and problems' (Fitzpatrick et al., 2006, cited in Fawcett et al., 2010, p. 7). Expanding on this idea, Bessant et al. (2006, p. 4) describe social policy as government activities that aim to improve the quality of people's lives. These policy actions are expressed through legislation and the provision of services and resources. Examples are the structured arrangements put in place to provide income security to certain groups (e.g. aged people, students, sole parents), to provide access for citizens to health care and education, and to address numerous social problems such as domestic violence and homelessness.

Governments are not the sole players in the policy-making process; many others are involved such as non-government organisations (NGOs), social movements (such as feminism and environmentalism), trade unions, individuals and groups affected by policies and proposed policies, and the media. Indeed, in thinking about feminism and social policy, attending to whose voices are heard and whose are silenced or marginalised within the policy process is important, as we will see later in this chapter.

There are many approaches to understanding the social policy process. For example, one perspective sees the process as a rational, problem-solving one with clearly defined sequential stages involving problem identification, selection of a solution through analysis of alternative solutions, implementation and evaluation. This approach has been critiqued as over-simplifying this contested process (Bessant et al., 2006). An alternative approach, located within the constructionist perspective, argues that social problems are not 'out there' awaiting discovery, but that they are constructed through discourse. For example, male violence to their female intimate partners has occurred across time and cultures, but the naming of these behaviours as domestic violence was an important step in creating this as a social problem. This approach to thinking about policy is exemplified by Carol Bacchi's (1999) approach to policy analysis, described as: 'What's the problem represented to be?' She argues for an approach to policy analysis that does not see policies as solutions to social problems but rather as 'competing interpretations or representations of political issues' (Bacchi, 1999, p. 2). Her approach involves analysing social policy solutions to identify their underlying assumptions and, importantly, identifying the effects of particular problem constructions.

Feminism and social policy

In addition to the discussion of policy actions, Fawcett at al. (2010) argue for a broader definition of social policy that includes government inaction, particularly in the face of strong advocacy about the importance of addressing a social need or problem. For example, Australia lagged behind most similar nations in only introducing a paid parental leave scheme in 2011. These authors note that this inaction or delay commonly occurs in relation to family policy, reflecting the contested issue of the extent to which the state should become involved in what are commonly regarded as 'private' family issues. Much feminist policy advocacy has been concerned with these very issues. Prior to the activism of second wave feminism in the 1970s, social policy was arguably largely gender blind to many barriers to women's equal citizenship with men. This activism played a key role in the move of governments into policy development around issues such as child care, reproductive rights, domestic and sexual violence, and sexual harassment. Continuing debates about policies addressing these issues highlight the contested and highly political nature of the social policy process.

The evolution of these policy issues over time provides an example of the ways in which developments in feminist thinking have continued to inform and influence the policy debate. For example, second wave feminists, drawing on radical feminist perspectives that emphasised gendered inequality under patriarchal social structures, argued that violence committed within the home should be treated in the same way as violence committed in public places, that is, as criminal behaviour. This advocacy successfully prompted law reform and other policies that overturned the previous reluctance of police and courts to intervene in violence within the family. However, feminist commitment to studying the ways in which policies are implemented in practice (e.g. Hunter, 2006) has been essential to identifying the unintended consequences of well-intentioned policies that can flow to some women. For example, criminalisation policies such as mandatory and preferred arrest and prosecution have been the subject of extensive feminist critique (e.g. Kim, 2013; Mills, 2003). Critiques have drawn on feminist intersectional perspectives to explore the effects of state intervention into the lives of women in marginalised social locations including women living with poverty (Goodman et al., 2009), immigrant and refugee women (Erez, Adelman & Gregory, 2009), women of colour (Snider, 1998) and Indigenous women. Feminist policy activism continues to call for more nuanced policies that, for example, evaluate policy effectiveness by examining the impacts on the most marginalised women (Coker, 2004) and that suggesting that domestic violence risk assessment incorporates the risks posed to women by systemic intervention, in addition to the risks posed by the perpetrator of violence (Laing & Humphreys, 2013). This brief example demonstrates the ways in which developing ideas within feminism can be applied to understand policy gaps and unintended policy consequences.

Social work and social policy

Social workers are inevitably engaged in social policy processes. Policies shape the roles and practices of social workers as they implement policies 'at the frontline' (Fawcett et al., 2010). Social work's emphasis on the person-in-context compels action spanning both the micro and macro spheres of policy and practice (Vodde & Gallant, 2002), responding to individuals, families and communities but always aware of the broader context. Inevitably an important part of this context is the ways in which policies affect people differentially. Social workers become aware of the effects of policies on the lived experience of people with whom they work; this makes them well placed to play a vital role in evaluating the impacts of policies and in advocacy aimed at modifying them. A good deal of social work practice involves resisting or attempting to ameliorate the harmful effects of policies that become visible through practice. In addition, social work research can also play a role in shaping and evaluating social policies. I discuss an example of this later in this chapter. In summary, social work's role in facilitating change through its commitment to social justice and the promotion of human rights requires active engagement in the social policy process, whatever the field or mode of practice.

The report of the Senate Inquiry into Forced Adoptions in Australia between the 1950s and early 1970s provides a stark example of the very real and long-term impacts that social policy can have on lives, and the inevitable involvement of social workers in this process. The report found that 'policies and practices resulting in forced adoptions were widespread throughout Australia in the post-war period' (Senate Community Affairs References Committee, 2012, p. 4). Negative attitudes towards young 'unmarried mothers' were shaped by gendered discourses that shamed women who had transgressed the boundaries of approved sexual expression (that is, within marriage) and that viewed white, married couples as providing the best environment for rearing children. The committee found that 'there was not appropriate government funding available to mothers prior to 1973 that would have provided the ongoing financial support necessary for mothers to keep their babies if they lacked any private source of income or family assistance' (Senate Community Affairs References Committee, 2012, p. 66). The testimony of women to the inquiry described the coercive pressures to relinquish their babies to which they were subjected, illegal practices that bypassed proper processes of consent and the long-term traumatic effects of these policies. Alongside the documentation of the involvement of social workers in implementing these policies are examples of resistance by some social workers and of advocacy efforts to overturn these harsh policies and to revise income support policy to provide access to financial support for single mothers (Senate Community Affairs References Committee, 2012, pp. 27, 112).

Rates of adoption dropped dramatically from the mid-1970s. While this can be attributed to factors such as increased access to contraception and falling birthrates, an important policy intervention was the introduction in 1973 by the Whitlam Labor government of the Supporting Mother's Benefit (renamed Supporting Parents Benefit and extended to single fathers in 1977). This policy extended the categories of women raising children who were eligible for income support (previously only widows); for the first time the federal government provided ongoing financial support for single women raising children.

This salutary example from the profession's history underscores the inevitability of social workers' involvement in social policy. As the introductory chapter makes clear, there are multiple feminisms. In my practice I have found that the common features of feminist approaches – including attention to inequalities based on gender and on gender's intersection with other social locations, attention to the operations of power in 'helping' relationships, and interrogating gender-related discourses – provide useful tools and a critical framework to assist in navigating complex and challenging policy terrains.

Contested problem representations

In this section of the chapter, I briefly describe policy changes to Australian family law over the last 20 years which provide a case study of contested problem representations (Bacchi, 1999). I also discuss the role of feminist policy analysis in uncovering the assumptions underpinning policy and presenting alternative representations, and the use of feminist research to identify the effects of particular problem representations and to inform policy advocacy.

Through a series of legislative changes in 1995 and 2006, Australia has moved towards a system of what is termed shared post-separation parenting arrangements, ideally established through negotiated agreements rather than litigation. Law reform processes typically involve extensive research and evidence of problems in the operations of the law. In this case, however, the major impetus for legislative change appears to have rested primarily with fathers' rights advocates who argued that men were the victims of inequality within the family law system (Flood, 2009; Kaye & Tolmie, 1998; Rhoades, 2000), despite little evidence to support these claims. Most couples make their own post-separation parenting arrangements, which largely reflect the gendered pattern of childrearing of intact families (Fehlberg, Behrens & Kaspiew, 2008). That is, despite the increased numbers of women in paid employment, and the cultural ideal of the 'new father' (Pleck, 1987, p. 358), patterns of child care have changed only minimally in recent decades and mothers continue to perform the major share of the work involved in the care of children (Flood, 2009; Maushart, 2001; Moloney, Weston & Hayes, 2013). Post-separation parenting arrangements reflect this pattern. Where arrangements are contested, fathers are equally as likely as mothers to gain residence of children (Rhoades, 2000). Helen Rhoades concluded from an extensive review of the evidence base for the initial changes to the law that 'Fathers' assertions of discrimination in custody litigation were statistically inaccurate, yet the perception of unfairness fuelled reform' (p. 13).

In brief, the initial changes in the Family Law Reform Act 1995 introduced the concept of 'parental responsibility', shared by both parents regardless of the child's residence arrangements, and introduced an objects clause which included the child's 'right to know and be cared for by both their parents' and the 'right to contact on a regular basis with both their parents and other [significant] people' (Kaspiew et al., 2009, p. 9) – colloquially referred to as the 'right to contact' principle.

Feminist analysis of these proposed changes brought to light the dangerous effects inherent in this policy for women and children separating from a relationship in which they experienced domestic violence and/or child abuse. Domestic violence does not necessarily end with separation and in fact may escalate in severity, including to lethal violence (NSW Domestic Violence Death Review Team, 2012). Separation may also lead to an intensification of 'nonviolent coercive tactics' (Frederick, 2008, p. 525), such as financial abuse and litigation abuse (Miller & Smolter, 2011). Further, children may be subjected to increased exposure to domestic violence after separation, since this may be the only context in which the violent partner has access to his victim (Hardesty & Chung, 2006; Jaffe, Crooks & Poisson, 2003). From a feminist perspective, the requirement that separated partners share parenting decisions was problematic because of the risks of post-separation violence and the coercive control (Stark, 2007) that is the core dynamic of domestic violence. Following intense advocacy by feminist groups who were concerned about the implications of these policy changes for women and their children escaping violence (Armstrong, 2001), the legislation was revised to include 'the need to ensure safety from family violence' as one of the considerations in decision making about parenting arrangements.

A raft of studies after the implementation of this legislation identified a trend to privileging the 'right to contact' principle over protection from family violence in subsequent Family Court decisions and the consequent ongoing exposure of women and children to violence (e.g. Dewar & Parker, 1999; Kaspiew, 2005; Kaye, Stubbs & Tolmie, 2003; Rendell, Rathus & Lynch, 2000; Rhoades, Graycar & Harrison, 1999; Shea Hart, 2004). These characterised the development of what was termed a 'pro-contact culture' (Fehlberg et al., 2008) in Australian family law. Despite the emerging evidence that this policy direction failed to protect many women and children from post-separation violence and abuse, further similar significant legislative changes were introduced in the Family Law Amendment (Shared Parental Responsibility) Act 2006.

Among the changes introduced in 2006 were compulsory mediation (termed family dispute resolution) prior to litigation except in cases of child abuse or family violence, through community-based Family Relationship Services, the presumption of equal shared parental responsibility and greater emphasis on the need to protect children from exposure to family violence and child abuse (Kaspiew et al., 2009, p. 4). The two primary considerations for decision makers in a complex, two-tier system were the 'meaningful involvement' of both parents in children's lives (an expansion of the previous concept of the 'right to contact') and the rights of the child to be protected from exposure to abuse, violence and neglect (Kaspiew et al., 2009). Where violence was an issue, there was clearly tension between these two key principles.

Using a feminist perspective: examining post-separation parenting arrangements

In this section, I draw on Bacchi's (1999) approach to policy analysis to explore the assumptions that underpinned these policy developments. Legislation enshrining children's right to contact and to a meaningful relationship with both parents reflected an assumption that this right was being inhibited. While the legislation was framed in gender-neutral terms and refers to 'parents', examination of some of the elements included in the 2006 legislation and the government's expressed rationale for the changes suggest that the problem of post-separation parenting was constructed as women who seek to limit relationships between fathers and children, often through false allegations of violence and abuse.

For example, in introducing the 2006 legislation, the then prime minister argued that there was a pressing need for 'cultural change' in the way in which post-separation parenting arrangements were decided and organised:

> The Government wants to bring about a cultural change in the way family breakdowns are handled. This $397.2 million package will give separating parents the support they need to sit down across the table and agree what is best for their children, rather than fighting in the courtroom.
>
> (Howard, 2004)

From a feminist understanding of domestic violence that sees it as intentional and as centred on the imposition of coercive control, this framing of the problem as primarily based in conflict is problematic for women who seek to limit an ex-partner's contact with children because of the risk of child abuse or exposure to domestic violence.

Despite the greater espoused emphasis on protection of children from exposure to violence and abuse, the legislation also included provisions that reflected scepticism about allegations of violence. These included what is termed the 'friendly parent provision', that is, the requirement for decision makers to take into account the extent to which a parent has facilitated the child's relationship with the other parent. Feminist analyses argued that this type of provision creates a problematic context making it difficult for women to raise allegations of violence and abuse (de Simone, 2008; Rathus, 2007). Despite the gender-neutral language of 'parenting', this type of provision primarily targets women because mother residence continues to be the primary post-separation arrangement (Hardesty & Chung, 2006). A further provision for costs to be awarded against a party who 'knowingly made false allegations or statements' was included, according to the legislation's Explanatory Memorandum, in order 'to address concerns that allegations of family violence may be "easily made" in family law proceedings' (cited in Kaspiew et al., 2009, p. 10). The assumptions underpinning these elements of the legislation appear to be that allegations of violence raised in family law proceedings are easily made and are commonly false.

An examination of other government statements introducing the legislation suggests that a core assumption is that it is women, rather than 'parents', who are most likely to make such false allegations. The then attorney general chose a conference of the Lone Fathers Association – vocal supporters of shared parenting and vocal in claiming that women make false allegations of violence in family law proceedings – to announce that claims of abuse would have to be 'independently verified' and that the new legislation would 'contain a number of measures as to how to make sure enforcement can be more effective' when orders have been 'deliberately disobeyed' (Peatling, 2005b, p. 3). In a similar vein, the chair of the parliamentary inquiry asserted that the proposed legislative changes heralded a 'more balanced' approach to family law and that 'children have a right to be protected from untrue claims of abuse that affected who had custody of them as well as from abuse' (Peatling, 2005a, p. 5). These political assertions reflect widespread community beliefs about women's propensity to make false allegations of violence and abuse in the context of divorce (VicHealth, 2014), which persist despite their lack of empirical basis (Brown & Alexander, 2007). They also reflect the problem representation advocated by fathers' rights groups.

The discourse of father absence that links it to poor outcomes for children, and particularly for boys (for example, Biddulph, 1997), also appears influential in shaping Australian family law policy, despite the contested nature of the evidence (Flood, 2003). In announcing the parliamentary inquiry that preceded the 2006 family law changes and the changes to the child support formula, the then prime minister drew on this discourse:

> I have expressed before, and I will say it again, that one of the regrettable features of society at the present time is that far too many young boys are growing up without proper male role models. They are not infrequently in the overwhelming care and custody of their mothers, which is understandable. If they do not have older brothers or uncles they closely relate to – and with an overwhelming number of teachers being female, in primary schools in particular – many young Australian boys are at the age of 15 or 16 before they have a male role model with whom they can identify.
>
> (Howard, 2003, p. 17278)

A substantial minority of children has minimal or no contact with their fathers after parental separation. Smyth cites data from the Australian Bureau of Statistics to the effect that 'more than one-quarter (28%) of the one million children under 18 years of age with a parent living elsewhere in 2007 saw that parent (mostly fathers) less than once a year or never' (2009, p. 41), a proportion that has been relatively constant for a decade. This problem of father absence has been framed in various ways, including as irresponsible fathering through the epithet of 'deadbeat dads' who fail to pay child support (Flood, 2003). However, the Family Law Pathways Advisory Group (2001), whose report was highly influential in shaping subsequent legislative change, and which received an overwhelming number of submissions from men and men's advocacy groups, provides examples of mothers being positioned as excluding men from post-separation parenting:

> It was evident that many men felt angry, frustrated and hopeless. Their anger was directed at both the system (particularly the law, lawyers, courts and the Child Support Agency) and ex-partners (who, they felt, deserved their anger for a range of reasons including leaving the relationship, denying contact or making false allegations).
>
> (p. 9)

These policy directions reveal the limitations of a problem-solving approach to social policy analysis, which emphasises a techno-rational weighing of evidence, since many core assumptions underpinning these policies did not reflect the available evidence. For example, the 1995 legislative changes resulted in an increase, rather than the anticipated decrease, in the numbers of contravention applications, that is, court hearings initiated by non-resident parents alleging that contact orders have been breached. Dewar and Parker's (1999) review of contravention applications found that the majority was brought by non-resident fathers, and that the majority was found to be without merit. Similarly, Rhoades' (2002) study of enforcement legislation found that only two of 100 cases matched the stereotype of the one-sided, unreasonable, contact-thwarting mother. The most common issue that emerged from analysis of these cases was domestic violence (in 55 of 100 cases). Despite findings such as these, the 2006 legislation included elements such as the 'friendly parent' provision that, as I have discussed, reflected assumptions about women's propensity to attempt to unfairly limit father–child contact after separation.

Bacchi's constructionist approach assists me to make sense of the competing and contradictory problem representations that are in the 2006 legislation. On one hand, the importance of dealing with abuse and domestic violence was recognised as a first-tier issue in decision making, yet aspects of the legalisation reflected scepticism about abuse allegations and created potential barriers to disclosure. Feminist analysis of the 2006 legislative amendments argued that the safety of women and children would be jeopardised in a system where the focus was on conflict rather than violence and that the 'friendly parent' and 'costs' provisions could inhibit women from seeking protection from violence (for example, de Simone, 2008; Rathus, 2007). In the final section of the chapter I describe a research project that explored the impacts of these policies from the perspectives of women attempting to establish safe post-separation parenting arrangements through the family law system in a context of domestic violence.

Feminist research: highlighting the effects of problem representations

Bacchi (1999) emphasises the importance of looking at the effects of particular problem representations. Following the implementation of the 2006 legislation, domestic violence workers, including many social workers, reported that women's and children's safety was being jeopardised by decisions about parenting arrangements that did not take adequate account of issues of domestic violence. Through a researcher–service provider collaboration, I undertook a qualitative study to explore women's experiences of negotiating the family law system following a relationship in which they experienced domestic violence (Laing, 2010). I conducted in-depth interviews with 22 women from diverse socioeconomic and cultural backgrounds who were at different stages in the family law process. This was a purposive sample with participants selected because of their expert knowledge of the family law system as participants in it. The aim was to give voice to a group who were deeply affected by the policy but whose experiences had been marginalised and silenced.

The women described violence that was severe, multifaceted and characterised by coercive, controlling tactics: 'Because our life was like living in a concentration camp, that's how I described it once' (Laing, 2010, p. 29). The violence did not end with the separation for the women, nor did the violence exposure of many of the children:

> I was severely assaulted, I was beaten unconscious … part of it happened in the flat while I was picking up the kids [at changeover] and then it sort of moved outside…. So my younger child saw him beating me and he was in the stairwell and he kept hiding his head … and he has told his counsellor that I wouldn't wake up – that he kept telling me 'mummy wake up'.
>
> (Laing, 2010, p. 33)

Despite a high rate of civil and criminal legal intervention in this sample, the women experienced considerable barriers to establishing safe parenting arrangements. Five of the women had 50:50 shared time arrangements, even though research contraindicates shared parenting in cases of domestic violence and high conflict (McIntosh & Chisholm, 2008). The majority had mother residence but with significant time spent in the care of fathers, including overnight. In three cases which involved very young children and allegations of both child sexual assault and domestic violence, the fathers' only contact was supervised; however, in all but one of these cases it was anticipated by the court that this would proceed to unsupervised contact through the passage of time, rather than through requirements that the men demonstrate changes that would make children safer in their care.

Here I will discuss several themes that were identified in the analysis. The women described *having to navigate a complex, fragmented and uncoordinated service system* marked by delays and barriers to accessing accurate information as they attempted to try to protect themselves and their children. They provided numerous examples of the ways in which the federal–state jurisdictional 'gap' (Higgins & Kaspiew, 2008), between the Family Court at federal level and state-based police and child protection services, thwarted their efforts to be safe.

> It's been really frustrating – like before I had Family Court orders and we had the cops involved and they didn't want to get involved because I didn't have Family Court orders. When I did have Family Court orders, the cops said they didn't want to get involved because I had Family Court orders.
>
> (Laing, 2010, p. 38)

However, beyond this systemic complexity, the women encountered *a climate of disbelief* from many professionals across the system. In response to their efforts to achieve safe parenting arrangements, they found that their motives in raising issues of violence were suspect:

> The duty lawyer [in the Family Court] said that DoCS [state child protection] was involved. The [Federal] Magistrate flew off the handle and she said: 'I have seen all this before where a mother feeds her story to DoCS, so of course they support her.'
>
> (Laing, 2010, p. 49)

Another woman's ex-partner had been convicted of assaulting her, and evidence of physical assault and abduction of the children had led the police to apply for a separate protection order on behalf of the children. Nevertheless, the Independent Children's Lawyer in the Family Court accused the woman of 'alienating' the children.

Alongside the reluctance to listen to women's concerns about the safety of themselves and their children, many professionals, including their own lawyers, explained to the women that *fathers were essential to children*, even when there was evidence of domestic violence and child abuse. One woman had experienced severe physical abuse that left her with a permanent physical disability when she was assaulted while holding her infant child. She found the emphasis on the children spending time with their father rather than on the violence and child abuse difficult to understand:

[A]nd they're saying to me but he has to have time with the children. And I'm saying 'but he's knocked me to the ground with a baby in my arms – why does he – and he's been charged, he's been found guilty of assault.'

(Laing, 2010, p. 9)

These experiences had serious consequences in the lives of the women and their children. The women described managing a very delicate balancing act as they made choices about whether, and how much, to raise issues of violence and abuse. They lived with the fear that they could be punished by losing the residence of their children if they were seen as 'unfriendly' or 'alienating' parents. As a consequence, they felt they had no choice other than to agree to arrangements that were not safe, for fear of a worse outcome: '[T]he Judge actually threatened to take [my child] off me and that I would have supervised care if he saw me in court again with such rubbish [allegations of domestic violence]' (Laing, 2010, p. 54).

In summary, the dominant discourses that had been influential in shaping the 2006 policy changes constructed women raising issues of violence as problematic participants in the family law process. Counter-discourses about the prevalence of violence and abuse in family breakdown appeared to remain marginal despite those elements of the law that attempted to address these issues.

Feminist policy advocacy

Several large-scale evaluations of the 2006 legislation found that, while there were many positive outcomes, the system was not dealing well with cases involving allegations of child abuse and domestic violence (Bagshaw et al., 2011; Kaspiew et al., 2009). While the findings of a non-representative sample in the qualitative study described cannot be generalised, they complement the findings of larger quantitative studies by highlighting the lived experience of women and the effects on the women and their children when safe parenting arrangements are not achieved. Continuing the collaboration that had initiated the research, I worked with the Alliance for Children's Safety, which comprises women's and children's services and advocacy groups and was established to advocate for changes to the 2006 legislation. We met with politicians, provided them with case studies based on women's and children's experiences, and held a rally at Parliament House advocating changes to the law that would better attend to the safety of women and children post-separation. The findings of my research also formed the basis of a submission to the senate committee established to review the legislation.

Legislative changes introduced following a highly contested review process in 2011 repealed the 'friendly parent' and 'costs' elements of the legislation, introduced a broader definition of family violence and gave priority to the 'protection from harm' over the 'meaningful relationship' principle when they were in conflict. Further research is needed to ascertain whether changing laws is sufficient to change practices that are deeply embedded in gendered discourses about parenting. What this example makes clear is that feminist policy analysis, research and advocacy provide social workers with the tools with which to interrogate and resist policies whose effects undermine human rights.

Further reading

Bacchi, C.L. (2009) Introducing a 'what's the problem represented to be?' approach to policy analysis. *Analysing Policy: What's the Problem Represented to Be?* Pearson, Frenchs Forest, NSW, pp. 1–24.

Coy, M., Perks, K., Scott, E. & Tweedale, R. (2012) Picking up the pieces: domestic violence and child contact. http://rightsofwomen.org.uk/wp-content/uploads/2014/10/Picking_Up_the_Pieces_Report-2012l.pdf (accessed 23 May 2015).

Elizabeth, V., Gavey, N. & Tolmie, J. (2012) '…He's just swapped his fists for the system': the governance of gender through custody law. *Gender and Society*, 26(2), pp. 239–260.

Fawcett, B., Goodwin, S., Meagher, G. & Phillips, R. (2010) *Social Policy for Social Change*. Palgrave, South Yarra.

Rivera, E.A., Sullivan, C.M. & Zeoli, A.M. (2012) Secondary victimization of abused mothers by family court mediators. *Feminist Criminology*, 7(3), pp. 234–252.

References

Armstrong, S. (2001) 'We told you so…': women's legal groups and the *Family Law Reform Act 1995*. *Australian Journal of Family Law*, 15(2), pp. 129–154.

Bacchi, C.L. (1999) *Women, Policy and Politics: The Construction of Policy Problems*. Sage, London.

Bagshaw, D., Brown, T., Wendt, S., Campbell, A., McInnes, E., Tinning, B. & Arias, P.F. (2011) The effect of family violence on post-separation parenting arrangements: the experiences and views of children and adults from families who separated post-1995 and post-2006. *Family Matters*, 86, pp. 49–61.

Bessant, J., Watts, R., Dalton, T. & Smyth, P. (2006) *Talking Policy: How Social Policy is Made*. Allen & Unwin, Crows Nest, NSW.

Biddulph, S. (1997) *Raising Boys*. Finch Publishing, Sydney.

Brown, T. & Alexander, R. (2007) *Child Abuse and Family Law: Understanding the Issues Facing Human Service and Legal Professionals*. Allen & Unwin, Crows Nest, NSW.

Coker, D. (2004) Race, poverty, and the crime-centred response to domestic violence. *Violence Against Women*, 10(11), pp. 1331–1353.

de Simone, T. (2008) The friendly parent provisions in Australian family law: how friendly will you need to be? *Australian Journal of Family Law*, 22, p. 56.

Dewar, J. & Parker, S. (1999) The impact of the new part VII *Family Law Act 1975*. *Australian Journal of Family Law*, 13(2), pp. 96–116.

Erez, E., Adelman, M. & Gregory, C. (2009) Intersections of immigration and domestic violence: voices of battered immigrant women. *Feminist Criminology*, 4(1), pp. 32–56.

Family Law Pathways Advisory Group (2001) *Out of the Maze: Pathways to the Future for Families Experiencing Separation*. Attorney-General's Department, Canberra.

Fawcett, B., Goodwin, S., Meagher, G. & Phillips, R. (2010) *Social Policy for Social Change*. Palgrave Macmillan, South Yarra, Vic.

Fehlberg, B., Behrens, J. & Kaspiew, R. (2008) *Australian Family Law: The Contemporary Context*. Oxford University Press, South Melbourne, Vic.

Flood, M. (2003) *Fatherhood and Fatherlessness*. Discussion Paper No. 59. Australia Institute, Canberra. www.tai.org.au/documents/downloads/DP59.pdf (accessed 21 October 2014).

Flood, M. (2009) 'Fathers' rights' and the defense of paternal authority in Australia. *Violence Against Women*, 16(3), pp. 328–347.

Frederick, L. (2008) Questions about Family Court domestic violence screening and assessment. *Family Court Review*, 46(3), pp. 523–530.

Goodman, L.A., Fels Smyth, K., Borges, A.M. & Singer, R. (2009) When crises collide: how do intimate partner violence and poverty intersect to shape women's mental health and coping? *Trauma, Violence and Abuse*, 10(4), pp. 306–329.

Hardesty, J.L. & Chung, G.H. (2006) Intimate partner violence, parental divorce, and child custody: directions for intervention and future research. *Family Relations*, 55(2), pp. 200–210.

Higgins, D.J. & Kaspiew, R. (2008) 'Mind the gap…': protecting children in family law cases. *Australian Journal of Family Law*, 22(3), pp. 235–258.

Howard, J. (2003) *Parliamentary Debates*, House of Representatives, Hansard, Vol. 10. Commonwealth of Australia, Canberra.

Howard, J. (2004) *Reforms to the Family Law System*. Media Centre, Prime Minister of Australia, Canberra.

Hunter, R. (2006) Narratives of domestic violence. *Sydney Law Review*, 28(4), pp. 733–776.

Jaffe, P.G., Crooks, C.V. & Poisson, S.E. (2003) Common misconceptions in addressing domestic violence in child custody disputes. *Juvenile and Family Court Journal*, 54(4), pp. 57–67.

Kaspiew, R. (2005) Violence in contested children's cases: an empirical exploration. *Australian Journal of Family Law*, 19, pp. 112–143.

Kaspiew, R., Gray, M., Weston, R., Moloney, L., Hand, K., Qu, L. & the Family Law Evaluation Team (2009) *Evaluation of the 2006 Family Law Reforms*. Australian Institute of Family Studies, Melbourne.

Kaye, M. & Tolmie, J. (1998) Fathers' rights groups in Australia and their engagement with issues in family law. *Australian Journal of Family Law*, 12(1), pp. 19–68.

Kaye, M., Stubbs, J. & Tolmie, J. (2003) Domestic violence and child contact arrangements. *Australian Journal of Family Law*, 17(2), pp. 93–133.

Kim, M.E. (2013) Challenging the pursuit of criminalisation in an era of mass incarceration: the limitations of social work responses to domestic violence in the USA. *British Journal of Social Work*, 43(7), pp. 1276–1293.

Laing, L. (2010) *No Way to Live: Women's Experiences of Negotiating the Family Law System in the Context of Domestic Violence*. University of Sydney and Benevolent Society, Sydney. http://hdl.handle.net/2123/6255 (accessed 8 July 2014).

Laing, L. & Humphreys, C. (2013) *Social Work and Domestic Violence: Developing Critical and Reflective Practice*. Sage, London.

McIntosh, J. & Chisholm, R. (2008) Cautionary notes on the shared care of children in conflicted parental separation. *Journal of Family Studies*, 14(1), pp. 37–52.

Maushart, S. (2001) *Wifework: What Marriage Really Means for Women.* Text Publishing, Melbourne.

Miller, S.L. & Smolter, N.L. (2011) 'Paper abuse': when all else fails, batterers use procedural stalking. *Violence Against Women*, 17(5), pp. 637–650.

Mills, L.G. (2003) *Insult to Injury: Rethinking our Responses to Intimate Abuse.* Princeton University Press, Princeton, NJ.

Moloney, L., Weston, R. & Hayes, A. (2013) Key social issues in the development of Australian family law: research and its impact on policy and practice. *Journal of Family Studies*, 19(2), pp. 110–138.

NSW Domestic Violence Death Review Team (2012) *Annual Report.* NSW Coroner's Court, Sydney. www.coroners.lawlink.nsw.gov.au/agdbasev7wr/_assets/coroners/m40160115/dvdrt_annual_report_final_october_2012x.pdf (accessed 9 December 2013).

Peatling, S. (2005a) Parents without custody to be given bigger say. *Sydney Morning Herald*, 19 August, p. 5.

Peatling, S. (2005b) Ruddock promises tougher family law. *Sydney Morning Herald*, 23 June, p. 3.

Pleck, J.H. (1987) American fathering in historical perspective. In M. Kimmel (ed.), *Changing Men: New Directions in Research on Men and Masculinity.* Sage, Newbury Park, CA, pp. 351–361.

Rathus, Z. (2007) Shifting the gaze: will past violence be silenced by a further shift of the gaze to the future under the new family law system? *Australian Journal of Family Law*, 21(1), pp. 87–112.

Rendell, K., Rathus, Z. & Lynch, A. (2000) *An Unacceptable Risk: A Report on Child Contact Arrangements where there is Violence in the Family.* Women's Legal Service, Brisbane.

Rhoades, H. (2000) Posing as reform: the case of the *Family Law Reform Act. Australian Journal of Family Law*, 14, pp. 1–18.

Rhoades, H. (2002) The 'no contact mother': reconstructions of motherhood in the era of the 'new father'. *International Journal of Law, Policy and the Family*, 16(1), pp. 71–94.

Rhoades, H., Graycar, R. & Harrison, M. (1999) *The Family Law Reform Act: Can Changing Legislation Change Legal Culture, Legal Practice and Community Expectations?* University of Sydney, Sydney.

Senate Community Affairs References Committee (2012) *Commonwealth Contribution to Former Forced Adoption Policies and Practices.* Parliament of Australia, Canberra. www.aph.gov.au/Parliamentary_Business/Committees/Senate/Community_Affairs/Completed_inquiries/2010-13/commcontribformerforcedadoption/report/~/media/wopapub/senate/committee/clac_ctte/completed_inquiries/2010-13/comm_contrib_former_forced_adoption/report/report.ashx (accessed 28 July 2014).

Shea Hart, A. (2004) Children exposed to domestic violence: undifferentiated needs in Australian family law. *Australian Journal of Family Law*, 18(2), pp. 170–192.

Smyth, B. (2009) A 5-year retrospective of post-separation shared care research in Australia. *Journal of Family Studies*, 15(1), pp. 36–59.

Snider, L. (1998) Towards safer societies: punishment, masculinities and violence against women. *British Journal of Criminology*, 38(1), pp. 1–39.

Stark, E. (2007) *Coercive Control: How Men Entrap Women in Personal Life.* Oxford University Press, New York.

VicHealth (2014) *Australians' Attitudes to Violence against Women: 2013 National Community Attitudes towards Violence against Women Survey – Research Summary.* VicHealth, Melbourne. www.vichealth.vic.gov.au/~/media/ResourceCentre/Publicationsand Resources/PVAW/NCAS/NCAS-ResearchSummary_2014.ashx (accessed 18 September 2014).

Vodde, R. & Gallant, J.P. (2002) Bridging the gap between micro and macro practice: large scale change and a unified model of narrative-deconstructive practice. *Journal of Social Work Education,* 38(3), pp. 439–458.

5 Feminism and the delivery of human services

Sue King and Deirdre Tedmanson

Introduction

Social policy in a number of countries, including Australia, is undergoing radical change through the implementation of new models of service delivery. These arise primarily from the trend towards the marketisation of human services and increased outsourcing of decision making, away from governments and towards end service users. The changes create new opportunities to put service users in positions of power in relation to the design and management of their services, but the changes also bring great risk. In this chapter we use a feminist ethics of care lens to examine the policy shifts that are being enacted by governments committed to either reducing or constraining the cost of social welfare through the development of both privatised and personalised service delivery models. For women, as service users, social workers and other human service workers, and informal carers, there are potential gains to be made under the new arrangements. However, we argue in this chapter that the risks accompanying new market-driven human service delivery models are understated, under-recognised and under-discussed.

Consumer-directed care or consumer-controlled care are terms frequently used in Australia to describe this shift away from government control; however the policy drivers and programmes developed are similar to those described in the United Kingdom as personalisation or direct payments (Lloyd, 2010), self-managed care in Canada and self-determination in the US (Fisher et al., 2010). Whilst the specific models developed in each country differ in both 'language and program design' (Crozier et al., 2013), the underlying principles remain the same. They have developed out of the now widespread new public management model in which governments reduce their role as a direct provider of services and instead create a competitive 'market' environment through which not-for-profit, for-profit and niche organisations are meant to compete to meet service needs.

These developments in the delivery of social policy have significant impacts on the lives of women as both recipients and providers of services, impacts which are felt most acutely by the most vulnerable in society, particularly those who are aged or living with disabilities. Proponents of the new approaches argue that they embed recognition of the support needed by many community members to live the life they wish, and that placing the individual at the centre of decision making about what services would be useful and how they should be provided can empower individuals, in accordance with fundamental social work values (AASW, 2010). However the uncritical promotion of this neo-liberal social policy discourse stifles insights about relations of power and gender inequities which, as Ball and Charles (2006, quoting Ferree, 2003) argue, renders 'gender invisible'. To date little attention has been given to the impact of the new service delivery environment on women. Here we consider what a feminist ethics of care lens can contribute to understanding these new policy developments.

Following a discussion of the ethics of care lens and the light it sheds on these social policy developments, we will examine the developments in human service delivery in a number of national contexts. In Australia two significant reports from the Australian Productivity Commission have mapped out the consumer-directed service delivery innovation and we will consider these alongside the ways in which the strategy has been implemented. We conclude by exploring the contribution of a feminist ethics of care perspective to the evaluation of the extent to which these policy initiatives advance the wellbeing of women as human service users, human service workers and designers of human services into the future.

Feminist ethics of care lens

The political and practical developments in the delivery of human services involved in the movement to consumer-directed care give expression to a particular neo-liberal philosophical position about the nature of social policy and human services. Debates about the appropriate positioning of the state in relation to citizens with specific needs, how we understand where the problem lies (Morris, 2001) and how concepts such as care are utilised have engaged the attention of feminist social workers and scholars over recent decades (Fawcett et al., 2010). Efforts to reconcile rights and issues of adequacy of care are particularly evident in the ethics of care approach, which has been widely written about since Gilligan's (1982) work first questioned how to balance these at times competing values (Barnes, 2011). Gilligan focused on gender differences by distinguishing between 'male rationality' and 'female caring'. By highlighting this imposed binary but at the same time asserting the importance of avoiding simplistic dichotomies (Gray, 2010) a feminist ethics of care approach has created a base for challenging hidden values and gendered assumptions. Although the focus of much feminist ethics of care analysis has been on the individual and professional relationships in care work, influential scholarship has also begun to take this feminist approach into the arena of social policy (Gray, 2010; Sevenhuijsen, 2003).

The feminist ethics of care perspective on social policy challenges the way in which dependence and care are constructed. In contrast to an emphasis on individual autonomy and independence, 'relationality and interdependence are core concepts in the ethic of care' (Sevenhuijsen, 2003, p. 183). The social context of human need is addressed by arguing that we are all interdependent and will need to give and receive support throughout a lifetime (Sevenhuijsen, 2003; Lloyd, 2010). An ethics of care approach makes visible both the giving and receiving of care over a lifetime and challenges the deficit construction of needing care and support which privileges a masculinist notion of independence and autonomy.

This overarching view of social relations has been treated with caution, however, by some feminists. Morris (2001), for example, argues that, whilst it provides a useful counter to the masculinist emphasis placed on individual coping, it must not be allowed to mask the recognition that for some people more adaptation and hence greater resourcing is required if they are to live full lives as citizens. Morris speaks for people whose lives are affected by impairment, for example, asserting that 'we need an ethics of care which, while starting from the position that everyone has the same human rights, also recognizes the additional requirements that some people have in order to access those human rights' (Morris, 2001, p. 15).

Sevenhuijsen (2003) argues that an ethics of care framework can be utilised to distinguish between self-sufficiency and self-determination. She argues that if autonomy is only thought of as self-sufficiency the full dimensions of care are made invisible, whereas if autonomy is conceptualised as relational it can be seen that self-determination can be achieved without denying human interconnection. Through this analysis, the feminist ethics of care provides a useful framework for exploring the potential marginalisation of care in social policy contexts (Gray, 2010) and in particular the positioning of care in contemporary moves to consumer-directed care.

Developments in the delivery of human services

In recent decades the focus of social policy has moved from a welfare state, in which services are seen as a right of citizenship, to be universally available and provided by centralised governments (Jamrozik, 2009), to the contemporary focus on the need to ration human services in the face of a purported increasing demand (Lymbery, 2010). While the scope of this chapter does not permit a full exploration of the twists and turns of the reduction in governments' commitments to universalist welfare provision and the discursive construction of the 'deserving poor' (Carson & Kerr, 2013, p. 28), this ideological repositioning of human services is associated with reducing the involvement of governments in providing for citizens and reducing the level of taxation needed to finance welfare provisions.

Accompanying a desire to reduce government outlays in social welfare is the associated commitment to market-like processes by which strictly targeted services are to be delivered through outsourced contracting arrangements with not-for-profit and for-profit organisations. This development has been justified by its proponents as a means to address what has been argued to be a growth in institutionalised service provision, captured by service providers' needs rather than those of the service user (Lloyd, 2010); along with an ideological belief that competition created by contracting out services will result in cost reduction and service delivery innovation.

As a result of this neo-liberal trend for governments to divest themselves of service delivery many not-for-profit organisations have grown into large agencies managing a range of government contracts to provide services. The growth of the 'for-profit' sector has been another major development. While the idea of profit-making human service organisations had previously been regarded with both ethical and financial scepticism, government tendering processes have made it possible for service delivery business organisations to develop to meet a particular niche in the market (Cunningham, Baines & Charlesworth, 2014).

The marketisation of human services has also had a significant impact on the reconceptualisation of service users. The idea that the person who uses a service should be provided with a choice of service provider is used to legitimise governments' desires to make organisations compete amongst themselves for the right to provide services. This concept is firmly rooted in rational choice theory (Buchanan, 2003) which in turn is firmly imbued with notions of a 'rational male' citizen subject. The service user is positioned as an empowered rational (male) person, who will have the agency and self-interest to make choices from a range of service options. This technocratic construction is in contrast to the feminist ethics of care conceptualisation of a service user as a community member whose wishes will direct the development of a range of relationships that will provide support and care.

Service user movements

Responsiveness to client needs is a value underpinning most models of service delivery in the human services. How such responsiveness can be achieved alongside an ethos of doing more with less is challenging. Debates about the appropriate way forward from a feminist perspective are commonly conceptualised as balancing the tension between feminist, democratic and consumerist models (Fawcett et al., 2010; Miller, 2004).

Lymbery suggests the key question is whether the person to be served is seen 'as a citizen with rights or a consumer' (2010, p. 15). A feminist lens adds the question: are services to be provided as if all citizens and consumers conform to an implicitly 'male' norm or is the woman seeking support entitled to service provision which takes account of the complexity of her roles as both giver and receiver of support?

Movements that emphasise the rights of service users are driving democratic models. They are particularly active in disability services, mental health and aged care. Their use of cooperative political processes tends to model a relational citizenship in which connection enables participation and social contribution. For example, in the disability sector the catchcry 'nothing about us without us' has resulted in service user involvement in the design of services, the management of consultation processes, the training of staff and the development of peer support programmes (Lord & Hutchison, 2003; de Miranda, 2004).

Considered from a feminist ethics of care perspective an important aspect of this citizenship of the service user is the position of the 'carer' in the political process. The voices of carers, particularly the parents of adults in need of support, have been an important component in gaining public and political attention for key service issues. However Lymbery (2010) argues that at any point in time the carer and the service user may have different, even potentially conflicting, interests. A feminist ethics of care lens can be responsive to this by encouraging a more nuanced exploration of the contributions and needs of both service users and carers.

International experiences and Australian developments

Changes in the delivery of human services have been a feature of the last decade, not only in Australia but around the world (Glasby, 2014). Although models vary, the principles underpinning the innovations and governments' expectations about increased service user satisfaction and containment of costs (Power, 2014) are common.

UK governments, for example, have redeveloped social care services to emphasise personal choice since 2007 (Lymbery, 2010). Glasby (2014) suggests that the implementation of this new model of service delivery has descended into a battle in which the interests of service users are opposed to the interests of service providers. He suggests that the consumerist model conceptualises the person being granted support as a microenterprise that employs workers and purchases technology needed for their support. In this process, the person being supported becomes 'the boss'. In this conceptualisation the worker is seen as vulnerable to exploitation by an 'employer' who is not experienced in staff management and certainly not informed about workers' rights. As discussed below, given that so many workers in the sector are women, such scenarios are concerning.

In Canada individualised funding has become the norm for some groups of service users, particularly those with a physical impairment (Lord & Hutchison, 2003; Fisher et al., 2010). In the United States similar contracted-out programmes are implemented at a state level and there is significant variation in models of delivery.

The movement to consumer-directed care in Australia, whilst arising from independent political processes, reflects similar discourses and goals to that of other countries. The Australian Productivity Commission has undertaken important work in developing the case for consumer-directed care in disability and aged care. In recent years much social policy development has been led by the Productivity Commission, reflecting the view that the financial management of social policy is central to the government's approach. Hughes (2011) argues that the research and public submission processes utilised by the commission have assisted in building the 'legitimacy' of an economic approach to future social policy. Certainly the commission's reports focus on funding challenges in the aged and disability sectors, while also exploring the demographic and cultural drivers of increased expectations of services (Productivity Commission, 2011a, 2011b).

Whilst arguing that community wellbeing is an important goal of social policy, and that a key objective of aged care is promoting people's connectedness to one another and the wellbeing of the network of people who provide formal and informal care for an elderly person, the commission has advocated funding models that place the responsibility for providing care on the individual and emphasise the importance of individuals making choices about the nature of service delivery and service provision. The reports do recognise the special needs of some populations in the community who will need block funding for resources (Hughes, 2011); however these are the exceptions in a model which emphasises self-reliance to avoid intergenerational inequity.

The introduction of the National Disability Insurance Scheme in 2013 formally embedded a choice and control model in social policy in Australia (Cortis et al., 2013). As with other such models the key elements of the model provide for service user control, choice and responsibility (Crozier & Muenchberger, 2013).

Whilst it is possible to appreciate and indeed celebrate the empowerment of individual service users arising from these developments, from a feminist ethics of care perspective it can be seen that the consumerist models are individualising risk which had previously been borne collectively (Scourfield, 2007). Scourfield argues that in these models the service user becomes a manager and entrepreneur not just in defining the service that they require but actually taking the steps to ensure that this service is delivered to them. Some studies have reported great benefits of this process, with shortages of qualified staff now being dealt with by the employment of friends and family (Crozier et al., 2013). However, as Scourfield also suggests, this very individualised method of achieving self-determination both denies the realities of dependence and interdependence and neglects the many benefits that can be found in the collective processes of innovation.

The risks of the individualised focus of these models can also be seen in the discussions about the vulnerability of service users to being exploited, either through fraud or forms of abuse, and associated with this the risk that the service user will misappropriate the funds allocated to them (Crozier et al., 2013). A feminist ethics of care lens leads to the construction of these risks in somewhat different terms. First it would note that the language in which these risks are discussed is a long way from the respectful emphasis on service user capacities that the new models are seeking to establish. Indeed it would seem that putting the spotlight on service users has enhanced their image as vulnerable rather than capable. Second, a feminist ethics of care lens would acknowledge that each of us has limitations and strengths in our ability to transact business and that it is our normal practice to utilise cooperative arrangements with organisations to conduct our business successfully.

Impact of the consumer-directed care model

The neo-liberal consumer-directed care model seeks to empower the service user by giving them purchasing power and entrepreneurial power to problem solve. It is derived from a belief that with these powers the service user will be able to dominate in their relationships with service providers, whether individuals or organisations, and thus get their needs met. A feminist ethic of care perspective pays attention to the fact that the service users' needs must be met in relationship with service providers and works from the basis that not domination but mutual respect and responsiveness will achieve the best outcomes for the service user.

Service users

Although consumer-directed care models emphasise the role of the service user as the decision maker and employer to ensure that their own needs are met, it can be argued that this description ignores the reality of both the individual and the social policy context. The resources devoted to meeting the needs of any individual are still determined through a centralised assessment and decision-making process in which the need to stretch a limited resource to meet the needs of a very large group of service users influences the allocation of resources to each individual. This then affects the rates of pay that the service user can provide to their carers and indeed the number of hours of support that they can afford to utilise (Lloyd, 2010).

It can be argued that the emphasis on consumer choice and control contributes to making invisible some of the real challenges of providing support to service users. Indeed it would be possible to see this as shifting responsibility for system-wide challenges to the individual consumer. There is also the risk that in becoming 'consumers' the distinct needs of individual service users are masked. Ottman et al. (2013) found from their systematic narrative review of relevant studies that the different life experiences and expectations of service users in addition to the broader contexts in which they live all affect people's ability to utilise and satisfaction with consumer-directed care.

Workers

Prior to the introduction of these important social policy changes the community services workforce was one of the lowest paid although fastest growing in the Australian economy. It was female dominated, with 87 per cent of these workers being women compared to 44 per cent in other industries (Australian Institute of Health and Welfare, 2013). More than half (57 per cent) of these workers worked part time, compared to only 34 per cent of workers in other occupations. In addition to the low salaries that result from this part-time work, workers in community service occupations are generally paid less than other workers, with some of the lowest paid being child-care workers ($22 per hour) and nursing support and care workers ($27 per hour) (Australian Institute of Health and Welfare, 2013). Not surprisingly, retention of staff, particularly in home care, is reported to be an issue for employers (Australian Institute of Health and Welfare, 2013).

The introduction of consumer-directed care cannot be expected to address these basic gender injustices arising from the lack of valuing of caring in our society. Not only is the willingness to undertake this supportive work shaped by cultural expectations of gender, the remuneration available reflects the undervaluing of these roles and the skills that they require. Whilst the individual service user may be quite willing to pay a more competitive rate of pay for a high-quality personal service, they will not be allocated a budget that allows for this without a reduction in essential hours of service. Alternatively some service users may feel the need for hours of support so acutely that they will want to pay an even lower hourly rate than previously in order to extend the service that they receive. Returning the negotiation of salary levels to the intimate service user–care provider relationship without support and oversight would seem to be a retrograde step both for workers and for the relationship.

Workforce shortages (Cortis et al., 2013) may be addressed through a consumer-directed care model by the expansion of the workforce to include friends and family of the service user. On the one hand this may be seen as the recognition of what was previously unpaid and invisible work. On the other hand, if the number of appropriately skilled workers available for this work is less than the need for service there is a risk that consumer-directed care contributes to making this problem invisible as service providers utilise friends and family who may or may not be appropriately skilled for the role and no one counts the job vacancy. There are undoubtedly a range of potential management issues that arise from the employment of your mother or cousin as your carer.

In community services, workforce shortages are not distributed evenly across the sector. Particular clients may need very specific worker skills relating to cultural and linguistic diversity and it has been noted that rural communities often cannot meet the needs of service users (Manthorpe & Stevens, 2010). Evidence that a market economy cannot necessarily address these issues can be found in the fact that even well-paid industries such as mining can have difficulty recruiting workers outside cities. Our feminist ethic of care lens would suggest that greater attention to workers as contributors in their own right and to the importance of the caring work that they do would be a more appropriate policy position to address this issue.

Service delivery organisations

The new service model has the potential to transform the relationship between service users and organisations. The movement from agency-directed services to consumer-directed, whilst foreshadowed and piloted for over a decade (Lord & Hutchison, 2003), has significant ramifications for those agencies committed to providing support in these areas. Although the research evidence about the effects on service users of personalisation, individual budgets and consumer-directed care is limited (Rabiee, Moran & Glendinning, 2009), in Australia (Crozier & Muenchberger, 2013) there is even less research available about the impact of this new model of service planning on organisations active in the human services.

There is much for social work to celebrate in the new changes. As Lloyd (2010) argues, they act as a counter to some of the more bureaucratic influences within organisations in recent years. However once again the very individualistic way in which the new relationships are conceptualised brings attendant risks. An individual service user may find themselves besieged by marketing initiatives from a range of organisations, all competing to 'win' a customer. Not only does one feel sympathy for this service user, it must be recognised that the cost of this very individualised marketing must be recouped in some way in the service provision – either the service user or the worker providing the service is going to need to receive less than if this intermediary had not intervened.

Conclusion

Women, over-represented as they are as service users, familial carers and human service workers, will be those most affected by the new service delivery models currently being implemented through the shift to neo-liberal marketisation. In the first instance this will be most felt in the disability and aged care service sectors, but it seems likely to spread throughout the human services.

Women have much to gain from the recognition through financial recompense of previously hidden caring and from the empowerment of service users and their carers in the definition of service need, management and provision of services. However exploration of this new system through a feminist ethics of care lens demonstrates that consumer-directed care also poses risks for women. The entrenched and stereotypical construction of a service user as a person whose needs can be met by the purchase of a series of services undervalues the complexity of the relationships and skills involved in providing support for someone with a significant disability. It distorts a relationship that must be based not in the market, but in the caring of community.

Service users and their networks of support are each distinct and will need to make choices, first, about the extent to which they engage with this new system. Evaluation and research informed by feminist theory clearly indicate that for many clients and carers new models of consumer-directed care can potentially provide increased levels of satisfaction, due to increased individual choice and greater system flexibility. However current research also identifies that some service users, particularly older people, express less satisfaction with the new arrangements (Ottman et al., 2013).

As a tool for social change the new consumer-directed care has the potential to disrupt established patterns of bureaucratic service delivery but the benefits achieved may be limited, especially in terms of the impact on women. There are some key questions about the provision of public resources that have not yet been answered. As Barnes asks, 'Does this mean we should abandon principles of universality of provision, geographical equity and public responsibility to ensure good co-ordination, and effective collaboration in services?' (2011, p. 165).

Furthermore there is an important question about the disruption of social networks that may result from this new service delivery model. Service user groups have over time found a voice that has enabled them to influence social policy. Will the individualised experience they now have reduce their common interests and ability to speak with one voice to decision makers? Who is accountable? Who will take responsibility for this system? Will politicians and bureaucrats see themselves as responsible for outcomes or will they see any difficulties as the result of inadequacies of the service user? How will the experiences of service users and their social networks be aggregated so that the systems and resourcing implications can be reviewed with a view to change and development? This chapter suggests that a feminist ethics of care provides a useful framework for a sustained deeper analysis of the new human service delivery system.

Further reading

Lloyd, L. (2010) The individual in social care: the ethics of care and the 'personalisation agenda' in services for older people in England. *Ethics and Social Welfare*, 4(2), pp. 188–200.

Scourfield, P. (2007) Social care and the modern citizen: client, consumer, service user, manager and entrepreneur. *British Journal of Social Work*, 37, pp. 107–122.

Sevenhuijsen, S. (2003) The place of care: the relevance of the feminist ethic of care for social policy. *Feminist Theory*, 4(2), pp. 179–197.

References

Australian Association of Social Workers (AASW) (2010) *Code of Ethics.* AASW, Canberra. www.aasw.asn.au/practitioner-resources/code-of-ethics (accessed 1 September 2014).

Australian Institute of Health and Welfare (2013) *Australia's Welfare 2013.* AIHW, Canberra. www.aihw.gov.au/publication-detail/?id=60129543825 (accessed 10 June 2015).

Ball, W. & Charles, N. (2006) Feminist social movements and policy change: devolution, childcare and domestic violence policies in Wales. *Women's Studies International Forum*, 29, pp. 172–183.

Barnes, M. (2011) Abandoning care? A critical perspective on personalisation from an ethic of care. *Ethics and Social Welfare*, 5(2), pp. 153–167.

Buchanan, J. (2003) *Public Choice: The Origins and Development of a Research Program.* Center for Study of Public Choice at George Mason University, Fairfax, VA.

Carson, E. & Kerr, L. (2013) *Australian Social Policy and the Human Services.* Cambridge University Press, Port Melbourne, Vic.

Cortis, N., Meagher, G., Chan, S., Davidson, B. & Fattore, T. (2013) *Building an Industry of Choice: Service Quality, Workforce Capacity and Consumer-Centred Funding in Disability Care.* Social Policy Research Centre, University of New South Wales, Sydney.

Crozier, M. & Muenchberger, H. (2013) 'It's your problem, not mine': does competence have anything to do with desire and aspiration to self-direct? *Australian Health Review*, 37, pp. 621–623.

Crozier, M., Muenchberger, H., Colley, J. & Ehrlich, C. (2013) The disability self-direction movement: considering the benefits and challenges for an Australian response. *Australian Journal of Social Issues*, 48(4), pp. 455–472.

Cunningham, I., Baines, D. & Charlesworth, S. (2014) Government funding, employment conditions, and work organization in non-profit community services: a comparative study. *Public Administration*, 92(3), pp. 582–598.

de Miranda, J. (2004) Coming to the addiction community: consumer-directed care. *Behavioral Healthcare Tomorrow*, 13(3), p. 25.

Fawcett, B., Goodwin, S., Meagher, G. & Phillips, R. (2010) *Social Policy for Social Change.* Palgrave Macmillan, Melbourne.

Fisher, K.R., Gleeson, R., Edwards, R., Purcal, C., Sitek, T., Dinning, B., Laragy, C., D'aegher, L. & Thompson, D. (2010) *Effectiveness of Individual Funding Approaches for Disability Support.* Department of Families, Housing, Community Services and Indigenous Affairs, Canberra.

Gilligan, C. (1982) *In a Different Voice: Psychological Theory and Women's Development.* Harvard University Press, Cambridge, MA.

Glasby, J. (2014) The controversies of choice and control: why some people might be hostile to English social care reforms. *British Journal of Social Work*, 44, pp. 252–266.

Gray, M. (2010) Moral sources and emergent ethical theories in social work. *British Journal of Social Work*, 40, pp. 1794–1811.

Hughes, M. (2011) The Productivity Commission Inquiry into Aged Care: a critical review. *Australian Social Work*, 64(4), pp. 526–536.

Jamrozik, A. (2009) *Social Policy in the Post-Welfare State: Australian Society in a Changing World*, 3rd edn. Pearson Education Australia, Frenchs Forest, NSW.

Lloyd, L. (2010) The individual in social care: the ethics of care and the 'personalisation agenda' in services for older people in England. *Ethics and Social Welfare*, 4(2), pp. 188–200.

Lord, J. & Hutchison, P. (2003) Individualised support and funding: building blocks for capacity building and inclusion. *Disability and Society*, 18(1), pp. 71–86.

Lymbery, M. (2010) A new vision for adult social care? Continuities and change in the care of older people. *Critical Social Policy*, 30(1), pp. 5–26.

Manthorpe, J. & Stevens, M. (2010) Increasing care options in the countryside: developing an understanding of the potential impact of personalization for social work with rural older people. *British Journal of Social Work*, 40, pp. 1452–1469.

Miller, C. (2004) *Producing Welfare: A Modern Agenda*. Palgrave Macmillan, Houndmills, Basingstoke.

Morris, J. (2001) Impairment and disability: constructing an ethics of care that promotes human rights. *Hypatia*, 16(4), pp. 1–16.

Ottman, G., Allen, J. & Feldman, P. (2013) A systematic narrative review of consumer-directed care for older people: implications for model development. *Health and Social Care in the Community*, 21(6), pp. 563–581.

Power, A. (2014) Personalisation and austerity in the crosshairs: government perspectives on the remaking of adult social care. *Journal of Social Policy*, 43(4), pp. 829–846.

Productivity Commission (2011a) *Caring for Older Australians*, Report No. 53, Final Inquiry Report. Productivity Commission, Canberra. www.pc.gov.au/__data/assets/pdf_file/0004/110929/aged-care-volume1.pdf (accessed 10 June 2015).

Productivity Commission (2011b) *Disability Care and Support*. Report No. 54. Productivity Commission, Canberra. www.pc.gov.au/__data/assets/pdf_file/0012/111270/disability-support-volume1.pdf (accessed 10 June 2015).

Rabiee, P., Moran, N. & Glendinning, C. (2009) Individual budgets: lessons from early users' experiences. *British Journal of Social Work*, 39, pp. 918–935.

Scourfield, P. (2007) Social care and the modern citizen: client, consumer, service user, manager and entrepreneur. *British Journal of Social Work*, 37, pp. 107–122.

Sevenhuijsen, S. (2003) The place of care: the relevance of the feminist ethic of care for social policy. *Feminist Theory*, 4(2), pp. 179–197.

6 Repositioning social work research in feminist epistemology, research and praxis

Lia Bryant

Introduction

The relationship between feminism and social work research is a strong one, producing powerful empirical research and scholarship. Despite this social work research, textbooks rarely engage deeply with critical feminist research methodologies (e.g. Rubin & Babbie, 2014; Shaw, 2010; Thyer, 2010). Further, texts focused on qualitative inquiry (e.g. Padgett, 2008; Carey, 2012) or with an applied focus (e.g. Becker, Bryman & Ferguson, 2012; Csiernik, Birnbaum & Decker-Pierce, 2010; Marlow, 2011) unexpectedly have limited or no discussion of feminist research approaches. While some texts include brief coverage of feminist research approaches, these are, however, often subsumed into other approaches such as participatory action research or 'anti-oppressive' enquiry (e.g. McLaughlin, 2012). Social work carves out its feminist research space in specialist academic journals, notably *Affilia*, as well as in mainstream qualitative social work journals like *Qualitative Social Work*. However, unlike similar social science disciplines, for example social geography (e.g. Moss, 2002) and sociology (e.g. Roberts, 1981), in social work there remains a lack of feminist research texts. As a feminist academic and social work teacher of research methods a recurring question for me is: why do the core sites of social work knowledge production especially for students exclude feminist methodologies as a legitimate site of research? It is clearly not due to a lack of engagement of social workers with feminism or a lack of published feminist social work research. At the same time there is also a lack of social work engagement in multidisciplinary feminist research handbooks (Gringeri, Wahab & Anderson-Nathe, 2010). In other words social workers appear not to be writing in feminist mainstream research textbooks and social work researchers appear not to be writing about feminism in social work research textbooks. In this chapter I will argue for the necessity of including what are uniquely 'feminist social work approaches' to the way social scientists teach, understand and do research that may also inform and give value to the broader multidisciplinary field of feminist research.

However, before progressing it is important to acknowledge that feminist research covers broad and contested theoretical terrains whilst commonly sharing the central precept that knowledge production is neither objective nor unsituated. Scholars like Susan Harding (1991) and Donna Haraway (1988) have challenged the male-dominated scientific view, which has determined knowledge claims including ways to undertake research. Haraway has aptly argued that

> all Western cultural narratives about objectivity are allegories of the ideologies governing the relations of what we call mind and body, distance and responsibility. Feminist objectivity is about limited location and situated knowledge, not about transcendence and splitting of subject and object. It allows us to become answerable for what we learn how to see.
>
> (p. 583)

Hence, Haraway has argued for a politics of location to identify how knowledge is produced, why and by whom. To identify the politics of location of both social work feminist research in social work, as well as social work's location in feminist research, this chapter begins by mapping how social workers methodologically use feminism. I provide an overview of dominant methodological choices which are predominantly based in intersectionality, narrative approaches and Foucauldian analyses. There is a robust body of social work feminist research that employs creative methods including arts-based research and creative writing, and I analyse these to identify whether broadening the methodological scope of research brings something that is specially *social work* to feminist inquiry. Specifically I am referring to research that encapsulates the values of social work and therefore is participatory for those engaging in it and transforms gender hierarchies and inequalities for subjects, groups or communities.

The contours of social work feminist research

For the purpose of this overview of feminist research in social work is research that is named as feminist or employs feminist theories and, similarly, social work research is research that is named as such by the authors or published in social work discipline-based journals. There are no research methodologies and methods that are specific to feminisms. However, feminist scholars and activists were central to the qualitative research movement in the 1970s, raising ethical questions about epistemology and in particular about whose knowledge is being produced, how and for what purpose. The concern driving the qualitative feminist movement was to produce knowledge that incorporated the voices of communities of people who had been marginalised, subjugated and oppressed. Further, feminists, like critical race and class thinkers, questioned research ethics that lacked reciprocity, asking: what did those who participated in research have to gain from their participation? Collaboration in research with participants was a central tenet in research design but one where there was and is often slippage in practice.

Contemporary social work feminist research often draws its focus from the broad rubric of post-structuralist approaches and theories and in particular Foucauldian discourse theories, narrative theories and intersectionality. I will begin with intersectionality and suggest that intersectionality is an approach, a methodological lens rather than a theoretical perspective, that can be used alongside multiple theories (Bryant & Pini, 2011).

Intersectionality

Intersectionality as an approach to feminist research was driven by the question: who is the subject of feminism? Over the last two decades under the rubric of post-structuralist approaches to feminism, understanding subjectivities as fluid, multiple and diverse has become a way of practising and knowing in research (Linstead & Pullen, 2006; Archer, 2004). Prior to this time feminism remained the province of white middle-class women. The universality of the category of 'woman' became increasingly contested over time but was called to account as early as the 1960s and 1970s by black feminists (Beale, 1970; Davis, 1981; hooks, 1984; Crenshaw, 1989). Hence it took several decades for feminism to problematise both gender and woman and take into account diverse divisions and intersections based on race, sexuality, class, ethnicity, (dis)ability and age. The intention of intersectional analyses is not to produce an additive account of disadvantage or to accord a binary between white middle-class women and 'others', thereby reproducing a normative white identity and ongoing institutional oppression (Valentine, 2007). Intersectionality is now commonly used but often in multiple ways and at times without definition (Nash, 2008; Jordan-Zachery, 2007; Phoenix & Pattynama, 2006). Brah and Phoenix (2004) provide a definition that allows for complexity. They argue that 'Intersectionality … [epitomises] the complex, irreducible, varied, and variable effects which ensure when multiple axes of differentiation – economic, political, cultural, psychic, subjective and experiential – intersect in historically specific contexts' (p. 76).

Bryant and Pini (2011) point to the gains and limitations of using intersectional analysis in feminist research. They argue that intersectionality focuses on power and as such enables the drawing of different theoretical perspectives including Foucauldian discursive analyses and performative analyses to mark and understand social divisions. Morris has suggested that 'a key insight of intersectional theory holds that modes of inequality, such as race, class and gender, can combine in ways that alter the meaning and effects on one another' (2007, p. 491). Intersectionality is limiting, however, if used without theoretical underpinning to give meanings to social categories and how they work to inform and shape the social world.

In the late 2000s a spate of feminist social work articles on intersectional analyses argued for an analysis of gender that was intertwined with 'other systems of oppression' (Mehrotra, 2010, p. 417). Social work feminist researchers building on this call for multiplicity, contextuality and positionality used intersectional analyses to examine a broad range of issues including domestic violence, welfare rights, education, critical and reflective social work practice, and a host of other issues (Mattsson, 2014; Ono, 2013; Netting, 2011; Vakalahi & Hardin Starks, 2010; Damant et al., 2008; Edmonds-Cady & Sosulski, 2012). Mehrotra (2010, p. 418) in particular has argued, following the scholarship of McCall (2005), that social work requires a continuum of intersectional analysis across a range of perspectives that moves beyond the core modernist categories of race, gender and class. For example, in her own research she draws upon postcolonial, queer and transnational feminism to understand queer women's experiences, practices and identities in the context of migration. This dynamic analysis of power is situated and contextual to intersectionality as a methodological lens and gives it value. It moves the feminist debate from the quagmire of grasping whether 'intersectionality is a concept, a theory, or a heuristic device for critical feminist theories' (Bryant & Pini, 2011, p. 13). As a methodological lens, intersectionality not only provides scope for ways of analysing and attempting to see complexity in the lives of women beyond the tripartite categorisation of gender, class and race (see Hulko, 2009) to focus on complex axes of subjectivity but also to extend analyses beyond marginalised groups to include those of power and privilege (Pease, 2012; Yuval-Davis, 2006), enabling examination of the reproduction of inequalities (Nash, 2008; Samuels & Ross-Sheriff, 2008). Understanding intersectionality as a methodological lens causes us pause to consider *how* to *do* research as social work feminist researchers. Intersectionality calls for an understanding of lived experience and equally a challenge to structural inequalities and oppressions (Sandberg, 2013; Fook, 2002). Complexities surround how to understand women's lives without necessarily privileging one category over another (usually gender) or subsuming multiple aspects of the self into neatly predetermined categorical interrelations (usually gender and class or gender and race) (see Bryant & Hoon, 2006) to include shifting and potentially changing subjectivities (see McCall, 2005) that are experienced differently according to place (Valentine, 2007).

Hulko provides a very clear example of the complexity associated with intersectionality and subjectivities that shift in relation to place and argues that 'a person may hold privileges that are because of his or her perceived Whiteness in one setting and experience discrimination as a "Black person" in another … and experience different "racial" statuses' (2009: 49). Badruddoja gives another keen example, demonstrating that 'women's positionalities are in flux, and through their identities, they "selectively accept and maintain certain definitions while rupturing others"' (2008, p. 181). Each of these examples reinforces the importance of different theoretical approaches and methods to examine intersectionality. Therefore the question of how to do intersectional research becomes a question of what methods and theories are most applicable in enabling complex intersectional analysis in social work. There is scope for social work research texts to include intersectional analyses to examine critically subjectivities, imaginaries, practices, privilege, marginalisation and oppression at multiscalar intersecting levels from the individual to the structural, from the global to the local.

Feminism, Foucault and social work research

The introduction of the vast body of work of Michel Foucault does not have a long tradition in social work feminist research, unlike for example feminist sociology, social geography and philosophy. There are pockets of feminist social work research drawing upon singular and multiple aspects of Foucault's work principally to understand power through archaeological discourse (Skehill, 2003; Carey & Foster, 2013; Shaw, 2015), knowledge (Gilbert & Powell, 2010; Scheyett, 2006; Eila Satka & Skehill, 2012), governmentality (Nissen, 2014; Bay, 2011), subjectivities and technologies of control (Hennum, 2012; Gilbert & Powell, 2010). In some ways social work's minimal engagement with Foucault (see Philip, 1979; Donzelot, 1980; Chambon, Irving & Epstein, 1999; Fook, 2002; Healy, 2000) is surprising given the historical and political nature of social work as a profession and its complementary and contradictory relation to the state especially in western economies. The profession is further complicated by engagement with and resistance to the state from the perspective of everyday practice as well as a body politic. The often-said and somewhat glib statement that social workers are instruments of the state fails to engage analytically with complex analyses of power. For Gilbert and Powell using Foucault to conceptualise power as a relational construct among subjects and between subjects and institutions means that for social work:

> The outcome is to produce dialectical relationships between knowledge, power and action that is productive in the sense of creating particular possibilities but which also maintains a level of uncertainty and unpredictability in terms of actions, providing opportunity for the exercise of discretion.
>
> (2010, p. 6)

Feminist social work researchers using Foucauldian theories have produced a varied research agenda focusing on, for example, the regulation and control of women's bodies/minds (e.g. Kokaliari & Berzoff, 2008; Scheyett, 2006). However, overall feminist social work research appears not to have progressed through a Foucauldian lens. Is this due to social work being, as

Gilbert and Powell posit, a 'disciplinary field depicted as "data-rich but theory-poor"' (2010: 4)? Or is it, as Scheyett suggests, due to criticism of Foucault for being 'anti-humanist and callous to the realities of suffering and for feeling no need to engage in or provide recommendations for action' (2006, p. 84)? There is likely to be merit in both positions and at the same time neither fully explains this lack of engagement as there is a plethora of social work research that is both theoretical and empirical, and social work like other disciplines engages with the work of theorists for their *generative* ability by using their concepts to interrogate the social world.

Foucault has a place in social work feminist research but, as Garrity (2010) has argued, perhaps in a more detailed and nuanced way. This is particularly the case in relation to perhaps the most overused of Foucault's concepts, discourse, which in social work is at times reduced and used interchangeably with language and/or narrative. Garrity explains:

> Foucault (1972 [2002]) explicitly distinguishes discourse from logic and linguistics and, through this, from the world of ideas and language; within a Foucauldian viewpoint discourse may include, but is not reducible to, language … discourse in The Archaeology of Knowledge is understood as a 'dispersion' (Foucault, 1972 [2002]: 121) – nor to a narrative – as discourse focuses not on personal experience but on the structural processes that enable someone to take up a particular 'subject position' (Foucault, 1972 [2002]: 221).
>
> (2010, pp. 196–197)

Since the 1980s there has been debate about what Foucault offers feminism and how and which dimensions of Foucault's work speak to feminist inquiry (McNay, 1992; Bordo, 1993). The notion of the lived body through technologies of the self has provided feminists with a medium for engaging with Foucault that allows an interrogation of both structures shaping subjects and the agency of subjects – thereby allowing analyses to move across and between questions of control, discipline, surveillance, regulation and autonomy, resistance and emancipation. Technologies of the self offer social work feminist research an avenue to interrogate the interstices between the formation and reproduction of institutional, structural, cultural and social dynamics and women's and men's responses, reactions, challenges and reconstitution of social norms and ways of being.

Feminism and narrative approaches to social work research

The power of narrative stemming from literary scholarship has become a prominent approach used in research across a broad range of social science disciplines. Riessman and Quinney (2005) suggest that narrative approaches to social work research, while growing, still remain limited in scope and take-up among researchers. Before turning to narrative approaches used in social work feminist inquiry it is important to note that the term 'narrative' has been used and defined in multiple ways and at times used obliquely to refer to stories. There is a breadth and variety of narrative approaches, adding to the complexity of pinning down the meaning of and approaches to narrative research (Spector-Mersel, 2010). However, there are specific analytical foci – or common ground – to take into account when employing narrative in research and these are: 'For whom was *this* story constructed, how was it made, and for what purpose? What cultural resources does it draw on – take for granted? What does it accomplish? Are there gaps and inconsistencies that might suggest altera-tive counter-narratives?' (Riessman & Quinney, 2005, p. 393).

Within narrative approaches data is presented in a variety of ways usually using long excerpts enabling personal reflections to speak to the reader. Thus, narrative research might include paragraphs or pages of words, far longer than the usual qualitative interview quotation. Narrative data may come from a range of data collection methods: an extensive interview, a series of interviews, a mix of written and verbal accounts, and the linking of fictional and personal talking and writing (e.g. Sermijn, Devlieger & Loots, 2008; Coombes & Morgan, 2004). Narrative may be temporal and linear or circular, sporadic or disjointed, and the extensive process of data collection is likely to reflect each of these ways of 'telling' (Cazden, 2001; Riessman, 1987; Coombes & Morgan, 2004).

In social work feminists have engaged with narrative approaches to examine a broad spectrum of issues including, for example, identity, mothering and disability (e.g. Mitra, 2011; Butler, Ford & Tregaskis, 2007; Urek, 2005; Tangenberg, 2003). Similarly to discourse analyses, in feminist social work research there is a lack of detail as to how narrative methods are employed and methodologically how narrative gives depth and value to feminist social work research. There are similar concerns across other disciplines about the nebulous use of narrative therapy, with Riessman and Speedy arguing that narrative 'has come to mean anything and everything' (2007, p. 428). On the whole feminist narrative research remains, like dis-course analysis, a generalised analysis of language and story. A narrative approach is often little different from a qualitative interview in process, analysis and presentation. To be clear, this is not to say that social workers are not using narrative approaches in research in detailed and complex ways but I am arguing that this work is not housed in *social work* research texts and journals. Riessman and Quinney said, after searching journals from 1990 to 2002 and again in 2005 for narrative research in social work, that 'We were disappointed with the size of the research corpus' (2005, p. 397). This remains the case in feminist social work research.

There is a small growing body of autoethnographic social work feminist publications that use a narrative approach to examine the interstices between the personal and the political (e.g. Averett, 2009; Butler et al., 2007). Autoethnography is a reflexive writing practice that requires the researcher to situate herself in her research, being critical and reflexive about her politics of location (Haraway, 1988; Ahmed, 2004). Her 'vision' and 'seeing' are embodied practices bound to shifting practices of privilege and/or subordination (Bryant & Livholts, 2015; Guillemin & Gillam, 2004; Lash, 2003). For Pillow, reflexivity produces discomfort and 'to be reflective does not demand an "other," while to be reflexive demands both an other and some self-conscious awareness of the process of scrutiny' (2003, p. 177). Bryant and Livholts have argued that 'autoethnography offers social work research the potential for critical engagement and social action' (2015). There are many examples of autoethnographic research that use personal stories to make visible the story of self and the other. As Pease has argued, situating oneself in research does not write away privilege; instead 'being critical about the structures of privilege and the oppression in the world can sit alongside writing in a personal voice. In fact, interrogating privilege from within requires it' (2012, p. 80).

Similarly, Butler (in Butler et al., 2007) uses autoethnography and in particular creative autoethnography to examine socially constructed meanings of femininity in relation to mental illness. She explains:

> The concept of creative autobiography originated for a critical evaluation of events in my own life and the meaning of them. In 1993, I produced an exhibition and accompanying theoretical analysis of a period of mental ill-health in my life. This work explored the social and psychological factors that had contributed to my ill-health and drew on feminist theory to explain the process of seeking external validation to the point of losing the capacity to self-validate.
>
> (2007, p. 288)

The examples above indicate that autoethnography as a social work narrative feminist approach is a theoretically informed and examined reflexive endeavour that may be emancipatory as well as producing new knowledge or ways of 'seeing' the social world (Bryant & Livholts, 2007; Averett, 2009).

Narrative approaches to feminist social work inquiry offer space for participants to speak and possibilities for greater understanding for self and others, allowing detailed and complex plots, events, experiences, practices and imaginaries to be brought to the fore. As Riessman and Quinney suggest, 'there is a relevant knowledge for social work that can be produced with diverse narrative approaches' which is 'vitally important in a time of evidence based practice' (2005, pp. 404–405).

Research in the seventh moment

The term the 'seventh moment', coined by Denzin (see Lincoln & Denzin, 2000; Denzin, 2002), refers to a new period of qualitative research that draws on the creative industries to interweave writing, analysis, data collection, empowerment and reflexivity. It is a moment and movement that focuses on 'previously silenced voices, a turn to performance texts, and an abiding concern with moral discourse, with conversations about democracy, politics, race, gender, nation, freedom and community' (Denzin, 2002, p. 26).

Cultural studies have been prevalent in shaping how to write ethnography using cultural tools like fiction, performance, autobiography and poetry. Denzin argued in 2002 that it was timely for social work to act in this moment to take up the call for critical and creative research methods. Over the last decade there has been an increasing array of social work research that uses critical and creative methods and that seeks to work alongside participants in the research journey (see Bryant, 2015). I have argued elsewhere (Bryant, 2015) that what makes this new wave in research exciting is not simply a transference of creative arts into social work feminist research but an understanding of creativity as a social phenomenon that emerges from the interaction between people, landscapes and objects. Doing social work research creatively is deeply tied to the values and ethics of social work and feminism, fostering greater collaboration with the communities involved in the study, ultimately moving towards positive social change (Denzin, 2002). The body of this work draws on arts-based methods (e.g. Huss & Cwikel, 2005), digital storytelling (e.g. Lenette, Brough & Cox, 2013; Matthews & Sunderland, 2013), photography and visual images (Russell & Diaz, 2013; Cruikshank, 2010) and fictional writing (Ungar, 2011; Hordyk, Soltane & Hanley, 2014; Taiwo, 2013). Feminist social workers have a history of using arts-based methods in practice and have been well placed to develop a strong body of research using creative methods. Research by Hordyk et al. (2014), Huss and Cwikel (2005), and Russell and Diaz (2013) are positive exemplars. Each of these studies uses different methods and approaches to data analysis. For example Hordyk et al. (2014, p. 205) used 'found poetry' or 'the data poem' to represent immigrant women's experiences of homelessness. Their rationale for using poetic inquiry is that it captures emotions and imagination in a non-linear way. Poetry provides alternative ways of knowing by using rhythm, imagery and other language devices and 'the *body* listens to poetry and in this listening, dualisms such as mind-body, intellect-emotion, self-other, researcher-researched on which science is based are collapsed' (Hordyk et al., 2014, p. 206). Their data poems emerged from transcripts, with researchers reading interview transcripts and placing aside repeated and significant phrases. For them, 'poetic inquiry is the interpretation of a verbal landscape' (Hordyk et al., 2014, p. 211), a way of interpreting which is similar to the placement of interview quotations in a text. Quotations and found poems share the re-representation of participants' voices; however, poetic enquiry aims to relate findings in ways that resonate with women in similar circumstances and with social workers in the community. Hordyk et al. (2014) are suggesting that found poetry is likely to have a greater social impact outside the academy.

Huss and Cwikel (2005) used arts-based research and therapy using drawings, paintings and clay work to understand Bedouin women's experiences of living in Israel. Huss and Cwikel, citing Save and Nuutinen (2003, p. 532), explain that arts-based methods create 'a field of many understandings … a "third thing" that is sensory, multi-interpretive, intuitive, and ever-changing, avoiding the final seal of truth' (Huss & Cwikel, 2005, p. 4). For example, women were able to express their experiences and emotions through art, with one woman sculpting an ashtray that represented her ageing embodiment as a feeling of being empty and discarded. Women's desires and future ambitions were also replicated in the art. One woman drew a home and flowers, stating, 'I want to a house; I want to build a house of my own. Most important, I want to plant a garden by the house' (Huss & Cwikel, 2005, p. 8).

Russell and Diaz (2013) in their study about lesbian cultural experience used photography to establish a visual record to complement their interview data. The photos of women at leisure, at work and with family captured the way women constitute their lesbian identities within heteronormative structures. For Russell and Diaz photography is a 'political endeavor of making a marginalized population visible … [and] photography can be empowering, give credit to their political efforts and validate their political concerns in transcending oppression' (2013, p. 449). Visual media have always been powerful political tools in bringing social issues to public consciousness. It is not difficult for us to recollect the black and white photos taken during the 1930s financial Depression in America as men stood in long queues hoping to obtain work or the power of the image of the GLBQTI (Gay, Lesbian, Bisexual, Queer, Trans, Intersex) flag used to promote and celebrate diverse genders and sexualities (Bryant, 2015).

There are multiple examples of social work feminist research turning towards creative tools, first, to enable a centralising of intersubjectivity and reciprocity (Bryant, 2015) and, second, to use academic writing 'as a form of activism and political practice' (Pease, 2012, p. 71). Turning attention to academic writing, Livholts (2012, p. 3) has argued that writing is also a method of inquiry, with multidisciplinary feminist researchers engaging in different ways of writing research (see for example Cixous, 1993). Nontraditional writing forms enable feminist social work researchers to resist privileging certain kinds of knowledge over other, subjugated knowledges. They allow ideas and findings potentially to reach beyond the academy but also allow researchers to experiment in ways of writing, enabling the complex embodied subjectivities of both 'participants' or more accurately co-researchers and academic researchers.

Critical and creative feminist social work research offers mainstream feminism methodologies that enable collaboration with those for whom for so long we have researched 'on' rather than 'with'. They provide ways of working with communities and fostering data that is accessible to our participants or co-researchers, allowing the potential for empowerment as well as reciprocity. Art, photography, film, poetry and stories have a power that interview transcripts alone cannot achieve – they activate our senses and emotions and imprint messages on our minds. Social workers have specific skills to bring to research by linking research and practice or undertaking research as a form of practice, that is, research as an enabling and political activity, providing feminism with innovative ways to engage in the research process.

Conclusion

On the whole, social work feminist researchers have minimally engaged with methodologies commonly deployed among feminists from other disciplines. Specifically, there is scope for social work feminist researchers to employ intersectionality, discourse analyses and narrative approaches to social work issues and problems. These approaches can add depth and rigour to research, allowing feminist social work researchers to speak to feminist social issues across disciplines. Moreover, for social work research to develop and grow it is imperative that research texts in social work include feminist methodologies and methods, that is, that through our production of knowledge our students learn how to 'do' feminist research.

This is an exciting time in feminist social work research, brimming with innovation and new ways of linking research endeavours to community needs. In Denzin's words, it is a 'period of explosion and ferment' (2002, p. 26). Social work has a place in feminist research. The values of social work align with feminism and with critical and creative research methodologies. In terms of disciplinarity in feminism, social work is unique in the ways we practice research, the way we work alongside our co-researchers to implement social transformation at the individual, community and societal level. It is now timely to document and advocate for the particularities of critical and creative social work research methodologies to inform ways of engaging in feminist research.

Further reading

Bryant, L. (ed.) (2015) *Critical and Creative Research Methodologies in Social Work.* Ashgate, Aldershot, UK.

Lincoln, Y.S. & Denzin, N.K. (2000) The seventh moment: out of the past. In N.K. Denzin & Y.S. Lincoln (eds), *The Sage Handbook of Qualitative Research*, 2nd edn. Sage, Thousand Oaks, CA, pp. 1047–1065.

References

Ahmed, S. (2004) Declarations of whiteness: the non-performativity of anti-racism. *Borderlands e-journal*, 3(2). www.borderlands.net.au/vol. 3no2_2004/ahmed_declarations.htm (accessed 26 May 2015).

Archer, L. (2004) Re/theorizing 'difference' in feminist research. *Women's Studies International Forum*, 27, pp. 459–473.

Averett, P. (2009) The search for Wonder Woman: an autoethnography of feminist identity. *AFFILIA: The Journal of Women and Social Work*, 24, pp. 360–368.

Badruddoja, R. (2008) Queer spaces, places, and gender: the tropologies of Rupa and Ronica. *NWSA Journal*, 20, pp. 156–188.

Bay, U. (2011) Unpacking neo-liberal technologies of government in Australian higher education social work departments. *Journal of Social Work*, 11, pp. 222–236.

Beale, F. (1970) Double jeopardy: to be black and female. In T.C. Bambara (ed.), *The Black Woman*. Washington Square Press, New York, pp. 109–122.

Becker, S., Bryman, A. & Ferguson, H. (eds) (2012) *Understanding Research for Social Policy and Social Work: Themes, Methods and Approaches*. Policy Press, Bristol, UK.

Bordo, S. (1993) *Unbearable Weight: Feminism, Western Culture, and the Body*. University of California Press, Berkeley, CA.

Brah, A. & Phoenix, A. (2004) Ain't I a woman? Revisiting intersectionality. *Journal of International Women's Studies*, 5, pp. 75–86.

Bryant, L. (2015) Introduction: taking up the call for critical and creative methods in social work research. In L. Bryant (ed.), *Critical and Creative Research Methods in Social Work*. Ashgate, Farnham, UK, pp. 1–24.

Bryant, L. & Hoon, E. (2006) How can the intersections between gender, class, and sexuality be translated to an empirical agenda? *International Journal of Qualitative Methods*, 5, pp. 67–79.

Bryant, L. & Livholts, M. (2007) Exploring the gendering of space by using memory work as a reflexive research method. *International Journal of Qualitative Methods*, 6, pp. 29–44.

Bryant, L. & Livholts, M. (2015) Opening the lens to see, feel and hear: using autoethnographic textual and visual methods to examine gender and telephony. In L. Bryant (ed.), *Critical and Creative Research Methods in Social Work*. Ashgate, Farnham, UK, pp. 109–130.

Bryant, L. & Pini, B. (2011) *Gender and Rurality*. Routledge, New York.

Butler, A., Ford, D. & Tregaskis, C. (2007) Who do we think we are? Self and reflexivity in social work practice. *Qualitative Social Work*, 6, pp. 281–299.

Carey, M. (2012) *Qualitative Research Skills for Social Work Theory and Practice*. Ashgate, Farnham, UK.

Carey, M. & Foster, V. (2013) Social work, ideology, discourse and the limits of post-hegemony. *Journal of Social Work*, 13, pp. 248–266.

Cazden, C.B. (2001) *Classroom Discourse: The Language of Teaching and Learning*. Heinemann, Portsmouth, NH.

Chambon, A.S., Irving, A. & Epstein, L. (eds) (1999) *Reading Foucault for Social Work*. Columbia University Press, New York.

Cixous, H. (1993) *Three Steps on the Ladder of Writing*. Columbia University Press, New York.

Coombes, L. & Morgan, M. (2004) Narrative form and the morality of psychology's gendering stories. *Narrative Inquiry*, 14, pp. 303–322.

Crenshaw, K. (1989) Demarginalizing the intersection of race and sex: a black feminist critique of antidiscrimination doctrine, feminist theory and antiracist politics. *University of Chicago Legal Forum*, 140, pp. 139–167.

Cruikshank, A. (2010) Empowering images: using photography as a medium to develop visual literacy. *Exchange*, September/October, pp. 53–56.

Csiernik, R., Birnbaum, R. & Decker-Pierce, B. (2010) *Practicing Social Work Research: Case Studies for Learning*. University of Toronto Press, Toronto.

Damant, D., Lapierre, S., Kouraga, A., Fortin, A., Hamelin-Brabant, L., Lavergne, C. & Lessard, G. (2008) Taking child abuse and mothering into account: intersectional feminism as an alternative for the study of domestic violence. *AFFILIA: The Journal of Women and Social Work*, 23, pp. 123–133.

Davis, A. (1981) *Women, Race and Class*. Random House, New York.

Denzin, N.K. (2002) Social work in the seventh moment. *Qualitative Social Work*, 1, pp. 25–38.

Donzelot, J. (1980) *The Policing of Families*. Hutchinson, London.

Edmonds-Cady, C. & Sosulski, M.R. (2012) Applications of situated learning to foster communities of practice. *Journal of Social Work Education*, 48, pp. 45–64.

Eila Satka, M. & Skehill, C. (2012) Michel Foucault and Dorothy Smith in case file research: strange bedfellows or complementary thinkers? *Qualitative Social Work*, 11, pp. 191–205.

Fook, J. (2002) *Social Work: Critical Theory and Practice*. Sage, London.

Garrity, Z. (2010) Discourse analysis, Foucault and social work research: identifying some methodological complexities. *Journal of Social Work*, 10, pp. 193–210.

Gilbert, T. & Powell, J.L. (2010) Power and social work in the United Kingdom: a Foucauldian excursion. *Journal of Social Work*, 10, pp. 3–22.

Gringeri, C.E., Wahab, S. & Anderson-Nathe, B. (2010) What makes it feminist? Mapping the landscape of feminist social work research. *AFFILIA: The Journal of Women and Social Work*, 25, pp. 390–405.

Guillemin, M. & Gillam, L. (2004) Ethics, reflexivity, and 'ethically important moments' in research. *Qualitative Inquiry*, 10, pp. 261–280.

Haraway, D. (1988) Situated knowledges: the science question in feminism and the privilege of partial perspective. *Feminist Studies*, 14(3), pp. 575–599.

Harding, S. (1991) *Whose Science? Whose Knowledge? Thinking from Women's Lives*. Open University Press, Milton Keynes, UK.

Healy, K. (2000) *Social Work Practices: Contemporary Perspectives on Change*. Sage, London.

Hennum, N.M.J. (2012) Children's confidences, parents' confessions: child welfare dialogues as technologies of control. *Qualitative Social Work*, 11, pp. 535–549.

hooks, b. (1984) *Feminist Theory: From Margin to Center*. South End Press, Boston, MA.

Hordyk, S.R., Soltane, S.B. & Hanley, J. (2014) Sometimes you have to go under water to come up: a poetic, critical realist approach to documenting the voices of homeless immigrant women. *Qualitative Social Work*, 13, pp. 203–220.

Hulko, W. (2009) The time- and context-contingent nature of intersectionality and interlocking oppressions. *AFFILIA: The Journal of Women and Social Work*, 24, pp. 44–55.

Huss, E. & Cwikel, J. (2005) Researching creations: applying arts-based research to Bedouin women's drawings. *International Journal of Qualitative Methods*, 4, pp. 1–16.

Jordan-Zachery, J.S. (2007) Am I a black woman or a woman who is black? A few thoughts on the meaning of intersectionality. *Politics and Gender*, 3, pp. 254–263.

Kokaliari, E. & Berzoff, J. (2008) Nonsuicidal self-injury among nonclinical college women: lessons from Foucault. *AFFILIA: The Journal of Women and Social Work*, 23, pp. 259–269.

Lash, S. (2003) Reflexivity as non-linearity. *Theory, Culture and Society*, 20, pp. 49–57.

Lenette, C., Brough, M. & Cox, L. (2013) Everyday resilience: narratives of single refugee women with children. *Qualitative Social Work*, 12, pp. 637–653.

Lincoln, Y.S. & Denzin, N.K. (2000) The seventh moment: out of the past. In N.K. Denzin & Y.S. Lincoln (eds), *The Sage Handbook of Qualitative Research*, 2nd edn. Sage, Thousand Oaks, CA, pp. 1047–1065.

Linstead, S. & Pullen, A. (2006) Gender as multiplicity: desire, displacement, difference and dispersion. *Human Relations*, 59, pp. 1287–1310.

Livholts, M. (2012) Introduction: contemporary untimely post/academic writings – transforming the shape of knowledge in feminist studies. In M. Livholts (ed.), *Emergent Writing Methodologies in Feminist Studies*. Routledge, London, pp. 1–24.

McCall, L. (2005) The complexity of intersectionality. *Signs*, 30, pp. 1771–1800.

McLaughlin, H. (2012) *Understanding Social Work Research*. Sage, London.

McNay, L. (1992) *Foucault and Feminism: Power, Gender and the Self*. Polity Press, Cambridge.

Marlow, C. (2011) *Research Methods for Generalist Social Work*. Brooks/Cole, Belmont, CA.

Matthews, N. & Sunderland, N. (2013) Digital life-story narratives as data for policy makers and practitioners: thinking through methodologies for large-scale multimedia qualitative datasets. *Journal of Broadcasting and Electronic Media*, 57, pp. 97–114.

Mattsson, T. (2014) Intersectionality as a useful tool: anti-oppressive social work and critical reflection. *AFFILIA: The Journal of Women and Social Work*, 29, pp. 8–17.

Mehrotra, G. (2010) Toward a continuum of intersectionality theorizing for feminist social work scholarship. *AFFILIA: The Journal of Women and Social Work*, 25, pp. 417–430.

Mitra, A. (2011) To be or not to be a feminist in India. *AFFILIA: The Journal of Women and Social Work*, 26, pp. 182–200.

Morris, E.W. (2007) 'Ladies' or 'loudies'? Perceptions and experiences of black girls in classrooms. *Youth and Society*, 38, pp. 490–515.

Moss, P. (ed.) (2002) *Feminist Geography in Practice: Research and Methods*. Blackwell, Oxford.

Nash, J.C. (2008) Re-thinking intersectionality. *Feminist Review*, 89, pp. 1–15.

Netting, F.E. (2011) Bridging critical feminist gerontology and social work to interrogate the narrative on civic engagement. *AFFILIA: The Journal of Women and Social Work*, 26, pp. 239–249.

Nissen, M.A. (2014) In search of a sociology of social problems for social work. *Qualitative Social Work*, 13, pp. 555–570.

Ono, E. (2013) Violence against racially minoritized women: implications for social work. *AFFILIA: The Journal of Women and Social Work*, 28, pp. 458–467.

Padgett, D. (2008) *Qualitative Methods in Social Work Research*. Sage, Los Angeles, CA.

Pease, B. (2012) Interrogating privileged subjectivities: reflections on writing personal accounts of privilege. In M. Livholts (ed.), *Emergent Writing Methodologies in Feminist Studies*. Routledge, London, pp. 71–82.

Philip, M. (1979) Notes on the form of knowledge in social work. *Sociological Review*, 27, pp. 83–111.

Phoenix, A. & Pattynama, P. (2006) Intersectionality. *European Journal of Women's Studies*, 13, pp. 187–192.

Pillow, W. (2003) Confession, catharsis, or cure? Rethinking the uses of reflexivity as methodological power in qualitative research. *International Journal of Qualitative Studies in Education*, 16, pp. 175–196.

Riessman, C.K. (1987) When gender is not enough: women interviewing women. *Gender and Society*, 1, pp. 72–207.

Riessman, C.K. & Quinney, L. (2005) Narrative in social work: a critical review. *Qualitative Social Work*, 4, pp. 391–412.

Riessman, C.K. & Speedy, J. (2007) Narrative inquiry in the psychotherapy professions: a critical review. In D.J. Clandinin (ed.), *Handbook of Narrative Inquiry: Mapping a Methodology*. Sage, Thousand Oaks, CA, pp. 426–456.

Roberts, H. (ed.) (1981) *Doing Feminist Research*. Routledge & Kegan Paul, New York.

Rubin, A. & Babbie, E.R. (2014) *Research Methods for Social Work*. Brooks/Cole and Cengage Learning, Belmont, CA.

Russell, A.C. & Diaz, N.D. (2013) Photography in social work research: using visual image to humanize findings. *Qualitative Social Work*, 12(4), pp. 433–453.

Samuels, G.M. & Ross-Sheriff, F. (2008) Identity, oppression, and power: feminisms and intersectionality theory. *AFFILIA: The Journal of Women and Social Work*, 23, pp. 5–9.

Sandberg, L. (2013) Backward, dumb, and violent hillbillies? Rural geographies and intersectional studies on intimate partner violence. *AFFILIA: The Journal of Women and Social Work*, 28(4), pp. 350–365.

Scheyett, A. (2006) Silence and surveillance: mental illness, evidence-based practice, and a Foucaultian lens. *Journal of Progressive Human Services*, 17, pp. 71–92.

Sermijn, J., Devlieger, P. & Loots, G. (2008) The narrative construction of the self: selfhood as a rhizomatic theory. *Qualitative Inquiry*, 14, pp. 632–650.

Shaw, I. (2010) *The Sage Handbook of Social Work Research*. Sage, Los Angeles, CA.

Shaw, I.F. (2015) The archaeology of research practices: a social work case. *Qualitative Inquiry*, 21(1), pp. 36–49.

Skehill, C. (2003) Social work in the Republic of Ireland: a history of the present. *Journal of Social Work*, 3, pp. 141–159.

Spector-Mersel, G. (2010) Narrative research: time for a paradigm. *Narrative Inquiry*, 20, pp. 204–224.

Taiwo, A. (2013) Relational poetry in the expression of social identity: creating interweaving dialogues. *Qualitative Social Work*, 12(2), pp. 215–228.

Tangenberg, K.M. (2003) Linking feminist social work and feminist theology in light of faith-based service initiatives. *AFFILIA: The Journal of Women and Social Work*, 18, pp. 379–394.

Thyer, B.A. (ed.) (2010) *The Handbook of Social Work Research Methods*. Sage, Los Angeles, CA.

Ungar, M. (2011) The social worker – a novel: the advantages of fictional representations of life narratives. *Cultural Studies↔Critical Methodologies*, 11, pp. 290–302.

Urek, M. (2005) Making a case in social work: the construction of an unsuitable mother. *Qualitative Social Work*, 4, pp. 451–467.

Vakalahi, H.F.O. & Hardin Starks, S. (2010) The complexities of becoming visible: reflecting on the stories of women of color as social work educators. *AFFILIA: The Journal of Women and Social Work*, 25, pp. 110–122.

Valentine, G. (2007) Theorizing and researching intersectionality: a challenge for feminist geography. *Professional Geographer*, 59, pp. 10–21.

Yuval-Davis, N. (2006) Intersectionality and feminist politics. *European Journal of Women's Studies*, 13, pp. 193–209.

7 Feminism and community development

Illustrating the rural

Margaret Alston

Introduction

Community development is a critical role for social workers but is often ill-defined and its purpose misunderstood. Good practice is dependent on an awareness of the ideological, political and social factors that shape communities in ways that are fundamentally gendered. In this chapter I focus on rurality to illustrate how a feminist consciousness enhances social work community development practice, based as it is on ideals of gender equality and social justice for all community members, not just those who hold recognisable power and influence. Without the insights such an approach provides, social workers may gain a false sense of community priorities and preferred actions and inadvertently act to cement established power relations and gender inequalities.

This chapter is designed to challenge this possibility. I examine broad processes of change underway in rural Australia and their implications for a feminist reading of social work. Adopting a feminist lens invites readers to unmask taken-for-granted gender inequalities that typify many communities and are reinforced by institutional structures, policies, programmes and professional practices. Hierarchical, patriarchal and highly gendered social structures are more overtly recognisable and appear more intransigent in rural areas than they are in urban areas, and, for social workers coming into these communities, this can be confronting. Older, usually Anglo, men dominate power structures and own or control most of the productive land and resources that constitute rural heartlands and agriculturally productive areas. The resulting gendered power relations appear so fixed and overt they are largely unremarked, ensuring that a dominant masculine hegemony is rarely challenged. These processes of power also mean that issues of significance to women – freedom from violence, child care, education and access to family planning – are rarely the subject of whole-of-community action.

Adopting a feminist perspective allows an examination of the gendered nature of rural lives and exposes the failure of policies and practices to address highly discriminatory gendered practices. In developing this perspective I draw on a number of research projects conducted in Australia over the past several years. In doing so I provide a focus for social workers working in rural areas to (i) critically examine the dominant framing of community life as normatively masculine, (ii) address gender-based disadvantage and (iii) advocate for policies and practices that not only advance gender equality but also improve women's safety and quality of life.

While much of what follows is necessarily truncated, it nonetheless may appear to imply that undifferentiated 'woman' (problematic in itself) is oppressed by dominant patriarchal structures, a position from which I do not necessarily resile. However there is a danger that the reader will assume therefore that women are powerless and must be 'saved'. This is not my position. Rather I agree with Deepak who writes in another context that we must 'caution against decontextualizing women's experiences and denying their agency in defining their own problems and participating in the design of proposed solutions' (2014, p. 161). What follows details the oppressive elements of a gendered culture. What must emerge is an energised feminist social work praxis that enables, empowers and facilitates women from diverse backgrounds living in very different contexts facing multiple challenges to be empowered to act on their own behalf.

Community development

Heenan (2004, pp. 800–801) defines a community development approach as one that establishes partnerships across the community, draws on local knowledge, assists the community to determine their priority of needs, distributes resources effectively, helps the community to own and control the process of renewal, fosters participation and strengthens social capital across the community. Heenan's work provides a comprehensive summary of community development practice. However workers should resist uncritically adopting this set of tasks without examining overt and covert power inequalities. A lack of political awareness will inevitably facilitate support for normative values, and potentially highly gendered outcomes. In this regard Freire's (1973) suggestion that 'conscientisation' should be the main focus of community development is significant. He defines this as raising awareness amongst people and communities of 'the social, economic and political realities of their oppression' (Powell, 2001: 77).

Rural community development

To begin to differentiate rural community development it is useful to reflect on the nature of 'rural community'. Unsurprisingly it is difficult to find an adequate definition of 'the rural' (Alston, 2009). What we do know is that rural areas in Australia are not homogeneous and in fact, as Miller, Farmer and Clarke note, 'if you've seen one rural community … you've seen one rural community' (1994, quoted in Raitano, 2010, p. 7). Rural areas are as diverse and complex as urban suburbs. Further, there are essential differences between Australian rural communities typified by diverse agricultural production, levels of poverty, governance structures, the type of climate challenges being faced and legal arrangements. These cannot be downplayed.

However there are similarities perhaps best encapsulated by Tönnies' (1957) original notion of *Gemeinschaft* – or the sense of belonging to a community, sharing common values and having a strong ethos of community support. What becomes evident when working in rural communities is the importance of connectedness to 'place' and community, or what Zapf (2010) describes as 'people as place'. The identity and wellbeing of rural people is bound up with rurality and thus, when place is damaged either by climate and environmental disasters or by more subtle processes described below, people's sense of wellbeing, community cohesion and connectedness are equally damaged.

Nonetheless there is a challenge in viewing *Gemeinschaft* or what others term 'the rural idyll' (Cloke, 2006; Smailes, 2006) as somehow morally superior. Elsewhere I have noted that 'The concept of a rural idyll also disguises the more sinister forces at play in relation to the rural – the power and gender imbalances, racism and conflicts and the powerful ideological forces that support inequalities and prejudices' (Alston, 2009, p. 8).

Adopting a feminist social work framework requires that this significant sense of place and belonging be understood, that the dark underbelly be acknowledged, and that any changes be addressed with a critical understanding of power and gender relations in the context of the restructuring taking place in rural communities across the world.

Social workers are drawn into rural community development work for a variety of reasons. These may include to work for one of the many NGOs dotted across the region, to provide outreach services for government social support services or to provide a crisis response during or following a disaster. Whatever the case, they are likely to have to do much with limited resources and to determine priorities for their distribution and therefore need to be critically aware of taken-for-granted inequalities.

How can feminism inform our understanding of community development?

Feminism provides a critical focus for social workers, incorporating as it does an overt attention to social justice and self-determination. It enables a questioning of traditional notions of power and leadership and views women as active agents making sense of their own experiences. It illuminates the way discourses shape our understanding of issues (including what is silenced and who is marginalised), thereby enabling collective action and assisting women to shape their own futures (Wendt & Boylan,

2014). At the heart of feminist inquiry is attention to power and how knowledge is built (Gringeri, Wahab & Anderson-Nathe, 2010, p. 392).

As Gringeri et al. (2010) note, feminist social work is openly political and liberatory; it fosters resistance and shines a light on power relations and the creation of knowledge. It allows us to understand whose know-ledge is valued, what other 'knowledges' are available and it brings in what Smith (1992, p. 17) describes as the 'everyday/everynight worlds' of women to ensure that knowledge is authentic.

Critical gender theorists such as Connell (2011) have advanced our understanding of a gender order – or an overarching system backed by tradition, customs, language, discourse, legislation and institutional structures that effectively creates significant inequalities and makes it more difficult for individual women and communities to effect change. By exposing the patriarchal dividend – or the benefit all men receive from keeping women oppressed – Connell allows a wider reading of gender/power relations and greater clarity concerning men's resistance to change. Enarson (2012) takes this somewhat further in her discussion of post-disaster sites, arguing that men will rush to re-establish things as they were, not only to restore a functioning community but also to ensure that power relations are not threatened and privilege is main-tained. A feminist perspective gives social workers a deep and critical understanding of what stands in the way of gender equality. Through our work in rural communities we have the capacity to foster and develop new ways of living where all can draw on the dividend of place. Critical to a politically aware and dynamic rural community develop-ment approach is an understanding of the drivers that underpin policy and practice.

While rural community development provides a link from local to national levels, and builds community capacity, a feminist approach requires us to adopt a more reflexive process (Wendt & Boylan, 2014). Such an approach enables workers to ensure that all groups are consulted, that vulnerable groups are supported, that a wide variety of local know-ledge is valued and incorporated, that advice is sought from all sections of the community, that a representative network of partners is built and that resources are distributed fairly and equitably. Such a perspective provides a solid basis not only to build the community but also to question gen-dered power relations and unequal resource distribution.

This approach requires us to ask ourselves a number of questions including: What values do we bring to our work? Are we facilitating neo-liberal policies that may not be inclusive or fair? Who are we consulting to gain an understanding of the community? Whose views, or local know-ledge, are we supporting? Whose needs are prioritised? How are we reach-ing out to vulnerable groups? What inclusive practices are being fostered?

If workers are brought into a post-disaster situation these questions are even more crucial. There is a strong desire in the immediate aftermath of a disaster to restore the community exactly as it was with all its inherent inequalities and prejudices. Aid is often given to re-establish livelihoods and women suggest that this is usually directed to landowners thus bypassing women and overlooking their particular issues. It is therefore critical that workers assess the processes of distribution and query on what basis priorities are being determined, who is being consulted and why, who is receiving the resources and why, and who and what is being neglected in this redistribution. The post-disaster space is an ideal site to develop new and more equitable ways of functioning and resourcing. In this space it is possible to question inherent gender inequalities and to advocate for, and support, more equitable processes.

Rapid structural changes: why community development is crucial

Australia's rural areas are changing in unexpected and challenging ways. Major processes of restructuring are occurring as a result of globalisation, neo-liberal policies, climate challenges, global financial crises, unstable political situations, eroding infrastructure and a declining political voice for rural people. These complex and intertwined factors are creating significant social consequences for the people who live in these vast, often remote spaces. These include large-scale movements of people from rural to urban areas, threatened food and water security, growing rural–urban wealth and opportunity differentials, changing livelihood strategies and complex challenges for family and community cohesion.

Agriculture

Rural communities tend to be dominated by, and reliant on, some form of agricultural production, and to a lesser extent mining and tourism. In Australia this includes broad acre farming in the more remote areas and irrigated/small acre farming closer to cities and regional centres. Further, as globalisation has accelerated, so too has the commercialisation of agricultural production. This had led to land being consolidated into larger holdings for commercial production particularly in more remote areas.

In Australia, by contrast with areas across the Asia-Pacific where agriculture is becoming increasingly feminised, restructuring has resulted in a more dominant masculinisation of agricultural work. This results from women moving into the paid workforce in large numbers seeking income for the family and to enable their partners to remain farming. In recent decades women's labour input, whether on the farm or in the paid workforce, has become crucial to the survival of family-based agricultural production. Yet women's input is often ignored when resources are allocated during times of crisis.

Climate challenges

As Molnar (2010) reminds us, rural areas are extremely vulnerable to climate-induced disasters – disasters that have led to major destabilisation not only of agricultural production and food security, but also of the rural communities reliant on these industries. The complexity of rural living has been compounded by new threats from climate challenges, challenges that do not recognise borders and national boundaries. Slow-onset changes such as droughts, erosion, salination of land, and sea and temperature rises, together with catastrophic events such as cyclones, storm surges, floods and bushfires are an increasingly unwelcome part of rural life. In many areas these have led to significant loss of lives, homes and livelihoods. In Australia the scale of the Black Saturday bushfires in 2009 and, across the Asia-Pacific region, the impact of the 2004 tsunami, and regular extreme weather events, indicate that these threats are not only more intense but appear to be more frequent, and that significant loss of lives, homes and livelihoods may result. In Australia's rural areas, uncertainty about climate challenges remains a dominant factor in the imaginations of rural people, eroding the sense of 'place' noted above.

These new threats have had major impacts on global water security and health. For example in many communities along the Bay of Bengal which formed the basis of a three-year research project (Alston, 2015), the impact of cyclonic activity, storm surges and ongoing salination has eroded water storage facilities and resulted in women having to go much further to collect fresh water. Similar situations are common in coastal regions across the Pacific, with major repercussions for women and girls, in some cases resulting in girls having to drop out of school.

Indeed the threat across the globe is so great that the UN Secretary-General, Ban Ki-Moon, has announced that the world is in danger both of running out of water (Parnell, 2013) and of food insecurity unless we enact 'policies that promote water rights for all, stronger regulatory capacity and gender equality' (Ban Ki-Moon, 2012). The link to gender equality in this context reinforces the critical input of women to global agriculture and food production and the need for this to be considered in community development projects.

Globalisation and neo-liberalism

A further opportunity/threat lies with globalisation and the opening up of world markets. This has exposed rural communities to the vagaries of market forces and to competitive practices that are far from fair and transparent. While there are enormous benefits of globalisation, many of which are evident in rural areas, including cultural exchanges, information flow and the spread of technological advances, the market-based neo-liberal philosophy underpinning the policies and practices of globalisation are focused on individual endeavour and privatisation. These expose rural communities to competitive practices that may undermine the rights of rural people to the full benefits of citizenship. One outcome of concern to social workers has been a reduction in publicly funded social supports to cushion rural areas.

In Australia at least, the dominance of neo-liberal ideologies has resulted in rural social issues being reduced to economic equations, profit being the overriding motive underpinning policy decisions, and economic language and solutions dominating discursive constructions of rural communities. Where neo-liberal principles dominate policy, gender equality and citizenship rights are superseded by market primacy. A good example has been the introduction of new water policies in Australia's Murray–Darling Basin, which were initially introduced in such a way as to exacerbate uncertainty and social disruption. The underlying premise that the market will be the determinant excuses governments from intervening in comprehensive socially just ways. Thus if policies introduced to address critical rural challenges are underpinned by neo-liberal principles, they may accelerate the social restructuring already underway in rural areas. In a very short period of time, these combined pressures have reshaped the population composition of rural areas and the social relations of rural community life.

Social support services

Most public services and corporate businesses closed their doors in rural areas decades ago. Many services have been privatised, while essential services such as hospital and specialist care have been centralised into regional growth centres. This privatisation has resulted in a patchy spread of social supports and an increasing reliance on charities and volunteers. The language and discourse underpinning service delivery hides the significant social problems and inequalities developing within rural communities and between rural and urban areas. The obvious consequence includes increasing rural–urban wealth divides and a rise in the numbers of socially excluded rural people unable to participate in society for reasons beyond their control (Burchardt, 2002). The link between rurality, poverty and escalating social exclusion is well established (Shucksmith, 2000; Alston, 2005).

Reduced government involvement in service delivery, the privatisation and centralisation of services, a reduction in public infrastructure and a laissez faire attitude to rural areas by governments has led to the positioning of these communities as problematic, unsustainable and on their own. The more remote a community from a major centre, the more likely it is to have little or no public service presence, reduced health, education and welfare services, poor or no mobile phone coverage, inadequate transport and telecommunications infrastructure and inflated costs for services.

Further, where male interests dominate local government, what financial supports are available are prioritised to areas such as football sports ovals rather than to child-care facilities or aged care services.

In one very evident example of the neglect of Australia's rural areas, research with women living in remote areas on the impacts of the closure of small maternity services across rural Australia led to the exposure of the significant hardships and indeed unsafe conditions in which many remote area women now give birth (Dietsch et al., 2008). Our final report on this project was titled *Luckily we had a Torch!*, a quotation from one woman's telling of her birthing experience, and one that aptly illustrates the situation of many of our participants having to drive hours to a hospital. This has on occasion resulted in women giving birth on isolated roadways, without the benefit of street lighting, and, if driving at night, running the gauntlet of kangaroos on the poorly maintained roads, reliant for assistance on their panicked partners.

The lack of mobile phone coverage across rural Australia is another example of service infrastructure linked to profit motives rather than social need. While this impacts all across rural Australia, research undertaken with rural women indicates that the lack of coverage affects their access to health services and information and results in them frequently travelling on isolated roads with no ready access to assistance (Alston, Kent & Kent, 2004).

While cities grapple with decisions about the most optimal large infrastructure projects to deal with their burgeoning populations, rural communities receive fewer benefits from public resources thereby increasing the differential access to a range of health, education, employment and income opportunities. The lack of political representation by and for rural people adds to their sense of being overlooked in the national imagination.

There is no doubt that rural restructuring has been broad and significant. Coupled with climate challenges and erosion of 'place' this has produced major social changes, many of which are highly gendered. The following section provides a brief snapshot of issues where gender is a visible and compelling element of change.

Social impacts

Demographic changes

The social impacts of the factors outlined above include declining or static populations in many rural areas, and poorly serviced communities, with increasing levels of extreme poverty and rising numbers of socially excluded people. In Australian rural communities in recent times there has been an influx of welfare-dependent people moving in to take advantage of cheaper housing and finding limited employment opportunities.

There is now a recognisably different social demographic in rural areas resulting from a significant outmigration of young people for work and/or education, leaving behind ageing populations that have higher mortality and morbidity rates, less access to education and who are more likely to work in insecure and casualised positions if they have jobs at all. Gendered population trends include the likelihood that remote communities will have a male-dominated population, that more young women will leave rural communities to pursue work or education opportunities and that there are greater numbers of women in older age categories.

Changing livelihoods and outmigration

There are also recognisable gendered social trends emerging as families change livelihood strategies. Many rural people are now seeking alternative income and this can include diversified agricultural production, home-based industries, small businesses and/or paid workforce participation. This critical need for alternative income has led to major processes of outmigration, either temporarily, seasonally or permanently. Outmigration is common across our region and is evident in young people moving, but also in the outmigration of women and/or men to earn income for the family.

In many Australian rural communities, as elsewhere, a complex set of circumstances has led to the significant movement of women into the paid workforce or seeking paid employment (Alston, 2000). Nonetheless the concurrent reduction of services has led to a loss of what have been traditionally female skilled jobs in schools and hospitals, banks and public service instrumentalities, and welfare and social support agencies. This has meant that women may have to travel away from their communities in search of work – forcing an involuntary separation of families that may over time become permanent (Alston & Whittenbury, 2012). Outmigration is a critical family livelihood strategy across the world involving the involuntary separation of families, relationship problems and health issues that are well documented elsewhere (Alston, 2012, 2015; Alston & Whittenbury, 2012).

Gender-based violence

There is growing evidence that violence against women is increasing in rural areas particularly as uncertainty grows over the viability of rural livelihoods and lifestyles. In research undertaken with communities in Australia affected by the long drought at the turn of the century, it became evident that violence is associated with structural changes (Whittenbury, 2012), and this supported evidence emerging from other rural sites affected by climate challenges (see for example Alston, 2015). Despite this there are few safe havens for rural women escaping violence, a lack of refuges and a lack of support from family and community (Alston, 1997).

Rural community development: localism, rural proofing and gender mainstreaming

Rural community development, advocacy and policy critique are critical to addressing these social and service delivery challenges. However rural community development has been shown to be ineffective if delivered through top-down processes and only partially successful if reliant on bottom-up, locally led initiatives (Shucksmith, 2013). Successful rural community development requires networked partners within and beyond the community at all levels of government and with active engagement in the affairs of the community. Rural communities have variable capacity and cannot be expected to develop on their own – and this is where social workers can be highly effective in linking partners and in developing active networks.

Across the world rural community advocates are challenging processes of decline and advocating new ideas to address the impacts of neo-liberal policies and austerity measures. In particular advocates argue that localism, rural proofing and gender mainstreaming, supported by resources provided by an 'enabling state' (Shucksmith, 2013), have the potential to arrest rural community decline.

In Europe and the United Kingdom where similar processes of rural decline are evident, rural community advocates have successfully argued that 'localism' and 'rural proofing' must become dominant drivers of policy initiatives. Localism refers to policies where power is devolved from national governments to local areas, allowing rural people to create new ways of working within their national contexts. Empowered communities have responded by attracting business opportunities. In Nordic countries there are also examples of rural parliaments being constituted with local area representatives and reporting on rural issues to their national parliaments. Shucksmith (2013) notes that the ability of rural places to adapt and thrive in the context of such changes is much greater because rural people can think about and influence how they change and develop. However the support of an enabling state is essential and it is here that rural community development workers must challenge neo-liberal policy drivers and advocate for greater state supports.

In introducing the Localism Act 2011 in the UK, Minister Greg Clark noted:

> For too long, central government has hoarded and concentrated power. Trying to improve people's lives by imposing decisions, setting targets and demanding inspections from Whitehall simply doesn't work. It creates bureaucracy. It leaves no room for adaptation to reflect local circumstances or innovation to deliver services more effectively and at lower cost. And it leaves people feeling 'done to' and imposed upon – the very opposite of the sense of participation and

involvement on which a healthy democracy thrives. We think that the best means of strengthening society is not for central government to try and seize all the power and responsibility for itself. It is to help people and their locally elected representatives to achieve their own ambitions.

(quoted in Shucksmith, 2013, p. 17)

This devolution to local power structures and local priority setting in order to empower rural communities has much to offer Australia provided we adopt inclusive decision-making structures and determine whole-of-community priorities.

'Rural proofing' is a further process adopted across Europe and the UK to ensure all policies are assessed for their impact on rural areas. As Short-all (2009, p. 5) notes, rural proofing is a commitment by government to review and examine all public policy to ensure it does not disadvantage rural areas.

Localism and rural proofing can provide a significant basis for advocacy by Australian rural development workers and would provide the basis for greater resourcing of vulnerable rural communities. However what these concepts appear to lack in their current conceptualisation and implementation in the UK and Europe is a gendered lens – a perspective that would ensure that all are included, that no voices are silenced and that women's voices and concerns are not subsumed into those of 'the family'. Gender mainstreaming provides an important additional policy principle, defined in the UN environment as

the process of assessing the implications for women and men of any planned action, including legislation, policies or programmes, in all areas and at all levels. It is a strategy for making women's as well as men's concerns and experiences an integral dimension of the design, implementation, monitoring and evaluation of policies and programmes in all political, economic and societal spheres so that women and men benefit equally and inequality is not perpetuated. The ultimate goal is to achieve gender equality.

(ECOSOC, 1997, p. 2)

Gender mainstreaming exposes gender inequalities and provides the basis to question who benefits from current policies and strategies and how these might be reshaped to effect greater equality. Localism, rural proofing and gender mainstreaming provide the basis for a new way of advocating for, and empowering, rural communities, providing as they do a challenge to neo-liberal centralist policies and returning power to local communities.

Shucksmith notes that rural community development requires capacity building at local levels to support 'networked action'; and 'rural proofing' of policies to ensure they do not contribute to 'persistent patterns of structural differentiation' (2013, p. 1). However, he adds that inequalities can be exacerbated by this approach. Thus localism and rural proofing are not sufficient. Gender mainstreaming and an overt feminist gaze are essential to ensure the rights of all rural community members are recognised in policies and practices.

Why gender matters

Bringing a feminist perspective to rural community development practice exposes the critical disadvantages and gender inequalities in rural communities. Gender differentials are evident across these areas and result in reduced access to supports that ultimately affect quality of life. A lack of violence support and crisis services, limited care services, a failure to recognise the critical economic contributions of women and reduced health and communications infrastructure have particular impacts for women. Further there are very evident gender differences in land ownership, health issues and care work. In many countries across the Asia-Pacific women are prevented under legislation from inheriting or owning property. By contrast, in Australia, patrilineal property inheritance practices reinforced by tradition and customs provide a more subtle form of exclusion that is nonetheless as effective in ensuring that the vast majority of productive land is owned by men. Such customs and practices are open to challenge.

Gender is also a critical health factor in areas where climate and environmental disasters have occurred (Alston et al., 2004; Alston & Whitney-Soanes, 2008) including in Australian areas experiencing drought conditions (Whittenbury, 2012), for example a significant rise in men suffering mental health issues and declining resilience (Alston, 2012) and critical increases in violence against women (Whittenbury, 2012; Enarson & Chakrabarti, 2009; Lynch, 2011). Women note the complex issues associated with maintaining the health and wellbeing of their families when water and food security are threatened after a disaster and when access to help is delayed or absent (Alston, 2015).

Care work in rural areas remains highly gendered, viewed as women's responsibility and complicated particularly as women's work has escalated at the same time as services have retracted. Juggling child, aged and disabled care is a distressing aspect of rural life, made more complicated during and after climate disasters when schools are closed or absent, where mobile phone coverage is patchy or non-existent and where transport services are limited. Gender inequalities are major factors in the social relations and resource distribution in communities. A feminist approach to community development allows us to critique these inequalities and to build capacity, expose disadvantage and empower women and girls to achieve equal access to the resources available.

Conclusion

Rural areas are undergoing significant changes due in large part to external factors beyond the control of the people who live there. The social impacts of restructuring and climate uncertainty have been made more difficult by neo-liberal policies that effectively have left rural communities to fend for themselves. I have drawn out the social complexity of 'the rural' by noting the deeply entrenched and highly gendered power relations that structure rural lives. I urge social workers working in rural community development not to ignore these normative processes. A feminist approach to community development work facilitates an examination of the 'taken-for-granted' aspects of rural life, exposes the power relations and brings the voices of those silenced by these constructions of knowledge in from the margins.

There has been little focus on rural areas in Australian social policy for much of the last two decades and a critical disregard for gender. If they are mentioned at all women are likely to be subsumed into 'family' policy, a position that reduces the services and supports available to women. In this chapter I have argued the need for Australia to adopt a different set of policy principles to assist the development of rural communities. Neo-liberalism has had particularly harsh consequences in rural areas, leading to significant decline in communities and a defraying of human capital. I argue that policy requires dedicated attention to rural areas and I introduce the notions of localism and rural proofing as important drivers of a more compassionate rural policy agenda. Nonetheless these are incomplete without attention to gendered factors that shape rural life and constrain the lives of rural women in significant ways. I therefore argue that gender mainstreaming is a necessary addition to these policy drivers to ensure equality in policy outcomes.

A feminist approach to rural community development enables social workers to bring a critical awareness to their work and not only to advocate for their communities, but also to foster and develop gender equality. Entrenched and normative gendered power relations will remain dominant unless challenged, exposed and questioned.

Further reading

Creese, G. & Frisby, W. (eds) (2011) *Feminist Community Research: Case Studies and Methodologies.* University of British Columbia, Vancouver.

Ledwith, M. (2005) *Community Development: A Critical Approach.* Policy Press, Bristol, UK.

Terman, R.A. (2009) Rural feminist community development in Appalachia. Appalachia State University, Boone, NC.

References

Alston, M. (1997) Violence against women in a rural context. *Australian Social Work*, 50(1), pp. 15–22.

Alston, M. (2000) *Breaking through the Grass Ceiling: Women, Power and Leadership in Rural Australia.* Harwood Publishers, Amsterdam.

Alston, M. (2005) Drought and social exclusion. In R. Eversole & J. Martin (eds), *Participation and Governance in Regional Development: Global Trends in an Australian Context.* Ashgate, Aldershot, UK, pp. 229–241.

Alston, M. (2009) *Innovative Human Services Practice: Changing Landscapes.* Pan Macmillan, Melbourne.

Alston, M. (2012) Rural male suicide in Australia. *Social Science and Medicine*, 74(4), pp. 515–522.

Alston, M. (2015) *Women and Climate Change in Bangladesh: Gender, Vulnerability and Resilience.* Routledge, London.

Alston, M. & Whittenbury, K. (2012) Does climatic crisis in Australia's food bowl create a basis for change in agricultural gender relations? *Agriculture and Human Values*, 30(1), pp. 115–128.

Alston, M. & Witney-Soanes, K. (2008) *Social Impacts of Drought and Declining Water Availability in the Murray Darling Basin.* Institute of Land, Water and Society, Charles Sturt University, Wagga Wagga, NSW.

Alston, M., Kent, J. & Kent, A. (2004) *Social Impacts of Drought: Report to NSW Agriculture.* Centre for Rural Social Research, Charles Sturt University, Wagga Wagga, NSW.

Ban Ki-Moon (2012) UN Secretary-General Ban Ki-moon's message on World Water Day 2012. *Water is a Human Right*, 17 April. www.right2water.eu/news/un-secretary-general-ban-ki-moons-message-world-water-day-2012 (accessed 11 June 2014).

Burchardt, T. (2002) Social exclusion: concepts and evidence. In D. Gordon & P. Townsend (eds), *Breadline Europe: The Measurement of Poverty.* Policy Press, Bristol, UK, pp. 385–406.

Cloke, P. (2006) Rurality and racialised others: out of place in the countryside. In P. Cloke, T. Marsden & P.H. Mooney (eds), *Handbook of Rural Studies.* Sage, London, pp. 379–388.

Connell, R. (2011) *Confronting Equality.* Allen & Unwin, Sydney.

Deepak, A.C. (2014) A postcolonial feminist social work perspective on global food insecurity. *AFFILIA: The Journal of Women and Social Work*, 29(2), pp. 153–164.

Dietsch, E., Davies, C., Shackleton, P., Alston, M. & McLeod, M. (2008) *'Luckily We had a Torch': Contemporary Birthing Experiences of Women Living in Rural and Remote NSW.* School of Nursing and Midwifery, Charles Sturt University, Wagga Wagga, NSW.

Economic and Social Council (ECOSOC) (1997) *Gender Mainstreaming: Extract from Report of the Economic and Social Council for 1997 (A/52/3, 18 September 1997).* www.un.org/womenwatch/daw/csw/GMS.PDF (accessed 18 June 2012).

Enarson, E. (2012) *Women Confronting Natural Disaster: From Vulnerability to Resilience.* Lynne Rienner Publishers, Boulder, CO.

Enarson, E. & Chakrabarti, P.G.D. (eds) (2009) *Women, Gender and Disaster: Global Issues and Initiatives.* Sage, Delhi.

Freire, P. (1973) *Cultural Action for Freedom.* Penguin, Harmondsworth, UK.

Gringeri, C.E., Wahab, S. & Anderson-Nathe, B. (2010) What makes it feminist? Mapping the landscape of feminist social work research. *AFFILIA: The Journal of Women and Social Work*, 25(4), pp. 390–405.

Heenan, D. (2004) Learning lessons from the past or re-visiting old mistakes: social work and community development in Northern Ireland. *British Journal of Social Work*, 34(6), pp. 793–809.

Lynch, K. (2011) Spike in domestic violence after Christchurch earthquake. *Stuff.co. nz*, 9 March. www.stuff.co.nz/national/christchurch-earthquake/4745720/Spike-in-domestic-violence-after-Christchurch-earthquake (accessed 14 March 2011).

Miller, M.K., Farmer, F.L. & Clarke, L.L. (1994) Rural populations and their health. In J.E. Beaulieu & D.E. Berry (eds), *Rural Health Services*. AUPHA Press Health Administration Press, Ann Arbor, MI, pp. 3–26.

Molnar, J.J. (2010) Climate change and social response: livelihoods, communities and the environment. *Rural Sociology*, 75(1), pp. 1–16.

Parnell, J. (2013) Ban Ki-Moon: world on course to run out of water. *Responding to Climate Change (RTCC)*, 23 May. www.rtcc.org/2013/05/22/ban-ki-moon-world-on-course-to-run-out-of-water/ (accessed 11 June 2014).

Powell, F. (ed.) (2001) *The Politics of Social Work*. Sage, London.

Raitano, F. (2010) Rural policy matters: rural issues, concerns, challenges and recommendations. *RCAC's Rural Review*, 28(2), pp. 7–13.

Shortall, S. (2009) *Does Rural Proofing Make Sense?* Presentation, School of Sociology, Social Policy and Social Work, Queens University, Belfast, Northern Ireland, 24 April.

Shucksmith, M. (2000) Endogenous development, capacity building and inclusion: perspectives from the UK experience of LEADER. *Sociologia Ruralis*, 40(2), pp. 208–218.

Shucksmith, M. (2013) *Future Directions in Rural Development*. Carnegie Trust, Fife. www.carnegieuktrust.org.uk/getattachment/545a7523-4da8-4ff7-95e6-dd912 abc6373/Future-Directions-in-Rural-Development-(Full-Repor.aspx (accessed 11 June 2014).

Smailes, P. (2006) *Redefining the Local: The Social Organisation of Rural Space in South Australia, 1982–2006*. PhD thesis, Flinders University, Bedford Park, SA.

Smith, D. (1992) Feminist reflections on political economy. In M.P. Connelly & P. Armstrong (eds), *Feminism in Action*. Canadian Scholars Press, Toronto, pp. 1–21.

Tönnies, F. (1957 [1887]) *Community and Society*, trans. Charles Price Loomis. Michigan State University Press, East Lansing, MI (originally published as *Gemeinschaft und Gesellschaft*).

Wendt, S. & Boylan, J. (2014) Feminist social work research engaging with post-structural ideas. *International Social Work*, 51(5), pp. 599–609.

Whittenbury, K. (2012) Climate change, women's health, wellbeing and experiences of gender based violence in Australia. In M. Alston & K. Whittenbury (eds), *Research, Action and Policy: Addressing the Gendered Impacts of Climate Change*. Springer, New York, pp. 207–222.

Zapf, M.K. (2010) Social work and the environment: understanding people and place. *Critical Social Work*, 11(3). www1.uwindsor.ca/criticalsocialwork/social-work-and-the-environment-understanding-people-and-place (accessed 22 April 2015).

8 'Do something, change something'
Feminist leadership in social work

Mel Gray and Leanne Schubert

> Leadership is a means, not an end. We build leadership capacity and skills *for something, to do something, or change something,* and not because leadership is a product or service for consumption. This is especially true in social justice contexts.
>
> (Batliwala, 2011, p. 5, emphasis added)

Feminist leadership within social work tends to be located within the contemporary environment of managerialist models of service delivery and management. However, pursuing this perspective alone denies an important historical discourse on feminist leadership, which has arisen outside social work, predominantly amid black feminists, among others, in the USA and the developing world. Not only is this feminist discourse on feminist leadership congruent with feminist principles, it also pursues pertinent domestic and global feminist issues, such as reproductive justice, eco-feminism, intersectionality and identity-based activism, violence against women and global women's rights to health.

In our view, feminist leadership has nothing to do with management. It needs to be understood as a collective force aimed at social transformation and social justice, particularly through empowering women's development. Mainly, it seeks to marry aspects of good leadership with feminist principles. But, as we shall see in this chapter, feminist leadership, as it has come to social work, has drawn too heavily on the management discourse. What results is an approach that seeks to marry feminist principles to management rather than leadership. There is an important difference and it is best understood by briefly reflecting on the roots of feminist leadership in change-oriented social movements.

Historical roots of feminist leadership

Historically, feminist leadership, particularly in the USA, flourished in key programmes within the civil and human rights movements, urban settlement houses, refugee settlements, suffrage movements, historical and cultural landmark preservation and environmental ecosystems protection (Rusaw, 2005; Stivers, 2002). Batliwala (2011) highlights the transformational nature of feminist leadership in undermining power inequalities. Its agenda is inherently political: it fights injustice and oppression wherever it results from discrimination due to people's gender, race, ethnicity, class and privilege. Feminist leadership inheres when feminists individually and collectively transform themselves to use their power, resources, strengths and skills to mobilise others around a shared agenda of social, cultural, economic and political transformation for equality and the realisation of human rights for all. Feminist leaders have a transformative, rights-based, social justice agenda: 'they lead differently, with feminist values and ideology ... to advance the agenda of feminist social transformation in a way that other forms of leadership do not and cannot' (Batliwala, 2011, p. 13). They pursue social justice feminism, which is structural in orientation, committed to a political agenda via an action-oriented, bottom-up, inclusive, participatory and empowering approach aimed at exposing and dismantling the sociopolitical structures and ideologies that perpetuate oppression and distributive injustice, such as neo-liberal capitalism.

Social justice feminists are mindful of historical hierarchies and inequities, the need for empowerment beyond the removal of oppression, and the co-existence and intersection of multiple oppressions that require a coalition of agendas. Social justice feminists are committed to advancing social justice through action-oriented social intervention strategies and action research (see Gray, Agllias & Davies, 2014). They look to history to understand subordinating structures so as to acquire knowledge with which to understand and then dismantle the bases of societal institutions that perpetuate hierarchies and inequities. They seek to uncover stories and experiences that have not been told or included in historical accounts and examine how they alter ways of seeing (Kalsem & Williams, 2010). They are acutely aware of the interrelationships between interlocking multiple oppressions and how issues of gender, race, class and other categories of identity and experience work together to create social injustice: they seek to identify 'the implications of race, class, and other subordinating structures' (Kalsem & Williams, 2010, p. 181). They are activists who are committed to making material changes to people's lives and consciously fashioning strategies for social change. They allow 'criteria of social justice to emerge from the identification of a broad pattern of societal injustice surpassing the discrimination of particular groups' (Azmanova, 2011, p. 143).

Social justice feminists favour feminist-informed research methodologies and intervention frameworks aligned with their social justice agenda. They prefer reflexive methodologies that involve engaged and fluid relationships between researchers and participants and that conceptualise participants as co-researchers and promote community involvement in problem conceptualisation, data collection and analysis, and knowledge distribution because they seek to undermine hierarchies of knowledge and power inherent in conventional research methods (Alkon, 2011). This type of research is political in nature and purpose; it aims to question, challenge, realign and illuminate the dimensions of power and privilege (Reid, 2004). It seeks to shift feminist inquiry 'to identify a larger systemic pattern of injustice, rooted in the key antinomies of capitalism' (Azmanova, 2011, p. 143). Social justice feminism is undergirded by a critical perspective that focuses on the structural aspects of social problems:

> Social injustice is not simply a matter of arbitrary unequal distribution of power that causes oppression; it is rooted in the specific structure of social relations for a given society and the particular types of institutions and norms these relations engender.
> (Horkheimer, 2002 [1937], quoted in Azmanova, 2011, p. 146)

Socialist and black feminists have come close to this perspective in highlighting how class, ethnicity, gender, race, sexual orientation and other dimensions of identity intersect in women's oppression. Their social justice feminism aims to take action to 'ameliorate ableism, ageism, classism, heterosexism, racism, sexism, transphobia, and other forms of injustice ... and to recognize the coexistence and intersections of these oppressive forces' (Moradi, 2012, p. 1136). However, 'endorsing pro social justice attitudes may not necessarily translate into engagement in social justice activism' (Moradi, 2012, p. 1136). What distinguishes social justice feminism from other forms of feminism is its strong links between social justice and social action (Kalsem & Williams, 2010; Moradi, 2012). Social action is a key focus and its transformational ideology guides action to challenge injustice and improve the social conditions for all members of society. Another important goal, beyond the removal of oppression, is empowerment.

Hence there is a strong correlation between feminist leadership and social justice feminism. For example, Porter and Henderson Daniel (2007) note that whether working with small groups, teams or communities, feminist leaders seek to empower people, while simultaneously working to improve their quality of life and the social conditions in which they live. Most of this discourse arises in the context of development, where there is a strong focus on building the capacity of women and women's organisations. The Disabled Women's Network Ontario emphasises the collective nature of feminist leadership, seeing it as '*women and women's organizations sharing power, authority and decision-making in our common pursuit of social, legal, political, economic and cultural equality*' (n.d., emphasis added). Hartman (1999) too sees a focus on building other *women's* capacities and confidence to be leaders in their communities. The challenge of feminist leaders is to enable *women* 'to be equipped as leaders in their own right' (Olusola, 2013, p. 32).

Early feminist leaders in Australian social work

Clearly then there is a close link between feminist leadership and social justice. This link was evident in the work of early feminist leaders within social work. One such leader is Norma Parker, who is regarded as a foundational figure within Australian social work. Parker specialised in social casework and pioneered psychiatric social work in Australia. She lived and practised during turbulent times, namely the 'economic depression, a World War, postwar reconstruction and widespread social unrest and discontent in the 1960s and beyond [during which] ... she was involved in developing a professional occupation that claimed to specialise in helping people with their social functioning' (Lawrence, 2004, p. 299).

Parker became an important contributor to Australian social work education at Sydney University and later the University of New South Wales. She also played an important role in reforming the Department of Child Welfare based on evidence gathered at the Girls' Industrial School at Parramatta. She was a central figure in forming the Catholic Trained Social Workers Association in 1940 and was also 'instrumental in the foundation of the Australian Association of Social Workers (AASW), serving as its inaugural president from 1946 to 1954' (Lee, 2012). Later she was influential in establishing 'the New South Wales Association for Mental Health in 1956, and ... the Australian Council of Social Services (ACOSS)' (Lee, 2012). As a founding member of St Joan's Social and Political Alliance, her feminist agenda was again at the fore to 'empower women to support social justice causes' (Lee, 2012). However, like many women leaders of her time, 'despite her achievements ... [Parker] was repeatedly passed over as head of department while less experienced younger men were appointed' (Lee, 2012). Nevertheless, Parker forged ahead: 'when there was something to be done, we did it. We were ... feminists' (quoted in Lee, 2012).

Another feminist role model in Australian social work, Margaret Whitlam, played a high-profile public leadership role. She began as a social worker in family welfare (Fife-Yeomans, 2012) and later was the sole social worker at Parramatta Hospital from 1964 to 1967 (Whitlam Institute, n.d.). She no doubt influenced her husband Gough Whitlam, Prime Minister of Australia from 1972 to 1975, whose Labor government set out a wide-ranging reform agenda following more than two decades of Liberal government (National Archives of Australia, n.d.). Margaret Whitlam was 'a political and prime ministerial wife. An outspoken public speaker, broadcaster and columnist ... [and] a qualified social worker ... particularly interested in social conditions' (National Archives of Australia, n.d.). In this high-profile public role, she became a 'champion of the less privileged' (Fife-Yeomans, 2012), promoting social justice and egalitarianism in Australian society. Appreciating the opportunity to influence change that her position afforded her, she saw her exemplary role as a prime minister's wife to be humane towards others and treat them with dignity and respect. As a feminist pioneer, Margaret Whitlam inspired Australian women everywhere (Fife-Yeomans, 2012). Nevertheless, she did not always agree with aspects of the feminist movement, airing her differences with outspoken radical feminist Germaine Greer, also an Australian though living in London from a young age (Fife-Yeomans, 2012).

Margaret Whitlam was a social justice feminist who influenced social reforms for women in the workplace and beyond. She fought for women's increased participation in the workforce, for equal pay and work conditions, and the removal of discriminatory and unjust policies, such as the no-fault divorce clause. She supported the foundation of the Family Court of Australia and support services for women. She served on the Australian National Advisory Committee and was a delegate at the associated world conference. She was instrumental in the 1975 International Women's Year, with the establishment of the single mother's benefit, appointment of a women's adviser to the Prime Minister, parental leave for female Commonwealth employees and the removal of restrictions on oral contraceptives. Her long-term commitment to, and ardent pursuit of, social justice was marked by the establishment of the Margaret Whitlam Chair of Social Work at the University of Western Sydney in 2010 (Whitlam Institute, n.d.).

These two Australian social workers are important role models for feminist leadership. Though they took different leadership approaches, they shared the understanding that they stood *for something, could do something, or change something* and highlighted the diverse ways in which this might be achieved.

Social justice feminism

From these roots, feminist leadership in social work had hoped to change women's conditions. It arose during the second wave of feminism when women were united in highlighting social injustices against women. It was distinctly partisan and critical, but, with the advent of postmodernism, lost this edge as the feminist agenda was challenged by multiple oppressions. Significantly, development-oriented feminist leadership has retained its gender focus. Being singularly committed to women's empowerment, it stands as a site of resistance to this postmodern trend. Definitions of development-oriented feminist leadership connect an amalgam of concepts – and their related principles – in various combinations:

- first, there is the idea it is informed by feminist principles;
- second, is its strong connection to social justice;
- third, especially in the context of social development, it is about amassing the collective power of women and women's organisations;
- then, fourth, it is tacked on to notions of leadership, especially transformational leadership.

These four areas – and their related principles – seem to inform most notions of feminist leadership to varying degrees. Thus Olusola notes the connection between social justice feminism and leadership in her definition:

> leadership from a feminist standpoint is informed by the power of [a] feminist lens which enables the feminist leader to identify injustices and oppression and inspires her to facilitate the development of more inclusive holistic communities … feminist leaders are motivated by fairness, injustice and equity and strive to keep issues of gender, race, social class, sexual orientation, and ability at the forefront.
>
> (2013, p. 29)

Batliwala too notes the strong links with social justice:

> feminist leadership is oriented to different arrangement of the human order, re-distribution of power and re-distribution of responsibilities, fighting societal inequalities, changing economic and social structures, beginning in the transformation of psychic structures, bridging personal freedom with collective freedom, aiming at cooperation instead of competition.
>
> (2008, p. 29)

It is clear to us that feminism has a historical presence in social work that is particularly linked to the principles and values of social justice. This is what feminist leadership has, in essence, been about. The question that remains, however, is whether this remains the case in contemporary social work. We do not have an answer for this question that is grounded in research, policy or practice, and this would require substantial further research than we are able to undertake for this chapter. Thus we are left to wonder whether this kind of momentum and leadership remains – or can remain – present in the highly regulated neo-liberally driven organisational contexts of contemporary social work practice. Similarly, we wonder about the influence of the diversification of feminism and the changed attitudes of young women towards an overtly political feminist agenda. While we have no doubt there is still much work for feminists to do, and the continuing unequal experiences of women remain just as present in this so-called post-feminist era, we wonder whether a feminist challenge can be effective within highly regulated, managerial organisations or whether, following the example of India's feminist leader Medha Patkar, feminists must move beyond these confines and become increasingly political to achieve their aims as social activists. Given the lack of political engagement by social workers (Gray et al., 2002), perhaps this stands as the profession's greatest challenge to feminist leadership in the contemporary climate.

Social justice feminist Medha Patkar is an Indian social activist, social reformer turned politician and graduate of the Tata Institute of Social Sciences. She left her faculty position there, as well as her unfinished PhD, to immerse herself in the fight for social justice for tribal and peasant communities and provide leadership to local people's organisations as National Convener of the National Alliance of People's Movements, an alliance of progressive people's organisations and movements fighting against social injustice in India. She has been a vocal environmental activist and led the struggle for the people affected by the controversial Sardar Sarovar Project on the Narmada River in Gujarat, India. She founded the Narmada Bachoao Andolan and National Alliance of People's Movements and is the recipient of numerous awards, including the Goldman Environmental Prize, Amnesty International's Human Rights Defender's Award and the BBC's Green Ribbon Award (see Patkar, 2012; PTI, 2013; Wikipedia, 2014).

Despite the evidence of social justice roots within the feminist movement more broadly, and within the practice of social work's role models, feminist leadership within social work discourse had quite different roots and it is to this we now turn.

How has feminist leadership arisen in the social work discourse?

Unlike development-oriented feminist leadership, feminist leadership as imported into social work has different origins and, to distinguish the two, we refer to it here as management-oriented feminist leadership. It connects an amalgam of concepts – and their related principles – in various combinations:

- first, it is described as consistent with social work values;
- second, it outlines the coherence of social work values with feminist principles and their strong connection to social justice;
- third, it looks to the management literature for theory on good leadership and leadership styles;
- then, fourth, it is tacked on to notions of leadership, especially transformational leadership.

As we shall see, consistency between feminist leadership and social work values is the starting point, with the distinctiveness of feminist leadership most obviously its feminist leanings rather than the promotion of women's interests or gender equality in the workplace. As Phillips and Cree (2014) note, in today's social work workplaces women are reluctant to call themselves feminists though they might follow inherently feminist values. While Lazzari, Colarossi and Collins (2009) acknowledge the importance of identification, they recommend a move away from labelling as a means of promoting inclusiveness, suggesting feminists should advocate feminism rather than label themselves 'feminist'. They see this as shifting the focus away from oneself towards the work that needs to be done. It is part of building shared responsibility through inclusiveness (Lazzari et al., 2009).

Unlike earlier periods in social work, where social workers strongly identified as feminists, today this label might be seen as problematic. For example, in the main, social work students see little resonance between feminism and social work. Thus the feminist label might alienate rather than engage them (Lazzari et al., 2009; Parnell & Andrews, 1994; Valentich, 2010; White, 2006). This position perhaps reflects the shifts in feminism evident in popular media, including the rejection of feminism by many women celebrities, though this might change in light of Emma Watson's recent speech on feminism at the United Nations, and Joseph Gordon-Levitt's pro-feminist stance. Such public statements might militate against negative stereotypes of feminists and the myth that feminists hate men, which have been attributed to a lack of education and the emergence of groups who feel feminism rejects them. This contrasts with increasing conversations in the digital world, where feminism appears in unexpected places; feminists have yet to exploit the growing potential for online activism supported by digital connectivity.

Despite the absence of a contemporary, straightforward definition of feminism, 'feminist' work continues to be produced that 'both interrogates the specific and general conditions of women's lives and explores the more ubiquitous construct of "gender", and in social work, feminist understandings remain central to practice, theory and research' (Phillips & Cree, 2014, p. 930). Phillips and Cree (2014) argue this may be due to the over-representation of women in social work or be related to the profession's pursuit of social justice. This may, in large part, reflect the continuing over-representation of women as providers and users of social work services. It may also echo social work's broader emancipatory, 'social justice' aspirations. Phillips and Cree identify the resurgence of feminism across the world, driven by the internet and the accompanying claim that we are witnessing a 'fourth wave' of feminism across the Global North (Cochrane, 2013).

Where does this fit in the social work cannon?

The influence of feminism

Social work places its values and ethics at its centre and accepts and adopts related theories and practices that support its values and ethical stance. Given social work is a female-dominated profession, it has long embraced feminism, which continues to be closely affiliated with its value base (Bricker-Jenkins & Hooyman, 1986; Lazzari et al., 2009; Van Den Bergh & Cooper, 1986), to the point where 'some would say ... social work is inherently feminist' (Lazzari et al., 2009, p. 349; see also Collins, 1986).

Feminism has had an important influence on social work's development, though there are diverse feminist identities within social work. While some social workers might have feminist leanings, they 'will not necessarily develop identities as feminist social workers, particularly if they have no well-established feminist practice context or role models' (Valentich, 2010, p. 221). This question of identification also extends to feminist social work leaders. From our own experience, we share in common, albeit to varying degrees and with different leanings, a connection with feminism that constitutes part of our respective social work identities.

North American feminists' early work framed discussions in terms of male dominance and sought alternatives to patriarchy and hierarchy. They established the first wave of feminism which sought equality – equal rights – for women (Gray & Boddy, 2010). Given feminists have consistently highlighted the domination of men and subordination of women at all levels of society, the conventional leader–follower model is anathema to feminists (Lazzari et al., 2009), who have struggled consistently to 'eradicate the ideology of domination that permeates cultures on various levels and in varying ways, as well as a commitment to reorganizing society so that the self-development of people can take precedence over imperialism, economic expansion, and material desires' (hooks, 2000, p. 26).

Feminists invited women and men to act with critical awareness of the impact of their behaviour on themselves and others (Lazzari et al., 2009). They turned the personal – the language we use, the decisions, judgements or choices we make, the actions we take and the relationships we form – into the political, because they were shaped by unequal hierarchical relationships and structures that disempowered women and needed to be changed. How our 'personal alliances, attitudes, biases, and emotions influence decision making' is an ever-present critical question for feminists (Lazzari et al., 2009, p. 353). This is particularly important in contemporary managerialist environments where outcomes and key performance indicators are prioritised over relationships and compliance is valued over critical questioning. Therefore, some believe feminist leadership is all the more important in managerial environments, where practitioners have to find creative ways to ensure service users' needs are met within increasingly punitive welfare regimes (Chin, 2004; Eagly, 2007; Lazzari et al., 2009).

Feminist social workers consistently promote a social justice agenda, where the key focus is change and empowerment, and intervene when power structures sustain injustice. They challenge multiple oppressions but prioritise gender justice and affirmative action where necessary (Batliwala, 2011; Chin, 2004; Chin et al., 2007; Kirton & Healy, 2012; Porter & Henderson Daniel, 2007). Feminist social workers also value:

- *relationships and relational practices*, such as nurturance as a means of engagement, communication and leadership, and coaching and mentoring by feminist role models;

- *inclusive participatory styles of engagement*, particularly of people who are socially and politically marginalised;
- *collaborative relationships and practices*, where there is clear, transparent, shared decision making that facilitates power sharing for, and draws on the strengths of, all parties involved;
- *reflective practice*, praxis and reflexivity;
- *choice* with shared responsibility and accountability;
- *non-violence* and championing the rights of women in abusive relationships.

These feminist principles, among others, are seen as important in how feminist leaders lead, whether or not they refer to themselves as feminist leaders. Though the term 'feminist leadership' might not feature prominently in the social work discourse, nevertheless feminist principles underlie the preferred style of social work leadership, as the following discussion shows.

Applying feminist principles to leadership

Phillips and Cree (2014) recommend several strategies for feminist social work education. First, they suggest the need to develop more nuanced approaches to feminism and to construct bridges to the 'new generation' that allow feminist insights to emerge rather than be imposed. This means taking a position where identifying with feminism does not 'require "being" a feminist' (p. 940) and refocusing on the structural issues of inequality clearly supported by evidence to promote further inquiry. Second, the need to build understanding through theoretical analyses influenced by feminist thinkers so as to reduce the confrontational elements of feminism but keep women's inequality and gender-based injustice at the forefront. This requires a willingness to critique the positive and negative aspects of the fourth wave of feminism.

Intemann et al. (2010) identify four common aims of feminist thinking that remain apposite. First, it challenges universalist and essentialist frameworks without ceding to relativism. Second, it centres coloniality and embodiment in critical analyses of the intermeshed realities of race and gender by shifting from oppression in the abstract to concrete struggles, particularly those of women of colour and women of colonised communities across the globe. In other words, it takes a historical, situated perspective. Third, it elaborates materialities of thought, being and community that must succeed atomistic conceptions of persons as disembodied, individually constituted and autonomous. Finally, it demonstrates what is distinctive and valuable about feminist philosophy, while fighting persistent marginalisation within it. However, Intemann et al. (2010) also acknowledge that diverse feminist identities and differing degrees of identification with feminism in social work often preclude a feminist inclination necessarily equating with becoming a feminist social worker or for that matter a feminist leader. They argue this is particularly so where there is an absence of an established feminist context, that is, an organisational environment that values feminist ideas and practices, and appropriate feminist role models.

Lazzari et al. (2009) are among the few theorists who have applied feminist principles directly to leadership in social work. They draw on mainstream theories of leadership in formulating their ideas rather than the literature on (development-oriented) feminist leadership per se. From their liberal feminist perspective, they highlight ongoing gender inequities: 'the current status of women still lags far behind that of men on numerous indicators' (p. 348). By implication, then, gender equality is a concern for them, and the absence of women in leadership roles, hence the subtitle of their article 'Where have all the leaders gone?' However, they see their feminist model of leadership as applying equally to men and women in leadership roles. Noting 'multiple feminisms' and disagreement about the right feminist theory in social work, their purpose is 'to discuss key (anchoring) principles and practices of feminist methodology and ethics and to apply them to possible contexts, forms, and functions of leadership and its relationship to social justice' (p. 351). The feminist principles they highlight – and that permeate the literature on management-oriented feminist leadership – have to do with:

- the critical analysis of power, domination and patriarchy;
- essentialism, gender, sex and difference;
- the relationship between the personal and the political;
- participation, representation and intersectionality;
- non-violence, relationality and growth;
- praxis and reflexivity.

Despite the challenges of today's work environments, the diversity of feminism and the changing nature of social work practice, these core areas of feminist leadership remain as current as ever. Cognisant of issues of power, race, gender, patriarchy and the like, feminist leaders favour a flattened hierarchy, where there are clearly demarcated roles and strategies to ensure that the same rights and standards apply to all members of the organisation. They prefer shared decision making and favour collaborative leadership styles (Chin, 2004). However, Kirton and Healy (2012) note there is disagreement between feminists about decision-making processes. While most see decision making as a collective or shared activity, more important than egalitarian leadership is the accountability of leaders. Also, given the situational perspective of feminists, collaborative, participatory strategies may not always be the best way of achieving our aims and sometimes independent or representative processes may be more effective and more equitable in ensuring everyone has an equal chance to participate

(Lazzari et al., 2009). However it is done, feminist leaders seek strategies that promote inclusion and collaboration.

Every opportunity is taken to question and speak up to 'support power with, shared and collective decision making' (Lazzari et al., 2009, p. 353). There is a strong belief among feminists that shared and empowering decision making is the best means to achieve the ends of empowerment and social justice (Chin, 2004; Fletcher & Kaufer, 2003). In 'committees, work groups, research teams, and teaching forums ... [feminist leaders] help change the environmental configuration [to this end]' (Lazzari et al., 2009, p. 353). Mel's experience in leadership within the academic environment would suggest this is a challenging proposition that is more easily applied within a social work team with a strong feminist orientation than in male-dominated university structures that do not share these cooperative values. It is easier to promote dialogue and action that reflects feminist values in mentoring and classroom environments within social work than beyond it in the broader university environment. Social workers feel comfortable engaging in discussions about power relationships and organisational structures. It is, however, not as easy to promote shared and collective decision making, empowerment and choice, or to question the status quo in powerful academic environments, where one is faced with an ever-present need to evaluate one's leadership activities and their congruence with feminist ethics, methods and experience (Lazzari et al., 2009). The discomfort arising from a lack of congruence between role-based organisational expectations and her feminist social work ethics led to Leanne's decision to opt out of management positions.

In contemporary managerial 'hierarchical organizations where patriarchal models of "power over" dictate structures and processes and "power with" is devalued and often punished' (Lazzari et al., 2009, p. 349) taking a feminist stance – or any value stance for that matter – is a risky business. Morley and Macfarlane highlight the importance of challenging neoliberal practices in contemporary social work environments that threaten feminist values of 'social justice, democracy, protection of human rights and equity' (2012, p. 688).

Thus there is dissonance between our feminist values and the organisational environments in which most of us work (Lazzari et al., 2009; White, 2006). However, little has been written on feminist leadership per se in social work and the only working model has come from Lazzari et al. (2009). Recently, however, Christensen (2011) reported on a study in which six college students used feminist leadership techniques in a sexual assault prevention programme based on Hawxhurst and Morrow's (1984) model. In reflecting on how feminist theory intersects with leadership practice, she draws on Lazzari et al. (2009). The main themes emerging from her study to deepen understanding of feminist leadership involve sharing, empowering and embodied knowledge (given this was a special theoretical focus for this study).

Influence of transformational leadership

The increasing number of women in managerial positions has 'created interest in the role of women as leaders' (Kark, 2004, p. 160). At the same time, there has been a growing engagement with the theory of transformational leadership. Kark explores how various approaches in feminist thought intersect with the study of gender and transformational (charismatic) leadership. The transformational leader 'empowers followers, and motivates them to perform beyond their expectations' (p. 161). This coincides with changes in management theory 'stressing the need for organisations to become less hierarchical, more flexible, team-oriented, and participative' (p. 161). This was a style of leadership associated with stereotypes of women and how they would be expected to behave as leaders, which may have influenced the study of the intersection between transformational leadership and gender. To date, there have been no conclusive studies that transformational leadership is a women's thing. Rather there has been more evidence on the effectiveness of transformational leadership.

Porter and Henderson Daniel (2007) outline the following characteristics of transformative leadership:

1   *inspirational motivation*: stirring others to action by communicating one's vision vividly, with optimism and enthusiasm;
2   *idealised influence*: modelling behaviours that reflect high ethical standards, which place the collective good above personal need;
3   *individualised consideration*: supporting, coaching and encouraging constituents;
4   *intellectual stimulation*: problem solving with constituents in collaborative and innovative ways.

Transformative leadership theory highlights participatory styles of leadership that challenge power hierarchies and attempt to equalise power through team building. Chin (2004) suggests it involves; (i) stewardship of organisational resources, (ii) vision creation, (iii) social advocacy and change and (iv) policy promotion. Both Lazzari et al. (2009) and Chin (2004) see transformative leadership as key to the feminist agenda of empowering others – by talking with kindred spirits, forming coalitions, collaborative decision making and supporting one another.

Finding synergies between diverse discourses

There would appear to be a disjunct between the way in which feminist leadership is discussed within (Bricker-Jenkins & Hooyman, 1986; Christensen, 2011; Lazzari et al., 2009; White, 2006) and outside (Batliwala, 2011; Chin, 2004; Chin et al., 2007; Olusola, 2013; Porter & Henderson

Daniel, 2007; Rusaw, 2005) social work. It seems that several strands of discourse are being brought together to theorise feminist leadership.

One strand of this discourse takes great pains to distinguish feminist leadership from management. This strand, however, tends to tack feminist principles on to characteristics of good leadership so that feminist leadership becomes a multi-layered entity. Thus, Chin et al. (2007) see feminist leadership as a goal and a style of leadership. This is reminiscent of the huge discourse on management styles. Key among these is a relational leadership style most often associated with a feminist approach (Chin, 2004, 2011). This then leads to discussions of the range of skills feminist leaders should have, such as skills in bringing people together, relationship building and communication, and in building consensus (Chin, 2004; Viezzer, 2001). Many of these are framed in relation to fostering a positive work environment, which is seen as critical to feminist leadership. Essentially this individualistic approach involves the feminist leader's use of self in setting direction, engaging in transparent collaborative decision making (Chin, 2004) and being accountable to colleagues and management alike (Lazzari et al., 2009). Paradoxically, Lazzari et al. then note that in feminist leadership 'what you do is not about you, but about the colleagues with whom you work and the clients or students you serve' (p. 354).

Another strand of the discourse equates feminist leadership with transformational leadership, which aims for a model in which leadership is exercised horizontally, in a non-competitive manner that is founded on trust building and group acceptance (Kark, 2004; Viezzer, 2001). This fits well with feminist principles regarding power inequities and the consequent preference for collaborative processes to equalise the power of the leader so as to create a more egalitarian environment through 'shared leadership' (Chin, 2004, p. 4). Hence, Lazzari et al. say, a feminist theory of leadership should

> apply to, and closely monitor or observe, all levels of leadership power and influence, both formal and informal; the sex differences that exist; gendered expectations; and the process and goals of leadership. This practice involves reconstructing power as empowerment, for example, making decisions with others, sharing control of resources and educational curricula, and generating ideas or ideologies and knowledge.
>
> (2009, p. 352)

Chin (2004) argues that feminist leadership models require goals directed at achieving feminist values; environments that do not attend to gender and power dynamics do not respect feminist goals. She draws attention to the need to challenge power structures and masculinised frameworks, including those within leadership itself. Further, she alerts us to the need to be wary of the gaps between the rhetoric and goals of organisations, noting that the power dynamics and associated stressors experienced by women leaders within masculinised environments have not been examined. Thus a feminist understanding of leadership locates behaviour within a context of power relationships (Chin, 2004, 2011) and a beginning point to implementing feminist leadership within an organisation might be as simple as initiating a discussion of the power relations within it (Lazzari et al., 2009).

Kirton and Healy observe that power is 'not only gendered but also racialized' (2012, p. 984), with men blind to gender privilege and white men and women blind to race privilege. Hence, Batliwala (2011) believes feminist leaders should consciously attend to their own use of power, though Viezzer (2001) claims neither feminists nor women who are transformative leaders seek power for power's sake. From another angle, Rao and Kelleher note that power is 'relational and unlimited in its potential to transform relationships ... human organisations and institutions' (2000, p. 77). This might be significant if the prediction that women will continue to ascend to greater authority and power across time were true (Eagly, 2007).

Another strand of the discourse focuses on values and seeks to find synergies between the values of social work, feminist values and the values of transformational leadership (Barker & Young, 1994). Porter and Henderson Daniel (2007) developed the *Values* schema for transformational leadership, which shares some synergies with feminist and social work values:

> *V*ision that is transforming, effectively communicated, and courageously executed;
> *A*ction that is collaborative, community-focused, and respectful;
> *L*earning that is empowering, reflexive, and lifelong;
> *U*nderstanding of power and boundaries issues that strive to empower;
> *E*thical practices that promote inclusiveness, integrity and responsibility;
> *S*ocial constructivism that informs one's practice of leadership.
>
> (p. 250)

Yet another strand of discourse attempts to disentangle the difference between feminist, feminine and women as leaders. For example, Chin (2004) distinguishes between women as leaders and feminist women leaders, given that not all women who are leaders are feminist. She acknowledges there are complex issues for women leaders who have a feminist leadership style in terms of handling perceptions and expectations that limit their role and behaviour, given that a narrower range of behaviours is considered acceptable for women than for men (Chin, 2004). Research suggests some women have changed their leadership behaviour to prevent men feeling intimidated by them (Holmes & Flood, 2013). Antrobus (2004) draws a distinction between transformational leadership concerned with causing social change and *feminist* transformational leadership concerned with achieving gender justice.

Following a trait approach, Loden (1985) sees the *feminine* leadership style as favouring cooperation over competition, intuition as well as rational thinking in problem solving, team structures where power and influence are shared within the group, interpersonal competence and participatory decision making. For Batliwala (2011), pointing to the (feminine) qualities women bring to leadership – collaboration, cooperation, collective decision making and relationship building – borders on essentialising women and, perhaps unintentionally, reinforcing gender stereotypes.

Then, finally, there is the hortatory strand of discourse where women are entreated to stand together as one, where every woman is seen as a leader in shaping justice for all and where women's organisations across the globe are seen to constitute a collective force for change. Feminist leadership will not manifest in one woman, but in a collective force and voice that will change the world:

> To create something that replaces and surpasses you, that has a life of its own because there are many people who will be drawn into it and who will give leadership to it as a group, even if you move on or go away. To me, that has always been the measure of leadership.... The point is that wherever we are as women, wherever we are situated in our lives, we can advance a feminist agenda if we stop thinking about how to be leaders and think rather about how to be doers, how to be agents.
>
> (Lerner, 1995, n.p.)

Further reading

Batliwala, S. (2011) *Feminist Leadership for Social Transformation: Clearing the Conceptual Cloud.* Creating Resources for Empowerment in Action (CREA), New Delhi.

Lazzari, M.M., Colarossi, L. & Collins, K.S. (2009) Feminists in social work: where have all the leaders gone? *AFFILIA: The Journal of Women and Social Work*, 24(4), 348–350.

Orme, J. (2003) 'It's feminist because I say so!' Feminism, social work and critical practice. *Qualitative Social Work*, 2(2), pp. 131–153.

References

Alkon, A.H. (2011) Reflexivity and environmental justice scholarship: a role for feminist methodologies. *Organization Environment*, 24(2), pp. 130–149.

Antrobus, P. (2004) *The Global Women's Movement: Issues and Strategies for the New Century (Global Issues).* Zed Books, London.

Azmanova, A. (2011) De-gendering social justice in the 21st century: an immanent critique of neoliberal capitalism. *European Journal of Social Theory*, 15(2), pp. 143–156.

Barker, A. & Young, C.E. (1994) Transformational leadership: the feminist connection in postmodern organisations. *Holistic Nursing Practice*, 9(1), pp. 16–25.

Batliwala, S. (2008) *Feminist Leadership for Social Transformation*. Resource commissioned for Building Feminist Leadership: Looking Back, Looking Forward, Cape Town, South Africa, 12–14 November 2008.

Batliwala, S. (2011). *Feminist Leadership for Social Transformation: Clearing the Conceptual Cloud*. Creating Resources for Empowerment in Action (CREA), New Delhi.

Bricker-Jenkins, M. & Hooyman, N.R. (1986) *Not for Women Only: Social Work Practice for a Feminist Future*. National Association of Social Workers, Silver Spring, MD.

Chin, J.L. (2004) 2003 Division 35 presidential address: feminist leadership: feminist visions and diverse voices. *Psychology of Women Quarterly*, 28, pp. 1–8.

Chin, J.L. (2011) *Women and Leadership: Transforming Visions and Current Contexts*. http://files.eric.ed.gov/fulltext/EJ944204.pdf (accessed 1 May 2015).

Chin, J.L., Lott, B., Rice, J.K. & Sanchez-Hucles, J. (eds) (2007) *Women and Leadership: Transforming Visions and Diverse Voices*. Blackwell, Oxford.

Christensen, M.C. (2011) Using feminist leadership to build a performance-based, peer education program. *Qualitative Social Work*, 12(3), pp. 254–269.

Cochrane, K. (2013) *All the Rebel Women: The Rise of the Fourth Wave of Feminism*. Guardian Books, London.

Collins, B. (1986) Defining feminist social work. *Social Work*, 31, pp. 214–219.

Disabled Women's Network Ontario (n.d.) *The Feminist Principle of Leadership*. http://dawn.thot.net/feminist html (accessed 1 October 2008).

Eagly, A.H. (2007) Female leadership advantage and disadvantage: resolving the contradictions. *Psychology of Women Quarterly*, 31, pp. 1–12.

Fife-Yeomans, J. (2012) Champion of the less privileged: Margaret Whitlam 1919–2012. *Sunday Telegraph*, 18 March.

Fletcher, J.K. & Kaufer, K. (2003). Shared leadership: paradox and possibility. In C.L. Pearce & J.A. Conger (eds), *Shared Leadership: Reframing the Hows and Whys of Leadership*. Sage, Thousand Oaks, CA, pp. 21–47.

Gray, M. & Boddy, J. (2010) Making sense of the waves: wipeout or still riding high? *AFFILIA: The Journal of Women and Social Work*, 25(4), pp. 368–389.

Gray, M., Agllias, K. & Davies, K. (2014) Social justice feminism. In M. Reisch (ed.), *The Routledge International Handbook of Social Justice*. Routledge, New York, pp. 173–187.

Gray, M., Collett van Rooyen, C.A.J., Rennie, G. & Gaha, J. (2002) The political participation of social workers: a comparative study. *International Journal of Social Welfare*, 11(2), pp. 99–110.

Hartman, M.S. (ed.) (1999) *Talking Leadership: Conversations with Powerful Women*. Rutgers University Press, Piscataway, NJ.

Hawxhurst, D. & Morrow, S. (1984) *Living our Visions: Building Feminist Community*. Fourth World, Tempe, AZ.

Holmes, S. & Flood, M. (2013) *Genders at Work: Exploring the Role of Workplace Equality in Preventing Men's Violence against Women*. White Ribbon Research Series No. 7. White Ribbon Australia, North Sydney, NSW. www.whiteribbon.org.au/uploads/media/Research_series/WRIB-470_Genders_At_Work_Paper_v03.pdf (accessed 21 September 2014).

hooks, b. (2000) *Feminist Theory: From Margin to Center*, 2nd edn. South End Press, Boston, MA.

Intemann, K., Lee, E.S., McCartney, K., Roshanravan, S. & Schriempf, A. (2010) What lies ahead: envisioning new futures for feminist philosophy. *Hypatia*, 25(4), pp. 927–934.

Kalsem, K. & Williams, V.L. (2010) *Social Justice Feminism*. Faculty Articles and Other Publications Paper 13. University of Cincinnati College of Law, Cincinnati, OH. http://scholarship.law.uc.edu/fac_pubs/13 (accessed 31 July 2014).

Kark, R. (2004) The transformational leader: who is (s)he? A feminist perspective. *Journal of Organizational Change Management*, 17(2), pp. 160–176.

Kirton, G. & Healy, G. (2012) 'Lift as you rise': union women's leadership talk. *Human Relations*, 65, pp. 979–999.

Lawrence, J. (2004) In memorium: a tribute to Norma Parker. *Australian Social Work*, 53(3), pp. 299–303.

Lazzari, M.M., Colarossi, L. & Collins, K.S. (2009) Feminists in social work: where have all the leaders gone? *AFFILIA: The Journal of Women and Social Work*, 24(4), pp. 348–359.

Lee, R. (2012) Norma Parker. *Australian Women and Leadership*, 6 August. www.womenaustralia.info/awal/tag/norma-parker/ (accessed 21 September 2014).

Lerner, G. (1995) Leadership: feminist, spiritual, political. *Woman of Power*, 24(44), n.p.

Loden, M. (1985) *Feminine Leadership*. Crown, New York.

Moradi, B. (2012) Feminist social justice orientation: an indicator of optimal functioning? *Counseling Psychologist*, 40, pp. 1133–1148.

Morley, C. & Macfarlane, S. (2012) The nexus between feminism and postmodernism: still a central concern for critical social work. *British Journal of Social Work*, 42, pp. 687–705.

National Archives of Australia (n.d.) Gough Whitlam. *Australia's Prime Ministers*. http://primeministers.naa.gov.au/primeministers/whitlam/ (accessed 21 September 2014).

Olusola, A.I. (2013) Exploring the relevance of feminist leadership in theological education of Nigeria. *International Journal of Philosophy and Theology*, 1(1), pp. 28–33.

Parnell, S. & Andrews, J. (1994) Complementary principles of social work and feminism: a teaching guide. *AFFILIA: The Journal of Women and Social Work*, 19(2), pp. 60–64.

Patkar, M. (2012) Medha Patkar refuses Basava Award from corruption-tainted Karnataka government. *Citizen News Service*, February. www.citizen-news.org/2012/02/medha-patkar-refuses-basava-award-from.html (accessed 29 April 2015).

Phillips, R. & Cree, V.E. (2014) What does the 'fourth wave' mean for teaching feminism in twenty-first century social work? *Social Work Education: The International Journal*, 33(7), pp. 930–943.

Porter, N. & Henderson Daniel, J. (2007) Developing transformational leaders: theory to practice. In J. Chin, B. Lott, J. Rice & J. Sanchez-Hucles (eds), *Women and Leadership: Transforming Visions and Diverse Voices*. Blackwell, Oxford, pp. 245–263.

PTI (2013) Land Acquisition Act has 'loopholes', says activist Medha Patkar. *Firstpost India*, 20 November. www.firstpost.com/india/land-acquisition-act-has-loopholes-says-activist-medha-patkar-1240725.html (accessed 29 April 2015).

Rao, A. & Kelleher, D. (2000) Leadership for social transformation: some ideas and questions on institutions and feminist leadership. *Gender and Development*, 8(3), pp. 74–79.

Reid, C. (2004) Advancing women's social justice agendas: a feminist action research framework. *International Journal of Qualitative Methods*, 3(3), pp. 1–15.

Rusaw, C. (2005) A proposed model of feminist public sector leadership. *Administrative Theory and Praxis*, 27(2), pp. 385–393.

Stivers, C. (2002) *Gender Images in Public Administration: Legitimacy and the Administrative State*, 2nd edn. Sage, Thousand Oaks, CA.

Valentich, M. (2010) Finding one's own identity as a feminist social worker. *Canadian Social Work Review*, 27(2), pp. 221–237.

Van Den Bergh, N. & Cooper, L.B. (eds) (1986) *Feminist Visions for Social Work*. National Association of Social Workers, Silver Spring, MD.

Viezzer, M.L. (2001) Feminist transformative leadership: a learning experience with peasant and gatherer women in Brazil. Paper presented at the 4th International Conference on Transformative Learning, Toronto, 1–3 November.

White, V. (2006) *The State of Feminist Social Work*. Routledge, London.

Whitlam Institute (n.d) *Mrs Margaret Whitlam OAM*. www.whitlam.org (accessed 21 September 2014).

Wikipedia (2014) Medha Patkar. *Wikipedia*. http://en.wikipedia.org/wiki/Medha_Patkar (accessed 10 September 2014).

9 Poverty alleviation in a globalised world

A feminist perspective

Lena Dominelli

Introduction

Globalisation is a contentious term. Hegemonic definitions portray it as a global economic system that links all modern nations together, and they ignore its differentiated effects (Soros, 2002). While this highlights the economic impact of globalisation and the spread of neo-liberal ideologies globally, the scope of these definitions is insufficient. I expand them by arguing that globalisation is a process of embedding capitalist social relations in everyday life practices throughout the world. It affects every aspect of life (Dominelli, 2009). Some impacts are positive, for example, cheap travel, facilitating rapid internet-based communications across time and space, increasing connectivities between people, promoting the growth of transnationalised families who feel 'at home' in more than one country and highlighting interdependencies between peoples, especially around climate change. Globalisation has given social workers a chance to network, as exemplified by the Global Agenda whereby the profession's three key international organisations, the International Association of Schools of Social Work (IASSW), International Council on Social Welfare (ICSW) and the International Federation of Social Workers (IFSW), combined forces to strengthen the voice of the profession around social issues internationally. Nonetheless, globalisation impacts negatively on; social institutions including the family, the labour market, universal services, programmes that reduce income inequalities and physical environments by subjecting everything to market mechanisms.

Globalisation has intensified the instability of the economic system by treating people and the ecosystem as means to economic ends and by increasing economic inequalities. Poverty becomes an internationalised social problem as wealth inequalities intensify both between countries and within them. Gender becomes a significant issue because estimates suggest that 70 per cent of poor people are women, women perform the bulk of low-paid work and women ensure family survival in straitened economic circumstances. This intensifies the multiple burdens women have had and continue to carry (Moghadam, 2005). Governments have allowed this to happen while a super-rich elite has benefited from this global polarisation of wealth and income. It is high time to ask why.

A crucial reason for disparities in income and wealth between men and women is the division of social relations into the public and private spheres and the allocation of women's roles primarily within the private domain of the home and caring (Walby, 1990). Women's lives have traditionally been structured around their responsibilities for caring for children, husbands and dependent relatives, especially older parents and disabled persons. These activities have formed the basis of women's dominance in the private realm of the home and their exclusion from the public sphere. Whilst this has been the hegemonic ideology of patriarchal ways of thinking, being and doing in the world, women's history has ample examples of resistance to these restrictions from ancient to contemporary times. Women who sought changes to improve women's lives have been called 'feminists'. Sometimes they have been pilloried or ridiculed for their aspirations. There are various schools of thought within this overall category: radical feminists, lesbians, queer/transgendered women, socialist feminist, Marxist feminists, liberation theology feminists, black feminists, Third World feminists and others (Banks, 1981; Jayawardna, 1986; Hill Collins, 1991).

Feminist understandings of globalisation's pervasiveness enable us better to understand power relations, structural inequalities manufactured through the marketplace and commodified caring relations. Additionally, social workers can highlight distorted labour processes that turn them into deprofessionalised workers subjected to corporate business practices (Clarke & Newman, 1997), the technocratisation of practice (Dominelli, 2004, 2009) and reduced services and resources to meet growing need as public expenditure cuts intensify poverty among service users and reduce benefits to pay for the aftermath of the 2007 recession.

In this chapter, I critically examine women's situation in relation to poverty and the impact of the Millennium Development Goals (MDGs): their gender-neutral approach, failure to engage with the limitations of neo-liberal forms of social development and incapacity to address structural inequalities. This will assist in better understanding why women and children are the main victim-survivors of such strategies. I will also examine how the current penchant for austerity measures that dominates social policy discourses internationally, especially in Western Europe where welfare states had cushioned many structural inequalities that adversely affected women, further reinforces existing inequalities rather than addressing them and makes women responsible for enhancing family wellbeing. Women lie at the heart of development and industrial modernisation strategies favoured by the UN and other international organisations including the World Bank and International Monetary Fund to *alleviate*, not *eliminate*, poverty. Feminists and social workers have important roles to play in challenging development discourses and assisting practitioners and students to co-work with women in their local communities to enhance wellbeing and promote community resilience. I also draw out the implications of this analysis for research and teaching in social work.

Theorising gendered structural inequalities: 'othering'

Poverty is important for social workers because the majority of their clients/ service users are poor children, women and men. Many problems practitioners encounter around helping women, especially mothers, are hindered by the lack of resources to support them as carers, and the low priority that governments accord to women's own needs as women. Caring as women's work is taken for granted, with men doing little of it. Poverty is a key structural inequality along with sexism, racism, ageism, classism and other 'isms' that oppress people and legitimate discrimination against specific groups of people. The dynamics of these forms of oppression are based on a hierarchy of superiority and inferiority that divides people into 'us' who are included and categorised as 'superior' and those characterised as 'them' who are excluded and considered inferior and less capable. These processes of inclusion and exclusion result in an 'othering' of those defined as 'inferior' so that relations of dominance or 'power over' characterise the relationships between them. Those labelled 'them' include women in an oppositional binary of male–female ('othering' binaries also apply to other social divisions). Women's responses to such categorisations range from accepting, accommodating or resisting these labels in and through their interactions with those deemed 'superior' (Dominelli, 2002a, 2002b). Woman's liberation struggles in whatever country or time period have resisted labelling and attempted to redefine social relations in terms of equality between men and women across all social divisions and geographical terrains.

Social divisions such as age, gender, ethnicity, class, 'race' and (dis) ability, on which structural inequalities are predicated, are interrelated and complex. Thus, disadvantage is poorly conceptualised if it is deemed to exist as a separate hierarchy of oppression. Poverty, which I define as a condition in which individuals have limited access to the basic necessities of life – food, clothing, shelter, education, health care, social services and secure incomes as enshrined in Articles 22 to 27 of the Universal Declaration of Human Rights (UDHR) – constitutes a human rights violation and undermines wellbeing and fulfilment. To the UDHR list, I would add ownership of property, access to communal resources such as land, technological innovations, roads, transportation structures, communication systems, energy supplies, clean water and sanitation facilities, financial resources, credit and information networks, because these are sources of power denied to poor people, especially women. For women, poverty is also about the lack of autonomy and the right to make decisions about one's own life, livelihood and body. Social workers can support women in asserting their authority and autonomy.

Gendering poverty

Inequalities of income and wealth have grown until, in the twenty-first century, an unaccountable, super-rich multinational elite runs global corporations to produce massive profits for the few and exerts enormous pressure on governments to reduce tax payments and receive corporate welfare grants (WEF, 2014). While millions of people across Europe and the United States are facing hardship; loss of their homes, welfare services and jobs; and bankruptcy of their nations during neo-liberalism's current fiscal crisis, the super-rich elite are growing in size and wealth.

In 2007 when the fiscal crisis began, there were 946 billionaires in the world, mainly men, and this has risen to 1,645 individuals holding $6.4 trillion in 69 countries by 2013 – a rise of 18.5 per cent over 2012. Of these billionaires, only 172 were women. Bill Gates, worth US$76 billion, resumed the role of richest man in the world after four years as second to Mexico's Carlos Slim Helu with US$72 billion. Amancio Ortega of Spain holds the third spot with his US$64 billion. Warren Buffet is now in fourth place with US$58.2 billion. To put it more graphically, in 2007 the world's richest three people had between them more than the total gross domestic product of the poorest 48 countries. And, within the US in 2005, Bill Gates had more money than 40 per cent of his fellow citizens combined. French-woman Liliane Bettencourt, the owner of L'Oréal, is the world's richest woman. But her US$34.5 billion is less than half of what Bill Gates, the richest man, has. While poverty might be relative, gender relations that disadvantage women prevail among the super-rich elite too.

The list has grown substantially since 1987 when the Forbes Billion-aires List was initially compiled with 140 billionaires spread across 24 countries. Of today's billionaires, 23 have been on the list since its inception. Americans (492 of them) are the most numerous national grouping, but billionaires are now located throughout the world. Mainland China with 152 billionaires, Russia with 111 billionaires and India with 56 billionaires, are catching up quickly. The UK has 47 billionaires and Hong Kong has 45 billionaires (Kroll & Dolan, 2014). Women are a small minority within all these countries. This excessive wealth intensifies poverty (Seery & Arendar, 2014).

In contrast, poverty affects more women than men, known as the 'feminisation of poverty'. The United Nations (UN) has defined absolute poverty as living on less than US$1.25 per day, recently updated from the 1980 figure of US$1 per day. There are 1.4 billion people living on less than $1.25 per day. Around three billion people live on less than US$2 per day. Around 70 per cent are women. These amounts are inadequate and a blot on humanity because how can anyone in the twenty-first century be expected to develop to their full potential, utilising their skills, talents and strengths, on so little? The few heroic women who manage to do so in the most appalling conditions of scarcity and restricted freedoms are exceptions. Even in the west, poverty levels are higher among women, especially those who are lone parents or older women. The UK's Office of National Statistics revealed that low-paid men earned 10 per cent more than low-paid women; highly paid men earned 20 per cent more than highly paid women.

Poverty is not just about inadequate incomes, but also about the right to experience fulfilled lives within one's community, share in a common sense of identity and belonging with other people, and control one's life oneself, albeit within a range of mutually agreed obligations to care for each other. Regardless of the size of the group, this includes the right to enjoy the rights of citizenship and entitlements that go with it, not the one-sided burden of providing the goods and services that enable wealthy people to enjoy all the fruits of life, or of providing essential but unvalued care to those one is responsible for, as women do within the family.

The feminisation of poverty is extensively explored in feminist literature, but the role of poverty alleviation strategies for women is rarely discussed on the world stage. Most discourses on poverty alleviation are optimistic, and highlight the potential of research on the topic to improve women's lives. Policies on poverty alleviation, not its elimination, have failed to reduce the increasing numbers of women drawn into poverty, even though they may have several low-paid jobs that draw them into the ranks of the working poor as in America, especially if lone mothers, or carry out unpaid work in the home with little economic security as recompense for their labours (Ehrenreich, 2001). Moreover, policy makers seem oblivious to the impact of the feminisation of poverty on the burdens that women already carry for family wellbeing, especially that of children and older people (Chant, 2006). Women's engagement in paid work is additional to these responsibilities.

Women's activism

Inequalities between men and women abound on the global stage, but it has not been through want of women trying to redress this imbalance. Feminist activism has a global pedigree and a centuries-old tradition including scholarship like Wollstonecraft's classic text (1792) and direct action. Our narratives around women's rights have ebbed and flowed with successes and failures, covering women's struggles for equality in all corners of the Earth at the interpersonal level within families, and through various social movements, many of which aim to combat poverty among women and their families because women have borne the brunt of it (Seery & Arendar, 2014). A turning point for western first-wave feminists was securing political representational rights, or the vote for women, with New Zealand being first in 1893 (Fraser, 1984; Daley & Nolan, 1994). Second-wave feminists demanded the right to work in the public sphere on the same basis as men and secure incomes for themselves and their children including Mother's Pensions in Canada (Guest, 2003), Family Allowances/Child Benefits in Western Europe and reproductive rights through *Roe v Wade* in the USA. Alongside these, feminists also prioritised domestic abuse and violence – emotional, physical and sexual, healthy old age, health services, education and the elimination of poverty. Space limitations mean I explore recent developments while specifically emphasising poverty.

Men, and the governments they lead, have been reluctant to pursue women's interests wholeheartedly and risk deprivileging men who form their bedrock support. Matters have become worse under the recent rise of religious fundamentalism across the major world faiths like Christianity, Islam and Hinduism (Rajavi, 2013) as men seek to reassert patriarchal relations (Almond, Appleby & Sivan, 2003). This shift is reflected in increased violence and assaults against women in countries where the majority population shares religious affiliations that reinforce patriarchal social relations and reaffirm male dominance. This trend rolls back feminist gains wherever possible, restricts women to the private realm, reasserts men's control over women's reproductive rights and fertility, holds women back educationally and enforces women's inactivity in the social sphere.

These reactions against women's liberation have also prompted further feminist action to defend past gains and encourage wider social change, including ending attacks on women's bodily integrity as exemplified by current actions around the elimination of female genital mutilation (FGM). This is a form of violence perpetrated against girl children usually through the hands of adult women for the benefit of adult men who can be assured of a woman's virginity and constraints to her sexual expression and enjoyment. It restricts women to the private sphere and encourages financial dependence on men. UNICEF (2014b) suggests that 30 million girls and women have undergone this form of bodily assault. It can cause psychological harm, illness and death. UKAid and the Department for International Development (DfID) have supported campaigns in diverse countries seeking to eradicate FGM practices, which affect poor women more than wealthy women.

Women's activism has also encouraged other government initiatives, especially at the global level through the UN and its key agencies, including CEDAW (Commission for the Elimination of Discrimination Against Women). The focus on education and health for women and children in the MDGs and the social protection floor to encourage minimal support for people can be considered in this light. Despite these initiatives, women continue to experience higher levels of poverty than men, and their overall life opportunities, especially in low-income countries, have diminished women's health and wellbeing, especially those aspects linked to pregnancy and giving birth (Seery & Arendar, 2014). Here I consider global initiatives that tackle poverty.

The Millennium Development Goals

The Millennium Development Goals (MDGs), agreed in 2000, provided eight targets that governments were to meet by 2015. Halving poverty by 2015 was one. Another, MDG 3, on education and gender equality contained seven strategic priorities and 12 indicators for gender equality and women's empowerment (UNDP, 2003, 2005). Although the UN General Assembly adopted these priorities in 2005, it failed to set benchmarks for assessing progress; consequently measurements of success do not appear in UN reports on the MDGs. I list these along with progress as assessed by the International Centre for Research on Women (ICRW, 2008).

1 Strengthen opportunities for post-primary education for girls

Indicator 1: Ratio of female-to-male gross enrolment rates in primary, secondary and tertiary education.
Indicator 2: Ratio of female-to-male completion rates in primary, secondary and tertiary education.
   ICRW (2008) claims there is reasonably good practice on this priority.

2 Guarantee sexual and reproductive health and rights

Indicator 3: Adolescent fertility rate.
Indicator 4: Proportion of contraceptive demand satisfied.
   Slow progress is unsurprising given that men's desire to control women's bodies has not been tackled as a priority in its own right (ICRW, 2008).

3 Invest in infrastructure to reduce women's and girls' time burdens

Indicator 5: Hours per day (or year) women and men spend fetching water and collecting fuel.
   Insufficient data prevented ICRW (2008) from assessing progress on this indicator, but women are time poor and rarely have leisure time in their own right. Gathering fuel and fetching clean water remain time-consuming tasks undertaken primarily by women.

4 Guarantee women's property and inheritance rights

Indicator 6: Land ownership by sex (male, female or jointly held).
Indicator 7: Housing title by sex (male, female or jointly held).
   ICRW also lacked data to assess progress on this contentious issue. Yet women globally are usually excluded from property ownership by tradition, lack of funds or both.

5 *Reduce gender inequality in employment*

Indicator 8: Gender differences in the structure of employment.
Indicator 9: Gender gaps in earnings in wage employment and self-employment.

Slow progress was achieved on this issue (ICRW, 2008). Women's contributions to household incomes, especially through unpaid work, were ignored. And the 'glass ceiling' remains in many industrial and financial sectors, even where women have made gains.

6 *Increase women's representation in political bodies*

Indicator 10: Percentage of seats held by women in national parliament.
Indicator 11: Percentage of seats held by women in local government bodies.

ICRW (2008) revealed limited progress in this arena. In some countries, for example Costa Rica, women hold 73 per cent of local government seats; in Rwanda 50 per cent of parliamentarians are women; in Mozambique women form 35 per cent of national representatives, indicating substantially higher figures than in many western countries, including the UK (ICRW, 2008, p. 17).

7 *Combat violence against women*

Indicator 12: Prevalence of domestic violence.

Despite the global attention given to this issue, ICRW (2008, p. 31) had insufficient data to assess progress on it. Nonetheless, incidence levels for intimate partner violence are high, for example 60 per cent in Peru and Uganda, and 70 per cent in Ethiopia. In western countries, Finland and New Zealand had the highest levels at 30 per cent.

Beijing Platform for Action

The Beijing Platform for Action covered action on the gendered effects of poverty, and adopted four strategic objectives:

1 Review, adopt and maintain macroeconomic policies and development strategies that address the needs and endeavours of poor women.
2 Revise laws and administrative practices to ensure women's equal rights and access to economic resources.
3 Provide women with access to savings and credit mechanisms and institutions.
4 Develop gender-based methodologies and conduct research to address the feminisation of poverty.

Progress on these objectives has been limited and poverty among women has both deepened and spread. Although specific figures are hard to come by, the UNDP (United Nations Development Program) estimates that 70 per cent of those living in absolute poverty are women. The Women's Environment and Development Organisation (2005), evaluating the targets of the 1995 Beijing Platform for Action following the Fourth World Conference on Women in Beijing, China, claims the targets have not been met, despite the passage of time and governments' commitment to their realisation (UNRISD, 2005; UNSD, 2005; UNMP/TFEGE, 2005).

The Beijing Platform for Action (UNIFEM, 2002) also recognised the importance of addressing men's violence against women and children in the home and on the streets. This is crucial to enabling women to transcend poverty by engaging in the public sphere where waged work and political participation are located. The public sphere must become a safe space for women, as Erin Pizzey argued in the 1970s when she opened the Women's Shelter in Chiswick, London, England (Pizzey, 1974). Feminist and social work conferences on men's violence and countless examples of lobbying for women's and children's rights to live free from this ('zero tolerance') highlight women and children as the largest casualties of violence perpetrated across gender divides. Women also experience violence and increased dependence on men for their livelihoods during armed conflicts, where women's bodies become symbols of nationhood as men fight each other, pillaging and raping women and children in total disregard of their rights. Sexual violence reflects men's violation of the rights of women and children to bodily integrity, and although women do occasionally commit physical and sexual violence against men and children their numbers are small (Straus, 2008). Sometimes women attack men because they have been subjected to years of hardship, and physical and sexual violence within the home, and they, not their systematic abuse, become the headline (Hope, 2010). I have previously described the potential for adult men and women to abuse their power over children because children are dependent upon them for their survival, emotionally, physically and economically, and I coined the term 'adultism' to describe this particular abuse of power (Dominelli, 1989).

Child marriages, another form of assault against children, can undermine women's capacity to earn independent livelihoods. Early marriage is particularly important to poor families seeking to reduce demands on family income. Most child marriages comprise young girls forced to 'marry' men many years older than them. This affects 700 million women globally. Of these, 250 million are married before the age of 15 (UNICEF, 2014a). This figure is predicted to rise as the planet's population increases, unless this practice is stopped. Child brides can have their health endangered by having children when too young, being infected with sexually transmitted diseases including HIV/AIDS and enduring high levels of social isolation because they become cut off from family and friends at a young age. They also face barriers to completing their education and acquiring the skills to earn their own living and rise out of poverty.

The rise of religious fundamentalism across the major world religions is linked to men's desire to re-establish patriarchal relations where they have lost them, and to enforce them where they have not. Keeping women dependent and incapable of earning wages outside the home becomes one way of asserting such control. In the USA, Gilder (1981) talked about the state's collusion in undermining men by giving women freedom through the provision of an income independent of men, and claimed that the state had 'cuckolded' men. Walby (1990) described the state's role in providing such financing including through the provision of benefits and employment opportunities for women in the welfare state as public patriarchy replacing private patriarchy. Now, with austerity measures in major industrial countries, particularly in Europe, whittling away at benefit levels, entitlement to benefits and employment opportunities, there is another shift again towards private patriarchy. This is linked to the commodification of welfare and the privatisation of public goods representing collective institutionalised solidarity through the welfare state. I call this new form of private patriarchy 'corporetarchy', because it involves global corporations reinforcing patriarchal relations whereby women are paid less to provide the same services made available through the welfare state. Most decisions taken by these multinationals are made by men. For example, women welfare assistants who work in Serco establishments in the UK earn less than they did when employed by a local authority to do the same work, and receive fewer benefits than they did previously. Thus, the ambitious Beijing Platform for Action has neither eliminated poverty nor ended violence against women.

The social protection floor

The social protection floor was recently devised internationally and promoted under the auspices of the International Labour Organization (ILO) to provide an income safety net for the world's poorest people. Women, as the bulk of this group, were expected to be the main beneficiaries. The social protection floor sets minimum guarantees determined nationally for income security and health care across the life cycle. It aims to create a platform of security below which no individual or family should fall (www.ilo.org/global/lang–en/index.htm). Caution needs to be exercised in seeing this as an effective poverty alleviation strategy because benefit levels can be set very low. Thus, it could entail the same trap that befell western welfare states, namely that benefit levels should not undermine low wages to compel people to accept low-paid work. This became the price for support exacted by those who control global markets and governments that ply the neo-liberal line that argues a minimal role for the state in ensuring the wellbeing of its populations. While earning less, the costs of goods and services have increased, so women find they must do more with less in meeting family needs by spending more time looking for bargains or making things from scratch (George, 2003).

Additionally, the majority of the policy makers lining up behind the 'social protection floor' are men. And while there is no justification for reifying men or seeing them as a monolithic group, the question of where the voices of women are in these deliberations has to be posed. Feminists in the second wave had asked for guaranteed incomes, equal pay for equal work, free high quality child care and health care, but none of these demands have been fully met, and feminism has entered its fourth phase. Even in one of the most gender-equal countries in the world, Sweden, a wages gap between men's and women's earnings exists. It is simply smaller than elsewhere, and child care, while of excellent quality, requires some form of parental input (Leitner, 2003).

Social development strategies: the overburdening of poor women?

Social development, primarily in the form of modernisation and industrialisation with its associated income generation projects, has been deemed a vehicle through which poverty alleviation strategies can reduce the number of poor people globally. Achieving this goal under the MDGs seems unlikely, so how can poverty be alleviated and women experience economic empowerment and who will create new initiatives for women? A problem with existing provisions is that many rely on women assuming traditional activities and doing them better and more effectively, often by receiving meagre sums of money, for example, sewing clothes for sale by acquiring a loan for a sewing machine through a microcredit scheme like the Grameen Bank. The Grameen Bank's Annual Report for 2013 reveals that it has helped countless women improve their livelihoods, and this is to be applauded. Mohamed Yunis was awarded a Nobel Prize for this initiative in 2006 and has become a millionaire. However, the poor women who have received loans through Grameen Banks have not reached this income level, and they pay high rates of interests – around 22 per cent, a substantial burden for them. Additionally, women become collectively responsible for repaying loans when a woman in their group cannot pay. This hardly seems an equitable deal, and women might do better creating a more traditional credit union.

The UN 2014 World Development Report indicates that 2.2 billion people continue to be poor or near poor, with about 70 per cent being women. Regardless of gains made through the MDGs, microcredit schemes or industrialisation strategies, progress in alleviating poverty has been slow. Consequently, improvements through poverty alleviation approaches cannot be considered sustainable. This highlights the importance of the development of a global holistic poverty *eradication* initiative that interrogates the dominance of global corporations in determining and running the world's business, usually to the detriment of women. Social workers can engage in public awareness and community mobilisations to raise these issues, discuss them locally and develop sustainable solutions that link caring for people with caring for the environment (Dominelli, 2012). Women – residents and social workers – could be at the centre of such ventures and draw men into the equation.

Social work roles in poverty elimination strategies

Social workers can act as advocates for the elimination of poverty at all levels from the local to the global. One of the pillars of the Global Agenda is eliminating socioeconomic inequalities, and feminist social work academics have highlighted the importance of feminist perspectives in understanding the world and contributing to shaping it. They can assist women in mobilising and empowering themselves to use existing strengths to innovate and develop creative solutions to problems that are rooted in sustainable conditions and enable women to help each other achieve together what would be impossible alone. Social workers can facilitate the processes of women accessing the information and external resources they need to follow their dreams of a better life for themselves and their children. They can also assist women to obtain the education and health care services to which they are entitled through the UDHR, which all UN member states have signed.

None of this work will be easy, nor is it without risk either for social workers or for the women involved. If their endeavours are unsuccessful, they will confirm stereotypes about women's incapacity to achieve things. If successful, they may antagonise traditionalists who do not wish to empower women. This lesson was forced upon Malala Yousafzai, a young girl whom the Taliban tried to kill on a school bus in 2012 for wanting to go to school in Pakistan's Swat Valley (Hussain, 2013).

Preparing social workers for a new role in poverty eradication and sustainable development strategies will require the classroom curriculum to include materials on social policy, law, holistic sustainable development, poverty, economics, community development, politics, power relations and anti-oppressive practice (Dominelli, 2002a, 2002b, 2012). Community-based practice placements could support sustainable development that analyses the gendered realities and oppressions women face. Safety considerations for social workers and women residents should also be covered.

Conclusions

Poverty and the oppression of women are socially constructed phenomena which can be eradicated. This needs courage and wisdom, a commitment to equality, political will, energy and resources. Social workers can help men and women unite to achieve this task. Men can also benefit by liberating themselves from their patriarchal chains.

Further reading

Dominelli, L. (2009) *Social Work in a Globalising World*. Polity Press, Cambridge.
George, S. (2003) Globalizing rights? In M.J. Gibney (ed.), *Globalizing Rights: The Oxford Amnesty Lectures 1999*. Oxford University Press, Oxford, pp. 15–33.
Moghadam, V.A. (2005) *Globalizing Women: Transnational Feminist Networks*. Johns Hopkins University Press, Baltimore, MD.

References

Almond, G.A., Appleby, R.S. & Sivan, E. (2003) *Strong Religion: The Rise of Fundamentalisms Around the World*. University of Chicago Press, Chicago, IL.
Banks, O. (1981) *Faces of Feminism*. Martin Robinson, London.
Chant, S. (2006) Re-thinking the 'feminization of poverty' in relation to aggregate gender indices. *Journal of Human Development*, 7(2), pp. 201–220. http://eprints.lse.ac.uk/2869/1/Re-thinking_the_feminisation_of_poverty_(LSERO).pdf (accessed 12 August 2013).
Clarke, J. & Newman, J. (1997) *The Managerial State*. Sage, London.
Daley, C. & Nolan, M. (eds) (1994) *Suffrage and Beyond: International Feminist Perspectives*. New York University Press, New York.
Dominelli, L. (1989) A betrayal of trust: an analysis of power relationships in incest abuse and its relevance for social work practice. *British Journal of Social Work*, 19, pp. 291–307.
Dominelli, L. (2002a) *Anti-Oppressive Social Work Theory and Practice*. Palgrave Macmillan, London.
Dominelli, L. (2002b) *Feminist Social Work Theory and Practice*. Palgrave Macmillan, London.
Dominelli, L. (2004) *Social Work: Theory and Practice for a Changing Profession*. Polity Press, Cambridge.
Dominelli, L. (2009) *Social Work in a Globalising World*. Polity Press, Cambridge.
Dominelli, L. (2012) *Green Social Work*. Polity Press, Cambridge.
Ehrenreich, B. (2001) *Nickled and Dimed*. Picador, London.
Fraser, A. (1984) *The Weaker Vessel*. Routledge, London.
George, S. (2003) Globalizing rights? In M.J. Gibney (ed.), *Globalizing Rights: The Oxford Amnesty Lectures 1999*. Oxford University Press, Oxford, pp. 15–33.
Gilder, G. (1981) *Wealth and Poverty*. Bell Books, New York.
Guest, D. (2003) *The Emergence of Social Security in Canada*, 3rd edn. University of British Columbia Press, Vancouver.
Hill Collins, P. (1991) *Black Feminist Thought: Knowledge, Consciousness and the Politics of Empowerment*. Routledge, London.
Hope, C. (2010) Women who murder partners after years of abuse could escape prison. *Telegraph*, 4 October. www.telegraph.co.uk/news/uknews/law-and-order/8041743/Women-who-murder-violent-partners-after-years-of-abuse-could-escape-prison.html (accessed 12 April 2013).

Hussain, M. (2013) Malala: the girl who was shot going to school. *BBC News*, 7 October. www.bbc.com/news/magazine-24379018 (accessed 20 December 2013).

International Centre for Research on Women (ICRW) (2008) *UN Millennium Project 2005. Taking Action: Achieving Gender Equality and Empowering Women.* Earthscan Publications, New York.

Jayawardna, K. (1986) *Feminism and Nationalism in the Third World.* Zed Books, London.

Kroll, L. & Dolan, K. (2014) Inside the Forbes 2014 Billionaires List. *Forbes Magazine*, 30 March. www.forbes.com/sites/luisakroll/2014/03/03/inside-the-2014-forbes-billionaires-list-facts-and-figures/ (accessed 1 August 2014).

Leitner, S. (2003) Varieties of familialism. *European Societies*, 5(4), pp. 352–375.

Moghadam, V.A. (2005) *Globalizing Women: Transnational Feminist Networks.* Johns Hopkins University Press, Baltimore, MD.

Pizzey, E. (1974) *Scream Quietly or the Neighbours Will Hear.* Penguin, Harmondsworth, UK.

Rajavi, M. (2013) *Women Against Fundamentalism.* Seven Locks Press, London.

Seery, E. & Arendar, C. (2014) Even it up: time to end extreme inequality. OXFAM International.

Soros, G. (2002) *George Soros on Globalization.* Public Affairs Publishers, New York.

Straus, M. (2008) Dominance and symmetry in partner violence by male and female university students in 32 nations. *Children and Youth Services Review*, 30(3), pp. 252–275.

United Nations International Children's Emergency Fund (UNICEF) (2014a) *Ending Child Marriage: Progress and Prospects.* UNICEF, New York.

United Nations International Children's Emergency Fund (UNICEF) (2014b) *Female Genital Mutilation/Cutting: What Might the Future Hold?* UNICEF, New York.

United Nations Fund for Women (UNIFEM) (2002) *Progress of the World's Women 2002, Volume 2.* UNIFEM, New York.

United Nations Development Program (UNDP) (2003) *Millennium Development Goals: National Reports Through a Gender Lens.* UNDP, New York.

United Nations Development Program (UNDP) (2005) *En Route to Equality: A Gender Review of National MDG Reports 2005.* UNDP, New York.

United Nations Research Institute for Social Development (UNRISD) (2005) *Gender Equality: Striving for Justice in an Unequal World.* UNRISD, Geneva.

United Nations Statistics Division (UNSD) (2005) *Special Report of the World's Women 2005: Progress in Statistics.* UNSD Department of Social and Economic Affairs, New York.

UNMP/TFEGE (2005) *Taking Action: Achieving Gender Equality and Empowering Women.* Earthscan, London.

Walby, S. (1990) *Theorising Patriarchy.* Basil Blackwell, Oxford.

Wollstonecraft, M. (1792) *A Vindication of the Rights of Woman.* Joseph Johnson, London.

Women's Environment and Development Organisation (WEDO) (2005) *Beijing Betrayed: Women Worldwide Report that Governments have Failed to Turn the Platform into Action.* WEDO, New York.

World Economic Forum (WEF) (2014) *Outlook on the Global Agenda 2015.* WEF, Geneva.

Part II

Social work practice

10 Talking up and listening well

Dismantling whiteness and building reflexivity

Deirdre Tedmanson and Christine Fejo-King

Eh Professor, big shot,
Big cheese, or whoever
You claim to be
You've really no idea.
Love to chat sister,
But there's faxes to send
And protest letters to write
… I turn and walk away
Preserving my dignity
Without humiliating hers.
> (Bellear, 1996, pp. 13–14, quoted in Brewster, 2007, p. 210. Reproduced
> with the kind permission of University Queensland Press)

Introduction

White privilege is pervasive and insidious. One of the most challenging and hard to change aspects of white privilege is how easily it infiltrates our everyday work and personal lives – operating silently, out of sight, at the perimeter of consciousness, often unspoken yet potent and poisonous. While institutionalised racism and overt discrimination stand out and easily offend our collective sense of social injustice, the covert everyday micro-racisms of white privilege are not as easily discerned or apprehended. The everyday taken-for-granted assumptions about who knows what is best for whom (and why), are more often quietly normalised and erased from view.

In this chapter we seek to expose and explore this subtle performance of everyday racism, legitimised by the invisibility which masks its disempowering, deleterious effects. This relentless (re)production of race privilege through the everyday 'micro-practices … that we fail to notice' enables 'white [people] varied by class and gender, to stuff their academic and social pick-up trucks with goodies not otherwise available to people of colour' (Fine, 2004, p. 245). As Applebaum reminds us, one of the most significant features of white ignorance 'is that it involves not just not knowing but not knowing what one does not know and believing that one knows' (2010, p. 6, quoted in Moreton-Robinson, 2011, p. 413). As Christine points out in some of her earlier work, 'examining the social construction of whiteness assists [us] in understanding the dominance of mono-cultural concepts that fail to consider a diversity of world views and ways of being' (Fejo-King & Briskman, 2009, p. 108).

Let us first begin by introducing ourselves and our purpose in this dialogue. Christine is the Chairperson of the National Coalition of Aboriginal and Torres Strait Islander Social Workers Association (NCAT-SISWA), and has been engaged in Aboriginal and Torres Strait Islander activism as a social worker for many years. She has been involved in the establishment of the Aboriginal Child Care Agency (Karu) in the Northern Territory as well as the Secretariat of National Aboriginal and Islander Child Care (SNAICC), and the peak Stolen Generation Alliance. Christine was also deeply involved in the background work for the apology to the Stolen Generations.[1] A proud and passionate social worker, she mentor other Indigenous social workers and students. Deirdre has worked together with a number of Aboriginal communities including homelands and 'remote'[2] communities on the Anangu Pitjant-jatjara Yankunytjatjara (APY) Lands in central Australia. This work has focused on a range of participatory action projects across the areas of social entrepreneurship, community development and human services over many years. Deirdre has over 20 years of experience in human services, community development, social policy and practice, and participatory action research and evaluation with a specific focus and deep ethical commitment to working in partnership and solidarity with Aboriginal communities and organisations.

In dialogue together in this chapter we explore how it is that 'white privilege' remains one of the most powerful, pervasive and under-discussed forms of contemporary racism(s). We identify some of the ways in which white privilege continues to impact adversely on Aboriginal and Torres Strait Islander women in particular, but also other Indigenous women and women of colour everywhere, and suggest strategies for dismantling whiteness and building greater reflexivity in professional practice around the intersections of gender and race issues.

Using critical race theory (Delgado, 1995; Delgado, Stefancic & Liendo, 2012) we argue for greater worker reflexivity, a conscious reversal of the gaze and a shared commitment to learning from Indigenous women's knowledges. By making room for others' standpoints, other ways of being and the production of new wisdoms in professional practice, a deeper dialogue between women can take place, past the usual sticking points of power and privilege. A shared sense of postcolonial feminist ethics challenges us to extend our concern for women's oppression to a deepening awareness of the multilayered oppressions experienced by Indigenous women whose knowledges, cultures and languages must be repositioned to the centre of *all* professional discourse.

First, we discuss whiteness in this chapter, exploring its place in both feminism and social work. We then consider how more critical reflexive approaches can contribute to the deconstruction of binaries, to open new conversations, new stories and new learning. We close our chapter by looking forward, to the 'unfolding relations' (Massumi, 2002, p. 9) and intersubjectivity of what we hope will be a more truly respectful and emancipatory cross-cultural feminism.

Whiteness

The cultural milieu of social work in Australia, as in most western societies, is 'predominantly white' and whiteness is 'an omnipresent reality within our practice and our profession' (Walter, Taylor & Habibis, 2011, p. 7). Whiteness in this context refers not so much to a racialised category (or skin colour) but rather to a 'set of locations that are historically, socially, politically, and culturally produced and moreover, are intrinsically linked with unfolding relations of dominance' (Frankenburg, 1997, p. 6). Early theorising on whiteness built on the postcolonial work of theorists like Edward Said (1978) and Frantz Fanon (1986) and gained added momentum through US civil rights anti-racist activism. Said's work (1978) for example was influential in deconstructing how cultural subordination was achieved by positioning people of colour as the 'other' while normalising the cultural practices of the dominant. Said shifted the focus from the 'ontological workings of racial dominance to its epistemological power in defining colonial relations' (Banerjee & Tedmanson, 2010, p. 148).

Elucidating the significance of 'whiteness' became a specific field of study in the 1990s (Allen, 1994; Dyer, 1997; Frankenberg, 1997; Hall, 1997; Hill, 1997). This body of scholarship revealed how 'whiteness' becomes 'the invisible norm against which other races are judged in the construction of identity, representation, subjectivity, nationalism and the law' (Moreton-Robinson, 2004, p. vii). 'White privilege' as part of the repertoire or tools of dominance refers to the spoils or benefits or unearned gains which accrue to the dominant culture by virtue of its domination of others but which remain invisible to the recipients. Rather than be viewed as unearned bounty, this process of racial privileging erases these gains from view, allowing its beneficiaries to consider as natural that which in effect is garnered at the expense of others.

When Aboriginal scholar Lillian Holt wrote her famous witty piece 'Psst ... I wannabe white' in 1999, she captured both the despair and the hope of Aboriginal women everywhere fervently wishing for a change in the racist dynamics of Australian society at the end of yet another century of struggle:

> Oh the arrogance of whiteness within these well-meaning white fellas. They exuded decency whilst being in denial. ... Yeah I wannabe white

... so that I don't have to be acutely aware every day of my 'otherness' in the eyes of the dominant whites.

(Holt, 1999, pp. 39–44)

Elsewhere McIntosh (1988) drew on her (white) feminist understanding of male gendered power to theorise ways in which white privilege eclipsed the needs and perspectives of women who are relentlessly and structurally positioned as less dominant or more marginalised. She listed some 46 easily identified practical and contextual privileges she gained directly through her 'whiteness' and considered the ontological implications of such inequities being normalised within the daily lived experiences of women of colour (p. 98).

An analysis of white privilege is thus an important way for us to interrogate the ways in which relations of power are insinuated into our everyday lives, serving to affirm some people while diminishing others. By reflecting on how white privilege operates we are enabled to see the means by which the subtle disadvantaging of others maintains systemic power. Understanding whiteness is not however just about identity politics or the superficiality of skin colour; rather it is about acknowledging the structural nature of hegemonic control and learning how to deconstruct it. As Bhabha suggests, such an understanding 'attempts to displace the normativity of the white position by seeing it as a strategy of authority rather than an authentic or essential "identity"' (1998, p. 21).

Adopting such a critical stance necessitates a reversal of the normative gaze. By examining ourselves – our privileges and *dis*privileges – and looking back at dominant cultural mores and deconstructing them, we can begin to see how readily whiteness is normalised. We can identify who is being advantaged and how such privileging operates, rather than simply and naively looking outward in a quest to 'help' those less privileged and more disadvantaged. Our focus needs to be the disruption of power, rather than the intervention of the power*ful* in the lives of 'others'.

Australian Indigenous feminist scholar Aileen Moreton-Robinson illustrates the power of this process of deconstruction and gaze reversal in her book *Talkin' Up to the White Woman* (2000). Here Moreton-Robinson elucidates the whiteness of Australian feminism and exposes the privileging of non-Indigenous women's experience and how this in turn underscores the patriarchal whiteness of the Australian state, with its underpinning of (ongoing) colonialism. By demonstrating how whiteness works within feminism to erase the standpoints and experience of Aboriginal and Torres Strait Islander women, Moreton-Robinson also demonstrates the power of whiteness to bend even self-styled 'progressive' narratives such as feminism and human rights discourses to its colonial ends. Further to this, others have similarly pointed out how the discursive regime of whiteness insidiously negates and subjugates, 'as it reinforces and naturalizes dominance' (Banerjee & Tedmanson, 2010, p. 149).

Aboriginal and Torres Strait Islander women, as Indigenous women everywhere, experience the combined oppression of racism and sexism in their lives as a result of the displacement, dispossession and violence at the heart of processes of colonisation in which all non-Indigenous Australians remain implicated (Moreton-Robinson, 2000, 2004; Fejo-King & Briskman, 2009; Fredericks, 2010; Wendt & Zannettino, 2015). We argue that whiteness still functions in the political economy of Australia today as an invisible regime of power that uses unmarked and unnamed culturally constituted and transmitted notions of everyday, commonsense, 'taken for granteds' – 'an epistemology of the West … that secures hegemony through discourse and has material effects in everyday life' (Moreton-Robinson, 2004, p. 75). It is essential, as Wendt and Zannettino (2015) argue, that as women concerned with feminism in social work we gain a deeper insight and build greater reflexivity into our understanding of gender relations through 'the stories of Aboriginal women themselves'. These stories challenge assumptions of Aboriginal women being 'incapable' and 'needy', which have grown from patriarchal whiteness paradigms and from within feminism itself (Wendt & Zannettino, 2015, p. 161).

Critical race theorists (e.g. Ladson-Billings & Donnor, 2005; Delgado, 1995; Delgado et al., 2012; Dixson & Rousseau, 2005; Riggs & Augoustinos, 2005; Riggs, 2007), along with whiteness theorists (e.g. Frankenberg, 1993, 1997; McIntosh, 1988; Fine, 2004, 2006; Kowal, 2011), and particularly the writings of a burgeoning cohort of talented critical Indigenous theorists (e.g. Tuhiwai-Smith, 2012; Behrendt, 1993; Rigney, 1997; Moreton-Robinson, 2000, 2004, 2011; Sinclair, 2004; Watson, 2007; Nakata, 2007; Martin, 2008; Wilson, 2008; Fredericks, 2010; Yellow Bird, 2013a, 2013b; Fejo-King & Briskman, 2009; Fejo-King, 2013) provide a sound basis for feminists to consider effective ways to recognise and dismantle whiteness within social work. The work of a growing group of Indigenous scholars, who are not only theorising but also continually subjected to the lived experiences of the ongoing effects of colonisation, provide powerful insights into the working of racialised power and its reproduction as 'structural, institutional, interpersonal and intra-psychic; outrageous and civilized; cultivated in the media, the market and the academy' (Fine, 2006, p. 85).

Arguing for space for the field of Indigenous feminisms to flourish in Joyce Green's edited collection (2007), Canadian Aboriginal scholar Verna St Denis provides a definition of Indigenous feminism as a critique of 'western patriarchy'. She suggests this is a powerful way to disrupt the internalisation of racialised power in the pervasive colonial discourse which permeates so much of our scholarship and social work context. St Denis (2007, p. 44) argues that when Indigenous feminists examine the intersections of race, gender and nation they can work towards undermining white western colonial patriarchy and assist in building national, pan-tribal and indeed international momentum towards decolonisation.

Locating whiteness in feminism and social work

With an understanding that whiteness lies at the very heart of the way in which Australia – along with many other western nations – was *un*settled (Tedmanson, 2008), and that the white conqueror's lie of *terra nullius*[3] enabled the founding of an Australian nation 'specifically built on the *non*-recognition of its Indigenous peoples' (Banerjee & Tedmanson, 2010, p. 149), comes the realisation that Australia's colonial history of violent invasion still shapes the context of Aboriginal and non-Aboriginal relations today. Structural relations of power between hegemonic whiteness and the law (Quayle & Sonn, 2013) have led to appropriation of Indigenous land, disruption of Indigenous livelihoods and the incarceration of Indigenous peoples in Australia (as elsewhere), and continue to entrench not only systemic disadvantage but also racially discriminatory practices, particularly in the area of social policy.[4]

One of the most troubling periods in Australia's social policy history, and of particular concern to social work, was the state-enforced mandatory removal of Aboriginal and Torres Strait Islander children in the 1950s, 1960s and 1970s. During this time many thousands of Indigenous children were forcibly removed from their families and communities, with the explicit intention of expunging their Aboriginality.

Many social workers throughout the nation were, by virtue of their positions working in child welfare and associated government and/or government-sponsored non-government roles, implicated in this genocidal policy regime and complicit in operationalising it in local contexts and communities. For Deirdre, a woman deeply engaged in Aboriginal and Torres Strait Islander social justice issues who identifies as non-Indigenous yet has past historical family intersections with Aboriginality largely whited out of view, this has a heart-breaking resonance – it is the 'whispering in the heart' that Reynolds (1998, p. 1) speaks of. For Christine, this period has a much deeper, more profound and lingering impact:

> I am a part of the Stolen Generations, and many others of my immediate family (mother, aunts, grandparents, and great grandparents) were also stolen children. Apart from representing the Australian Capital Territory's Stolen Generations and the NCATSISWA, I was asked to offer the support of the NCATSISWA to the Stolen Generations Alliance. I did what had been requested of me, and it seems almost as though I blinked at an important moment, and when I opened my eyes, I found myself in the position of National Indigenous Co-Chair of the Stolen Generations Alliance.
>
> (Fejo-King, 2011, p. 133)

Christine's journey and that of the women in her family – most notably the indomitable Nanna Fejo who became a human face of the nation's formal apology to Aboriginal peoples – is a most inspiring and profound story, epitomising many other Aboriginal women's stories. It highlights the importance of family, of the power of kinship, of the extraordinary pain of loss, of heartbreak and struggle, and of survival, strength and reconnection.

Christine says: 'As a social worker traversing the healing process for myself, my family and for others, while simultaneously being a pivotal part of the leadership of this emotional national event, a pinnacle moment in Australia's history, I have found it important to share my story with other women and with other social workers, in the hope they will reflect on the oppressions so easily acceded to still'. Deirdre says: 'I view Christine's skill and generosity in sharing this deeply personal journey, so core to her own family, as part of a process of learning and healing for the social work profession, to be truly remarkable' (see for example Fejo-King & Rae, 1996; Fejo-King & Briskman, 2009; Fejo-King, 2011, 2013).

What the NCATSISWA and many thousands of Indigenous Australians had wished for across the generations was a definitive moment of recognition in which Australia acknowledged the pain the policies which gave rise to the Stolen Generations had caused – acknowledged and apologised. As Freire (1972) wrote and taught, by not recognising and honouring the humanity of the colonised, the coloniser loses his or her own humanity in turn. Recognition and an apology is a first stage in finding the right words to build a story of reconciliation together.

For over ten years the Stolen Generations and their supporters fought to have the recommendations of the *Bringing Them Home Report* (Human Rights and Equal Opportunity Commission, 1997) implemented. NCAT-SISWA, other social workers and many other supportive people worked on the ground in every state and territory to bring to pass a much hoped for dream. On 13 February 2008 then Prime Minister of Australia Kevin Rudd made a pivotal speech of apology to Australia's Indigenous peoples on behalf of the Australian Parliament and all Australians, to 'reflect on their past mistreatment', in particular the Stolen Generations.

> For the pain, suffering and hurt of these Stolen Generations, their descendants and for their families left behind, we say sorry. To the mothers and the fathers, the brothers and the sisters, for the breaking up of families and communities, we say sorry. And for the indignity and degradation thus inflicted on a proud people and a proud culture, we say sorry.[5]

This was an important step, not just for Christine's family, who were especially proud to have our Nanna Fejo's words and story featured as part of the Prime Minister's apology, but for all Indigenous Australians, indeed all Australians – and all social workers. The apology encompassed the positive elements of critical reflexivity and was an attempt to re-right our nation's narrative by including recognition of the violence of colonisation and its ongoing effects. It aimed to dismantle (at least in part) the fictional white 'lies' and structural silence surrounding Australia's Indigenous–non-Indigenous engagement. It was also an attempt to recognise the power of critical Indigenous standpoints – which necessitate the inclusion of Indigenous perspectives told through Indigenous eyes. This was the power of Nanna Fejo's story.

Dismantling whiteness through deep listening and Indigenous standpoints

A critical Indigenous perspective encompassing Indigenous standpoint theory brings alternative ways of being and alternative epistemologies to the existing bodies of knowledge we have about feminism and social work. Standpoint theory is a means of denoting the situated nature of all knowledge. According to Harding, feminist standpoint theory was proposed 'not just as an explanatory theory but also ... as a method or theory of method (methodology)' (2004, p. 1). Feminist standpoint theory developed in response to the primacy always accorded to male subjectivity – as if men's experience was the defining norm and the production of knowledge always needed to be understood from a patriarchal perspective. Women in this dynamic are subordinated to men and women's differing experiences are also rendered invisible in this process, relegated to that of the non-male 'other' – the subsidiary or 'different' subjectivity. Men's knowledge, particularly 'white' western men's knowledge, and their perspective on the world have historically been continually privileged by such a dynamic.

However works by Smith (1974), Hartsock (1998), Haraway (1988) and Harding (1993, 1997, 2004) have carved out a space for feminist standpoints and have exposed the gendered connection between relations of power and the production of knowledge. As Moreton-Robinson explains, feminist standpoint theorists have 'assisted in mapping feminism's epistemological boundaries ... [and] challenged dominant patriarchal paradigms which discursively privilege men as knowing subjects by exposing the partiality of the universal male standpoint' (2013, p. 332).

A feminist standpoint, however, is also primarily a white western standpoint, predicated on giving primacy to the lived experience of non-Indigenous women whose lives have been historically shaped by events such as the Industrial Revolution, the growth of British and other European colonialisms, suffragette struggles for the vote and populist pan-European notions of 'enlightenment' and human superiority (over the environment, non-human animals and Indigenous civilisations). The female subject within a feminist standpoint theory is generally taken for granted as one shaped by her everyday life under capitalism. For example the gendered division of labour, relations to private land and financial ownership, and advancement (or lack thereof) within the political, civil and economic domains of the nation-state are common preoccupations within much feminist literature.

This is not the lived experience of many Indigenous women however, for whom the struggle to live free of racism, with equal access to resources and/or recognition within a state that has been the agent of Indigenous people's dispossession, will likely take priority over or at least share importance with struggles common to all women for agency and independence in daily familial, economic and social relations. Freedom from the violence of colonialism sits alongside (and is implicated in) the quest of all women to live free of the threat of family violence. As Nakata argues, 'Indigenous people are entangled in a very contested knowledge space at the Cultural Interface ... [and one's] social position is discursively constituted within and constitutive of complex sets of social relations as expressed through the social organization of everyday life' (2007, p. 216).

Indigenous people's sense of belonging, or as Christine puts it 'Aboriginal ways of knowing, being and doing' (Fejo-King, 2013, p. 74), are often derived quite differently from that of their non-Indigenous counterparts. Identity for example is not as readily centred on an individuated 'self' but rather is relational and interconnected in nature, with people made aware from their earliest days (in culture) of a series of complex and intrinsically powerful interconnections – with land, with non-human animals, with relations and extended kinship networks – with whom we are integrally and reciprocally bound. This knowledge about the world view and cosmology of Aboriginal and Torres Strait Islander peoples has only comparatively recently begun to be considered as essential to an anti-racist, culturally responsive and culturally safe feminism that is informed by Indigenous standpoints, a feminism that is relevant and attentive to Indigenous women's experiences. Australian Indigenous feminist scholars like Moreton-Robinson (2000, 2004, 2011, 2013) and Watson (2007, 2015; Watson & Heath, 2004) have been at the forefront of this emergent Indigenous feminist scholarship. Similarly Green (2007), Smith and Kauanui (2008), Blackstock (2009), Goeman and Denetdale (2009), Mikaere (1999), Tamburro (2013) and Stewart-Harawira (2007) amongst others are providing inspiring leadership for Indigenous feminist perspectives emerging in Canada, the US and New Zealand.

In addition, works by Christine as well as others have identified ways in which both an understanding of whiteness and the importance of Indigenous standpoints, combined with the unique qualities embodied in Indigenous women's feminisms, can inform improvements to social work education and practice (see for example Atkinson, 2002; Bennett, Zubrzycki & Bacon, 2011; Bessarab, 2012; Fredericks, 2010; Fejo-King & Briskman, 2009; Fejo-King, 2013; Gray, Coates & Yellow-Bird, 2008; Gray et al., 2013; Hart, 2008; Tedmanson, 2008, 2012, 2015; Walter et al., 2011; Wendt & Baker, 2013; Zufferey, 2012). This is what Watson and

Heath (2004) refer to as our collective opportunity for 'growing up' the space for conversation.

It is in this space of conversation, the crucial space of 'cultural interface' (Nakata, 2007), that creative change can grow. For Aboriginal women, the respect of deep listening is of paramount importance. As Irene Watson (2007) argues, Indigenous women's law needs to be revalued and restored to its rightful place as the centre of women's knowledge and power. As Christine points out, (our) knowledge as Indigenous women is learned from parents and grandparents who learned it from our ancestors:

> It is knowledge I have passed on to my children who will ensure that my grandchildren also learn. This is knowledge that will guide their lives so they too, can be firmly grounded within their kinship and totemic systems and never become separated from them or from who they are.
>
> (2013, p. 74)

By privileging Indigenous experience, stories and knowledge in all aspects of the education and supervision of current and future social workers 'the lived, historical experiences, ideas, traditions, dreams, interests, aspirations and struggles of Indigenous peoples' (Rigney, 1997, p. 117) become the central focus of learning. Gradually these qualities will align to strengthen non-Indigenous people's learning. What follows will be the subtle but hopefully also lasting counter-hegemonic, decolonising and empowering effects that result from improvements in mutual understanding. From the standpoint of 'radical Indigenism' (Garroutte, 2003, p. 101) adopting Indigenous knowledges, wisdoms and stories is an essential part of repositioning power, reversing the gaze and reframing how knowledge is conceived and shared.

Centring Indigenous women's voices acknowledges the personal, oral, experiential, local and holistic power of Indigenous epistemologies, often conveyed in narrative through storytelling using metaphorical language (Wilson, 2008). Tuhiwai-Smith articulates storytelling as key to decolonisation:

> Telling our stories from the past, reclaiming the past, giving testimony to the injustices of the past are all strategies which are commonly employed by Indigenous peoples struggling for justice … the need to tell our stories remains the powerful imperative of a powerful form of resistance.
>
> (2012, pp. 34–35)

As well as appreciating the importance of storytelling as a means of sharing knowledge, recognition of a deep cultural affiliation to land is also shared by many Indigenous peoples around the world. Such interconnection between people, and also between people and place, embodies a respect for forms of human and non-human or spiritual forms of agency quite distinct from less spiritual and more linear western rationalities (Tedmanson, 2012). Mahood (2000) explains this attachment to country as a quality of being many non-Indigenous people find difficult to comprehend, as 'to revisit country is not only to reanimate it but to walk the contours of one's own deep self, both individual and shared' (p. 12).

Giving voice or providing opportunities for conversation in this context can also mean non-Indigenous practitioners learning to sit with silence. From an Indigenous feminist standpoint, silence can demonstrate respect, a rich space of reflection and inward pause, a recognition that not all emotions and thoughts can be (or need be) verbalised (Ryan, 2011). Silence can be part of a rich, deep dialogue reaching beyond western notions of conversation (Mahood, 2008; Ryan, 2011).

Learning to listen deeply and to appreciate, acknowledge and respect diverse Indigenous world views is not always an easy journey. It is especially complex when we seek to incorporate new feminist perspectives in social work and social work education. As Indigenous (Canadian) social worker Cindy Blackstock points out:

> The notion of improving other people is endemic to social work. It is both a source of moral nobility and trepidation. It implies an ability to define accurately another's deficit, to locate an importance in his/her life and assumes the efficacy of external motivations and sensibilities to change.
>
> (2009, p. 31)

Recognising that the change we seek may need to start with a reversal of the gaze to focus on whiteness and its role in the relations of power that perpetuate domination is an important beginning. As Christine points out in her book *Let's Talk about Kinship* (2013, p. 150), the goal of 'improving' others, especially Aboriginal Australians, by making us more like white Australians has been embedded in the ideology, policies and practices of this country since invasion. As Deirdre also points out (2012, p. 249), non-Indigenous Australians need to build their capacity for engagement before intervening in Indigenous lives. In the end we need to work from a sense of feminist solidarity with a commitment to capacity sharing and reciprocity, not assumptions of knowing. As Indigenous feminist academic Moreton-Robinson (2004) puts it, Indigenous women are often the 'known' and seldom the 'knowers'. As Wendt and Zannettino (2015) also suggest, any perpetuation of images or discourses which position Aboriginal women as inferior to and servants of their men, for example, need to be replaced or at least balanced with discussion of and insights into the inherent power of women in Aboriginal cultures. By working from a strengths approach, intrinsic in feminism's role in empowering women to be seen and heard, as well as a commitment to listening and learning from anti-racist and reflexive practice, dialogue at the cultural interface can continue to mature.

Conclusion

Walter et al. suggest that 'Australian social work is predominantly white' and that this privileging of the dominant culture's perspectives is an 'omnipresent reality within our practice and our profession' (2011, p. 7). In this chapter we have together traversed some of the key thinking on 'whiteness' and its impact in the context of social work and feminism. Focusing in particular on the direction of much of Christine's work, which employs narrative and storytelling to explicate the importance of relationships, family and kinship to Aboriginal peoples, the chapter charts how Australia's colonial history and the pervasiveness of structural racism as well as the privileging of everyday whiteness has had a profound impact on the context of social work in Australia. Against this backdrop we have explored Indigenous feminist standpoints for the important diversity of views they offer both to educate and to enrich feminist understandings. The chapter is part of an ongoing conversation, not just between the two of us as women deeply committed to growing social justice in ourselves and for our families and communities, but also we hope as part of a longer, deeper dialogue taking place between women across our countries and beyond.

In closing, we return to our opening focus on Lisa Bellear's powerful poem 'Feelings', and its portrait of the absurdity of white 'expertise' in action. As Brewster cleverly notes, however, in analysing the poem's political motif, it remains less concerned 'with the issue of defining *who* we are … than [with] imagining *how* we can live together' (2007, p. 218) in order to realise greater egalitarian and socially just relations as women. It is to this beautiful emancipatory vision that we dedicate our chapter.

Notes

1 In 2008 Prime Minister Kevin Rudd apologised on behalf of Australia to the Stolen Generations, Aboriginal and Islander peoples who as children endured forced separation from their families and communities, and to the families who lost their children (Fejo-King, 2011) The 1997 Inquiry into the Separation of Aboriginal and Torres Strait Islander Children from their Families found that between one in ten and three in ten Aboriginal and Torres Strait Islander children were forcibly removed from their families and communities between 1910 and 1970. For more information, see www.reconciliation.org.au/wp-content/uploads/2013/12/Apology-fact-sheet.pdf.

2 The word 'remote' is a contestable term, as for some people on the APY Lands for example regional centres and cities may be alienating and 'remote' places. To paraphrase a witty comment Professor Lillian Holt was once anecdotally reported as saying, I too work in a 'remote' community, it's called a university!

3 *Terra nullius* or the claim that the continent was unoccupied was a basis on which Australia's land mass was claimed for the British Crown at the time of invasion. This grand 'lie' was not overturned until the 1992 *Mabo* High Court judgement which upheld Indigenous man Eddie Mabo's claim he and his antecedents had occupied the land at the time of invasion.

4 See, for example, the Northern Territory Emergency Response Intervention (NTER) of 2007 during which the then Howard Government amended Australia's Racial Discrimination Act 1975 to enable it to enact specific policies designed to target the NT's Aboriginal communities.

5 The full apology speech by Australia's then Prime Minister Kevin Rudd can be viewed at www.australia.gov.au/about-australia/our-country/our-people/apology-to-australias-indigenous-peoples.

Further reading

Bessarab, D. (2012) The supervisory yarn: embedding Indigenous epistemology in supervision. In B. Bennett, S. Green, S. Gilbert & D. Bessarab (eds), *Our Voices: Aboriginal and Torres Strait Islander Social Work*. Palgrave Macmillan, South Yarra, Vic, pp. 73–92.

Fejo-King, C. & Briskman, L. (2009) Reversing colonial practices with Indigenous peoples. In J. Allan, L. Briskman & B. Pease (eds), *Critical Social Work: Theories and Practices for a Just World*, 2nd edn. Allan & Unwin, Crow's Nest, NSW, pp. 105–116.

Green, J. (ed.) (2007) *Making Space for Indigenous Feminism.* Zed Books, London.

Hart, M. (2008) Critical reflections on an Aboriginal approach to helping. In M. Gray, J. Coates & M. Yellow-Bird (eds), *Indigenous Social Work around the World: Towards Culturally Relevant Education and Practice.* Ashgate, Farnham, UK, pp. 129–140.

Moreton-Robinson, A. (2011) The white man's burden: patriarchal white epistemic violence and Aboriginal women's knowledges within the academy. *Australian Feminist Studies*, 26(70), pp. 413–431.

Moreton-Robinson, A. (2013) Towards an Australian Indigenous women's standpoint theory. *Australian Feminist Studies*, 28(78), pp. 331–347.

Watson, I. (2007) Aboriginal women's law and lives: how might we keep growing the law? *Australian Feminist Law Journal*, 26, pp. 95–107.

References

Allen, T.W. (1994) *The Invention of the White Race.* Verso, London.

Applebaum, B. (2010) White: on the possibility of doing philosophy in good faith. In G. Yancy (ed.), *The Centre Must not Hold: White Women Philosophers on the Whiteness of Philosophy.* Lexington, Lanham, MD, pp. 5–16.

Atkinson, J. (2002) *Trauma Trails, Recreating Song Lines: The Transgenerational Effects of Trauma in Indigenous Australia.* Spinifex Press, North Melbourne.

Banerjee, S.B. & Tedmanson, D. (2010) Grass burning under our feet: Indigenous enterprise development in a political economy of whiteness. *Management Learning*, 41(2), pp. 147–165.

Behrendt, L. (1993) Aboriginal women and the white lies of the feminist movement: implications for Aboriginal women in the rights discourse. *Australian Feminist Law Journal*, 27(1), pp. 27–44.

Bellear, L. (1996) *Dreaming in Urban Areas*. University of Queensland Press, St Lucia, Qld.

Bennett, B., Zubrzycki, J. & Bacon, V. (2011) What do we know? The experiences of social workers working alongside Aboriginal people. *Australian Social Work*, 64(1), pp. 20–37.

Bessarab, D. (2012) The supervisory yarn: embedding Indigenous epistemology in supervision. In B. Bennett, S. Green, S. Gilbert & D. Bessarab (eds), *Our Voices: Aboriginal and Torres Strait Islander Social Work*. Palgrave Macmillan, South Yarra, Vic, pp. 73–92.

Bhabha, H. (1998) The white stuff. *Artforum International*, 36(9), pp. 21–23.

Blackstock, C. (2009) The occasional evil of angels: learning from the experiences of Aboriginal peoples and social work. *First Nations Child and Family Review*, 4(1), pp. 28–37.

Brewster, A. (2007) Brokering cross-racial feminism. *Feminist Theory*, 8(2), pp. 209–221.

Delgado, R. (ed.) (1995) *Critical Race Theory: The Cutting Edge*. Temple University Press, Philadelphia, PN.

Delgado, R., Stefancic, J. & Liendo, E. (2012) *Critical Race Theory: An Introduction*, 2nd edn. New York University Press, New York.

Dixson, A.D. & Rousseau, C.K. (2005) And we are still not saved: critical race theory in education ten years later. *Race, Ethnicity and Education*, 8(1), pp. 7–27.

Dyer, R. (1997) *White*. Routledge, New York.

Fanon, F. (1986 [1952]) *Black Skin, White Masks*. Pluto, London.

Fejo-King, C. (2011) The National Apology to the Stolen Generations: the ripple effect. *Australian Social Work*, 64(1), pp. 130–143.

Fejo-King, C. (2013) *Let's Talk Kinship: Innovating Australian Social Work Education, Theory, Research and Practice through Aboriginal Knowledge*. Christine King Consulting, Brisbane.

Fejo-King, C. & Briskman, L. (2009) Reversing colonial practices with Indigenous peoples. In J. Allan, L. Briskman & B. Pease (eds), *Critical Social Work: Theories and Practices for a Just World*, 2nd edn. Allan & Unwin, Crow's Nest, NSW, pp. 105–116.

Fejo-King, C. & Rae, C. (1996) *Strong Women, Strong Babies, Strong Culture*. Northern Territory Health Service, Darwin, NT.

Fine, M. (2004) Witnessing whiteness/gathering intelligence. In M. Fine, L. Weis, L. Pruitt & A. Burns (eds), *Off White: Readings of Power, Privilege and Resistance*. Routledge, New York, pp. 245–256.

Fine, M. (2006) Bearing witness: methods for researching oppression and resistance. A textbook for critical research. *Social Justice Research*, 19(1), pp. 83–108.

Frankenberg, R. (1993) *The Social Construction of Whiteness: White Women, Race Matters*. Routledge, London.

Frankenberg, R. (1997) *Displacing Whiteness: Essays in Social and Cultural Criticism*. Duke University Press, London.

Fredericks, B. (2010) Re-empowering ourselves: Australian Aboriginal women. *Signs: Journal of Women in Culture and Society*, 35(3), pp. 546–550.

Freire, P. (1972) *Pedagogy of the Oppressed*, Penguin Books, Harmondsworth, UK.

Garroutte, E. (2003) *Real Indians: Identity and the Survival of Native America*. University of California Press, Berkeley, CA.

Goeman, R. & Denetdale, J.N. (2009) Native feminisms: legacies, interventions, and indigenous sovereignties, *Wicazo Sa Review*, 24(2), pp. 9–13.

Gray, M., Coates, J. & Yellow-Bird, M. (eds) (2008) *Indigenous Social Work around the World: Towards Culturally Relevant Education and Practice.* Ashgate, Farnham, UK.

Gray, M., Coates, J., Yellow Bird, M. & Hetherington, T. (eds) (2013) *Decolonizing Social Work.* Ashgate, Farnham, UK.

Green, J. (ed.) (2007) *Making Space for Indigenous Feminism.* Zed Books, London.

Hall, S. (1997) *Representation: Cultural Representations and Signifying Practices.* Sage, London.

Haraway, D. (1988) Situated knowledges: the science question in feminism and the privilege of partial perspective. *Feminist Studies,* 14(3), pp. 575–599.

Harding, S. (1993) Rethinking standpoint epistemology: what is 'strong objectivity'? In L. Alcoff & E. Potter (eds), *Feminist Epistemologies.* Routledge, New York, pp. 575–599.

Harding, S. (1997) Comment on Hekman's 'truth and method: feminist standpoint theory revisited': whose standpoint needs the regimes of truth and reality? *Signs: Journal of Women in Culture and Society,* 22(21), pp. 382–391.

Harding, S. (2004) *The Feminist Standpoint Reader.* Routledge, New York.

Hart, M. (2008) Critical reflections on an Aboriginal approach to helping. In M. Gray, J. Coates & M. Yellow-Bird (eds), *Indigenous Social Work around the World: Towards Culturally Relevant Education and Practice.* Ashgate, Farnham, UK, pp. 129–140.

Hartsock, N. (1998) *The Feminist Standpoint Revisited and Other Essays.* Westview Press, Boulder, CO.

Hill, M. (1997) *Whiteness: A Critical Reader.* New York University Press, New York.

Holt, L. (1999) Pssst … I wannabe white. In B. McKay (ed.), *Unmasking Whiteness: Race Relations and Reconciliation.* Griffith University Press, Brisbane, pp. 39–51.

Human Rights and Equal Opportunities Commission (1997) *Report of the National Inquiry into the Separation of Aboriginal and Torres Strait Islander Children from their Families.* Commonwealth Government Press, Sydney.

Kowal, E. (2011) The stigma of white privilege: Australian anti-racists and Indigenous improvement. *Cultural Studies,* 25(3), pp. 313–333.

Ladson-Billings, G. & Donnor, J. (2005) The moral activist role of critical race theory scholarship. In N.K. Denzin & Y.S. Lincoln (eds), *The Sage Handbook of Qualitative Research,* 3rd edn. Sage, Thousand Oaks, CA, pp. 279–302.

McIntosh, P. (1988) White privilege: unpacking the invisible knapsack. *White Privilege and Male Privilege: A Personal Account of Coming to see Correspondence through Work in Women's Studies,* Working Paper 189. Wellesley College Center for Research on Women, Wellesley, MA.

Mahood, K. (2000) *Craft for a Dry Lake.* Anchor, Sydney.

Mahood, K. (2008) Listening is harder than you think [online]. *Griffith Review,* 19(Autumn), pp. 163–177. http://search.informit.com.au.ezlibproxy.unisa.edu.au/documentSummary;dn=301737631979177;res=IELLCC (accessed 25 June 2014).

Martin, K. (2008) *Please Knock Before You Enter: Aboriginal Regulation of Outsiders and the Implications for Researchers.* Post Pressed, Teneriffe, Qld.

Massumi, B. (2002) *Parables for the Virtual.* Duke University Press, Durham, NC.

Mikaere, A. (1999) Colonisation and the imposition of patriarchy: a Ngati Raukawa woman's perspective. *Te Ukaipo,* 3, pp. 7–19.

Moreton-Robinson, A. (2000) *Talkin' Up to the White Woman: Indigenous Women and White Feminism.* University of Queensland Press, St Lucia, Qld.

Moreton-Robinson, A. (2004) Preface. In A. Moreton-Robinson (ed.), *Whitening Race.* Aboriginal Studies Press, Canberra, pp. ix–x.

Moreton-Robinson, A. (2011) The white man's burden: patriarchal white epistemic violence and Aboriginal women's knowledges within the academy. *Australian Feminist Studies*, 26(70), pp. 413–431.

Moreton-Robinson, A. (2013) Towards an Australian Indigenous women's standpoint theory. *Australian Feminist Studies*, 28(78), pp. 331–347.

Nakata, M. (2007) *Disciplining the Savages: Savaging the Disciplines*. Aboriginal Studies Press, Canberra.

Quayle, A. & Sonn, C. (2013) Explicating race privilege: examining symbolic barriers to Aboriginal and non-Indigenous partnership. *Social Identities*, 19(5), pp. 552–570.

Reynolds, H. (1998) *The Whispering in Our Hearts*. Allen & Unwin, St Leonards, NSW.

Riggs, D. (ed.) (2007) *Taking up the Challenge: Critical Race and Whiteness Studies in a Postcolonising Nation*. Crawford House, Belair, SA.

Riggs, D.W. & Augoustinos, M. (2005) The psychic life of colonial power: racialised subjectivities, bodies and methods. *Journal of Community and Applied Social Psychology*, 15(6), pp. 461–477.

Rigney, L.I. (1997) Internationalisation of an Indigenous anti-colonial cultural critique of research methodologies: a guide to Indigenist research methodology and its principles. *Journal for Native American Studies*, 14(2), pp. 109–121.

Ryan, F. (2011) Kanyininpa (Holding): a way of nurturing children in Aboriginal Australia. *Australian Social Work*, 64(2), pp. 183–197.

Said, E. (1978) *Orientalism: Western Representations of the Orient*. Routledge, London.

Sinclair, R. (2004) Aboriginal social work education in Canada: decolonizing pedagogy for the seventh generation. *First Peoples Child and Family Review*, 1, pp. 49–61.

Smith, A. & Kauanui, J.K. (2008) Native feminisms engage American studies. *American Quarterly*, 60(2), pp. 241–249.

Smith, D. (1974) Women's perspective as a radical critique of sociology. *Sociological Inquiry*, 44, pp. 1–13.

St Denis, V. (2007) Aboriginal women on feminism: exploring diverse points of view. In V. Green (ed.), *Making Space for Indigenous Feminism*. Zed Books, London, pp. 33–51.

Stewart-Harawira, M. (2007) Practicing Indigenous feminism: resistance to imperialism. In J. Green (ed.), *Making Space for Indigenous Feminism*. Zed Books, London, pp. 97–117.

Tamburro, A. (2013) Including decolonization in social work education and practice. *Journal of Indigenous Social Development*, 2(1), pp. 1–16.

Tedmanson, D. (2008) Isle of exception: sovereign power and Palm Island. *Critical Perspectives on International Business*, 4(2–3), pp. 142–165.

Tedmanson, D. (2012) Whose capacity needs building? Reflections on capacity building initiatives in remote Australian Indigenous communities. In A. Prasad (ed.), *Against the Grain: Advances in Postcolonial Organization Studies*. Copenhagen Business School Press, Copenhagen, pp. 249–275.

Tedmanson, D. (2015) *Ngapartji Ngapartji*: narratives of reciprocity in 'yarning up' participatory research. In L. Bryant (ed.), *Critical and Creative Research Methodologies in Social Work*. Ashgate, Farnham, UK, pp. 75–92.

Tuhiwai-Smith, L. (2012) *Decolonizing Methodologies: Research and Indigenous Peoples*. Zed Books, London.

Walter, L., Taylor, S. & Habibis, D. (2011) How white is social work in Australia? *Australian Social Work*, 64(1), pp. 6–19.

Watson, I. (2007) Aboriginal women's law and lives: how might we keep growing the law? *Australian Feminist Law Journal*, 26, pp. 95–107.

Watson, I. (2015) *Aboriginal Peoples, Colonialism and International Law: Raw Law*. Routledge, Oxford.

Watson, I. & Heath, M. (2004) Growing up the space: a conversation about the future of feminism. *Australian Feminist Law Journal*, 20, pp. 95–111.

Wendt, S. & Baker, J. (2013) Aboriginal women's perceptions and experiences of a family violence transitional accommodation service. *Australian Social Work*, 66(4), pp. 511–527.

Wendt, S. & Zannettino, L. (2015) *Domestic Violence in Diverse Contexts: A Re-Examination of Gender*. Routledge, London.

Wilson, S. (2008) *Research is Ceremony: Indigenous Research Methods*. Fernwood, Halifax & Winnipeg.

Yellow Bird, M. (2013a) Neurodecolonization: applying mindfulness research to decolonizing social work. In M. Gray, J. Coates, M. Yellow Bird & T. Hetherington (eds), *Decolonizing Social Work*. Ashgate, Farnham, UK, pp. 293–310.

Yellow Bird, M. (2013b) Preface: United Nations Declaration on the Rights of Indigenous Peoples through Indigenous eyes. In M. Gray, J. Coates, M. Yellow Bird & T. Hetherington (eds), *Decolonizing Social Work*. Ashgate, Burlington, VT, pp. xix–xxiii.

Zufferey, C. (2012) 'Not knowing that I do not know and not wanting to know': reflections of a white Australian social worker. *International Social Work*, 56(5), pp. 659–673.

11 'Something is missing here'

Weaving feminist theories into social work practice with refugees

Laurie Cook Heffron, Susanna Snyder, Karin Wachter, Maura Nsonwu and Noël Busch-Armendariz

I'm not afraid of nobody here. Nobody is gonna kill me in the middle of the night or anything. I just feel like I like to live with people. Why am I alone? I miss that time where we would sit like 7:00 pm or 8:00 pm, before going to bed. People are talking. Kids are running around. I have my little one, only one year. I'm lookin' at her; she can't even talk. I feel like something is missing here. We just go to bed. We have to go to bed early because we have nobody to talk to. We used to live in a place full of people. People come over in the night. You will talk before going to bed. I just don't feel good because that's not there. It's gone. I find myself, I feel I'm alone.

(Congolese refugee mother)

Introduction

The number of forced migrants has reached its highest global levels in 20 years. By the end of 2012 over 45 million people were displaced by war, conflict and other crises, including 15.4 million refugees and 28.8 million internally displaced persons (UNHCR, 2013a). Women account for approximately one-half of those displaced, and face an array of challenges. However, only recently has the refugee regime recognised that women have needs and concerns specific to their gendered identities (Hajdukowski-Ahmed, Khanlou & Moussa, 2008). Each year, approximately 60,000–70,000 people arrive in the United States through the UNHCR resettlement programme. According to the US Office of Refugee Resettlement, the US resettles refugees into more than 250 local communities per year, engaging approximately 1,500 non-profit organisations, 49 states and countless volunteers from local civic organisations, churches, synagogues and other religious and community-based institutions (ORR Director, personal communication, 28 March 2012). Resettlement programmes provide various services, including housing, food, medical care, employment preparation and English as a second language (www.acf.hhs.gov/programs/orr).

The social work profession plays a key role in supporting refugee women as they navigate and respond to their shifting circumstances during resettlement in the US. The foundation of any refugee resettlement agency is the provision of case management services related to basic needs, employment and complex medical issues. Some agencies also provide mental health counselling services. Federal and state funded refugee resettlement programmes draw tremendously from the social work profession in terms of human resources, and social work values help to ensure the wellbeing of clients as well as staff. Former refugees and other migrants play a significant role in carrying out aspects of social work practice in the field of refugee resettlement, as do paraprofessionals (those without formalised social work training) working as case managers and interpreters.

In this chapter we focus on the experiences of refugee women[1] resettled in the US and explore the ways in which feminist approaches may enhance social work practice with them. Following an introduction to the causes of and responses to forced migration from a feminist perspective, we discuss the gendered nature of resettlement experiences in the US. While gender was long neglected in the literature surrounding refugees (Busher, 2010; Martin & Tirman, 2009), scholars and practitioners have increasingly been recognising that 'every stage of displacement ... is gendered' (Mertus, 2003, p. 252). We then explore four aspects of feminist theory and articulate their implications for social work practice with refugees: we seek to weave theory with practice. Our own qualitative study of Congolese refugee women undertaken in 2013 (Wachter et al., 2015) offers concrete examples of these implications.

Caveats should be highlighted at this point. While we recognise the spectrum of gender and sexual identities and expressions – a reality crucially affirmed by feminist theorists – we do not explore the implications of these within social practice with refugees in a systematic fashion (Fiddian-Qasmiyeh, 2014). Second, although we do not explicitly address the needs of internally displaced persons, asylum seekers, asylees and undocumented immigrants, or detail the implications of feminist theory in relation to these groups, we hope that the discussion in this chapter will offer insights for social workers allied with these populations. Furthermore, we offer this chapter as feminists, advocates and scholars who have worked in the areas of forced migration, humanitarian assistance and refugee resettlement. None of us have personal experience as refugees, and thus we risk speaking 'for' rather than 'with' those whom we wish to stand alongside (Alcoff, 1991, p. 23). Likewise, we occupy positions of power and privilege related to race, class and formal education. What follows is therefore offered as a contribution to ongoing conversations concerning the role feminisms play in social work practice with refugees, and one upon which we hope that many others will build.

Experiencing forced migration as a woman

A foundational insight of feminist theory is the need to foreground the experiences of women and enhance their visibility as actors, honouring their unique experiences and insights. In this section, we explore the complexity of causes and experiences of forced migration, focusing particularly on aspects that pertain to women.

Root causes, flight and global regime responses

Familiarity with causes and experiences of forced migration as well as the responses of the global refugee regime can directly enhance the quality of social work practice.[2] People migrate for a range of complex, interwoven reasons, and the experiences refugees face before and during their journeys continue to have significant impact as they seek to rebuild their lives in a new place. At a macro level, historical, social, political and economic factors – such as wide wealth disparities between the Global South and North – are structurally significant (Snyder, 2012). Mezzo-level factors, including interpersonal relations and transnational networks (of family, kin and smugglers) that provide resources and information about the migration process, can also impact on decisions to migrate as well as destinations (Castles & Miller, 2009). At the individual or micro level, desire to escape poverty or domestic violence and to seek a better life elsewhere come into play. Turning specifically to forced displacement, political push factors are central. Immediate precipitating factors for movement – political and ethnic conflicts, persecution and violence, war, economic insecurity, natural disasters, food insecurity, disease and environmental degradation – all take place within larger historical, political and environmental contexts (Loescher, 2000; Snyder, 2012). According to the 1951 United Nations Convention Relating to the Status of Refugees, refugees are those who flee their home countries due to a well-founded fear of persecution due to 'race, religion, nationality, membership of a particular social group or political opinion'.

Experiences of forced migration are invariably marked by trauma and duress. Women, men and children may face the sudden loss of home, family members and friends, rape, torture, witnessing atrocities and food insecurity or starvation (Balgopal, 2000; Gerard & Pickering, 2014; Potocky-Tripodi, 2002). Gender-based violence – and sexual violence in particular – is a pervasive danger for women in all violent conflicts and humanitarian crises, and is often used as a strategic tool of war, colonisation and genocide (Nawyn, Reosti & Gjokaj, 2009). While sexual violence does not define what it means to be a refugee woman (Fiddian-Qasmiyeh, 2014), the bodies of many women can 'become sites of symbolic struggle between opposing sides, and also sites of repression because women are seen as bearers of national identity, producers and reproducers of national boundaries, identities and cultures' (Freedman, 2007, pp. 49–50).[3]

Many of the reasons causing women to flee tend to fall outside the narrow and essentially political categorisations allowed by those who constructed refugee laws, definitions and processing apparatus in the post-Second World War era. Indeed, violence against women is usually considered to take place in the personal or 'private' sphere (Crawley, 1999, p. 321), and where women are recognised as political agents they are usually seen as secondary – being dependents of persecuted men. Acts such as female genital mutilation, honour killing or forced sterilisation are regularly attributed to 'cultural differences' rather than human rights violations (Freedman, 2007; Sadoway, 2008). While the persecution of men is often related to state violence, 'women who are persecuted more often are targeted by family members, neighbors, or other acquaintances, and the violence is often sexual' (Nawyn et al., 2009, p. 193). Domestic violence is similarly regarded as private rather than public. Thus, not only do women have to survive and manage their traumatic experiences of gender-based violence in addition to the struggles that all refugees face, but they may also find it difficult to prove that these experiences constitute a convincing legal reason for receiving refugee status (Fiddian-Qasmiyeh, 2014). Our experience suggests that repeated requirements to retell their stories to officials can add to the trauma women experience.

Refugee resettlement in the US

Contemporary global responses to refugees, coordinated by UNHCR, aim to provide protection and humanitarian assistance to those who are displaced. For those who have fled across international borders, the ultimate goal is to repatriate refugees to their country of origin. When repatriation is not possible, UNHCR, host governments and other stakeholders consider local integration in the country of displacement, and lastly resettlement to a third country as a durable solution. Only 1 per cent of refugees registered by UNHCR are selected for resettlement, and a complex set of policies and agendas govern decision making around who is chosen (UNHCR, 2013b).

Reflective of the 1980 Refugee Act, the US Refugee Admissions Program (USRAP) is based on the goal that refugees should integrate into US society and become economically self-sufficient as quickly as possible. The social services and benefits available to refugees resettled through the USRAP mirror these priorities.[4] Consequently, the success of refugees' adaptation to the US context is measured in terms of their employment, and all other aspects of their experience are seen through the lens of economic self-sufficiency.

Resettlement in the US brings stressors to refugee individuals and families. Language, employment and transportation barriers complicate efforts to adapt to the new environment, and the continuing impact of pre-migration and/or flight trauma, torture, violence and hardships present further medical, social and economic challenges (Benson et al., 2012; Choi et al., 2015; Fozdar & Hartley, 2013). Where family, social and community systems have broken down due to war or violence, refugees often lose key support structures and social status that may have previously served as protective factors from stress and psychological distress (Miller & Rasco, 2004).

During the process of resettlement, refugee women tend to face a greater number of stressors and different stressors from their male counterparts (Deacon & Sullivan, 2009). While female refugees often shoulder the burden of providing for their families, they rarely benefit from the status, social support or economic opportunities afforded to men that could assist them in carrying out these responsibilities. Finding employment and developing social support networks may be particularly challenging, as language and cultural barriers keep refugee women isolated, inhibit interactions with receiving communities and hinder connections with other refugees. Traditional family power structures may be challenged when women are obliged to work or find employment outside the home before their husbands do (Mayadas & Segal, 2000; Potocky-Tripodi, 2002), and as children act as interpreters or cultural brokers for their parents (Pipher, 2002). Norms regarding parenting, discipline and conflict resolution may also radically shift (Balgopal, 2000; Puig, 2002). In addition to the *tasks* of resettlement – from finding employment to attending English language classes – women have unique experiences in terms of negotiating a new sense of identity especially in relation to shifting roles and expectations related to gender, race and class. Experiences of flight and exile often lead to the questioning and transformation of personal and group identity (Binder & Tošić, 2005; Deacon & Sullivan, 2009), and migration can simultaneously reaffirm traditional gendered power dynamics and provide opportunities for their transformation (McDowell, 1999; Walton-Roberts, 2004). Structural oppression can be newly or re-inscribed: as Fiddian-Qasmiyeh states, 'integrating into a host state, resettlement state or country of origin may equally lead to new or repeated forms of exclusion and marginalization' (2014, p. 405). For example, the resettlement context may present continued structures of patriarchal oppression, in addition to new forms of discrimination, not least Islamophobia or racism.

Weaving feminist concepts with practice

How, then, might feminist theories enhance social work practice with resettled refugee women? Translating theory into practice is not a straightforward process and we do not intend to offer simple 'how-to' guidelines. Instead, in this section, we invite consideration of a range of possible implications of key feminist insights in social work practice. We host a conversation between theory and practice, exploring interweavings between the two and implications for social work practice. In recognition of the diverse richness of feminist thought, we draw from postcolonial, Chicana, anti-oppression and black feminist scholarship. While there are many conceptual feminist elements that may inform social work practice, we identify and describe four key constructs: (1) valuing intersectional and fluid identities, (2) recognising heterogeneity, (3) affirming agency and (4) sharing power. These concepts are all inherently interrelated. For each, we make suggestions for practice and outline examples from our research on the experiences of Congolese refugee women in the US. While our examples focus on Congolese refugee women, feminist insights have value for work with people along the gender spectrum, including men.

Valuing intersectional and fluid identities

The notion of intersectional and fluid identities is identified by a range of feminist theories and is crucial in considering refugee resettlement practice. The concept of intersectionality recognises that race, gender, religion, ethnicity, age, sexual orientation and class co-exist to shape social identity, behaviour, opportunities and access to rights. Critical race theorist Kimberle Crenshaw (1991) introduced intersectionality as a framework to understand the way multiple forms of oppression are interrelated. Social constructions of age, gender and race do not independently inform identity, discrimination and social inequality, but rather 'mutually construct one another' (Collins, 1998, p. 63). With regard to forced migrant women, social identities may all combine to create unique individual experiences of oppression. In addition, feminists point out that social identities are neither fixed nor static: disparate identities and experiences instead collide and shift over time. Chicana feminists explain that we should not be concerned with the split itself, or choosing one identity over the other, or about shifting between identities. Rather, the challenge lies in making sense of and synthesising the disparate aspects of social identities into non-fragmented, whole (albeit not homogeneous) beings (Moya, 2001). Cherrié Moraga eloquently states, 'I am a woman with a foot in both worlds, and I refuse the split' (Moraga & Anzaldúa, 1981, p. 34). Chandra Talpade Mohanty, a postcolonial and transnational feminist with experience of migration, similarly describes consciousness as 'simultaneously singular and plural' (2003, p. 81).

Two concepts developed by Chicana feminists as elements of mestiza (or mixed-race) consciousness serve as additional lenses through which to consider refugee women's multiple identities: *la facultad* and *nepantla* (Moya, 2001). According to Aída Hurtado (1998), exposure to multiple identities may entail a synthesis of colliding cultures or opposing frameworks. In doing so, those who are marginalised develop *la facultad* – the 'ability to hold multiple social perspectives while simultaneously maintaining a core center' (p. 150) – a transformative survival skill that allows individuals to adjust quickly to changing or threatening circumstances. Gloria Anzaldúa's concept of *nepantla* refers to a sense of in-betweenness and ambiguity experienced by Mexican-American women (Anzaldúa et al.,

2003). *Nepantleras* are the 'supreme border crossers' and, in addition to navigating and managing multiple identities, spaces and realities, are able to construct new meanings and new identities.

Feminist transnationalist perspectives also argue for the dismantling of dualistic thinking of here-versus-there, and value the nuance in the in-between. Linkages between and across time and space are complex, and the notion of transnationalism implies an expansive and fluid sense of place, belonging, identity and responsibility that many individuals and families feel. According to Schiller, Basch and Blanc-Szanton, 'immigrants live their lives across borders and maintain their ties to home, even when their countries of origin and settlement are geographically distant' (1992, p. ix). Economic responsibilities, parenting roles and communication often continue to exist across boundaries after an individual has migrated (Furman et al., 2008). Refugee women's experiences of migration are often quite complex and include many periods and locations of flight and displacement. Literature around transnational motherhood, in particular, examines the ways in which motherhood is socially constructed and altern-ative notions of motherhood are built through migration (Falicov, 2007; Hondagneu-Sotelo & Avila, 1997; Vervliet et al., 2014). Furthermore, 'transnational separations cannot be viewed solely as affecting mothers and children as isolated individuals but, rather, as impacting the intimately experienced bond between them' (Horton, 2009, p. 22).

In the face of assimilationist undercurrents beneath the rhetoric of refugee 'integration' (Balgopal, 2000), feminist affirmations of intersec-tional and fluid identities challenge any assumptions that refugee women prioritise or maintain a single, static identity. They provide support to resist the pressure inherent in refugee resettlement to leave previous iden-tities and transnational relationships and responsibilities at the border in order to integrate into the resettlement community. Social workers are often faced with holding the tension between the resettlement system's goal of household economic self-sufficiency and the importance forced migrants place on financially supporting family in the home country or country of asylum. For example, many refugee women send money, or remittances, to support family and communities back home. Meanwhile, refugee resettlement programmes work towards the aim of refugees cover-ing all their household expenses on a meagre salary before families' resettlement financial resources come to an end.

Recognising heterogeneity

Just as individual refugee women do not possess singular or static identi-ties, we must also recognise the complex diversity within *and* across groups of refugees. Feminist theories encourage us to recognise that women are not homogeneous, and cannot therefore all be responded to in identical ways. It is common for social work practitioners, in misguided attempts towards cultural competence, to make assumptions about refugee women as a whole. Mohanty perceives 'the crux of the problem [to live] in that initial assumption of women as a homogenous group or category ("the oppressed"), a familiar assumption in Western radical and liberal feminisms' (2003, p. 39). Social workers may be easily drawn to making assumptions about the experiences of refugee women, their racial and ethnic identities, class contexts and other elements of social identity. We must strive to challenge the dehumanising myth of homogeneity and to recognise the heterogeneity of *all* refugees – both within refugee groups and within refugee subgroups (Chang-Muy & Congress, 2008; Lenette, 2015).

Mohanty (2003) also articulates global power dynamics that can sometimes lead us to consider refugee women as one homogeneous group. Noting the First–Third World imbalance of power, Mohanty suggests that the hegemonic notion of the superiority of the west produces 'a corresponding set of universal images of the Third World woman', and 'images of the veiled woman, the powerful mother, the chaste virgin, the obedient wife, and so on' (p. 41). She points out that 'besides being normed on a White, Western (read: progressive/modern) or non-Western (read: backward/traditional) hierarchy', we may 'freeze Third World women in time, space, and history' (p. 48).

Today, cultural competence within the social work profession is squarely situated and discussed within a social justice framework, inviting practitioners to resist conceptualising refugees as a homogeneous group (Chang-Muy & Congress, 2008; Lenette, 2015). We need intentionally to cultivate our own understanding of 'diversity' in relation to forced migration and recognise the variety among refugee women we encounter. In addition to understanding the sociocultural contexts they currently inhabit, it is imperative to improve our understanding of the contexts from which individuals come, the crises that caused them to flee and their countries of first asylum. Practitioners and policy makers tend to conflate *nationality or country of origin* with *ethnicity*, disregarding diverse ethnic identities within a resettling group from one country of origin and potential inter-ethnic dynamics at play.

During our study with resettled Congolese refugee women, we observed how identity dynamics could play out in women's resettlement experiences in detrimental ways. For example, we observed that service providers were often not aware of existing tensions among Congolese ethnic groups that were exacerbated by the conflict they were fleeing. Service providers were discouraged from inquiring into this complex and sensitive aspect of people's identities, and lack of information hindered their ability to understand such dynamics. As a result, the refugee resettlement community mistakenly assumed that incoming Congolese would always connect and find support with existing Congolese or other African communities already settled in the US.

While social workers do not need to understand all dynamics and sens-
itivities at play, and we only have so much capacity/time, it is important
for us to go deeper, to invoke questions and interest, and to develop
opportunities to enhance our knowledge. Solid understanding of the
context and circumstances from which refugees fled and were resettled
may help us to anticipate particular needs. For example, gender-based
violence in humanitarian crises and overseas refugee contexts should be
on the radar of resettlement agencies preparing to receive any group. It is
possible that refugee women, men, adolescents and children may be survivors of sexual violence, or otherwise impacted by having witnessed or been
forced to participate in the sexual violence perpetrated against others
(Wachter et al., 2015).

Affirming agency

A third key element stressed by feminist theorists is that people who are
oppressed exercise agency, resilience and courage in the midst of the challenges they face: they – and women in particular – are not simply passive
victims. As Elena Fiddian-Qasmiyeh highlights, 'displaced women [can]
simultaneously be victim*ized* and yet remain active agents deserving of
respect, and not simply pity' (2014, p. 398). While oppression may equate
in large part to 'the absence of choices' (hooks, 2000, p. 32), it is crucial
to recognise the ways in which women and indeed all refugees manage
and negotiate extremely difficult experiences and circumstances creatively
and successfully. Many not only survive but also thrive. During resettlement, however, refugees may find themselves in the damaging position of
needing to identify as vulnerable or traumatised in order to access adequate resettlement support (Westoby & Ingamells, 2010).

Social workers should therefore be careful not to represent refugee
women as being 'needy' while lacking freedom to act: they are *subjects*
rather than passive *objects* in their own migration stories. Women negotiate
a maze of force and opportunity with nuance and deftness and may frequently resist and challenge the injustices and persecution they face. As
Mohanty puts it, 'defining women as archetypal victims freezes them into
"objects-who-defend-themselves," men into "subjects-who-perpetrate-
violence," and (every) society into powerless (read: women) and powerful
(read: men) groups of people' (2003, p. 24). Women are 'agents who
make choices, have a critical perspective on their own situations, and think
and organize collectively against their oppressors' (Mohanty, 2003, p. 72).
If social workers and other well-intentioned refugee supporters fail to
recognise the ingenuity and strength of the women among whom they are
working, they will only succeed in exacerbating their disempowerment.
Too many of us 'refer to the supposed "vulnerability"' of women on the
move without seeking to understand their real needs (Freedman, 2007,
p. 124). Refugee women's voices need to be at the centre of service

provision, programme development and policy making in refugee resettlement, and the multiple strengths, diversity and contributions women bring to the process should be honoured. What is more, whatever legal categorisations might imply, no movement is entirely voluntary or entirely forced: this conventional dichotomy is illusory. While the official refugee definition promotes the notion that refugees migrate against their will, 'almost no movement is entirely voluntary and motivated solely by pull factors or wholly forced and affected only by push factors' (Snyder, 2012, p. 59). All migration is both constrained *and* enabled (Richmond, 1993), and forced migrants make decisions along a continuum that recognises the full complexity of force, choice and agency.

This approach echoes strengths-based perspectives and empowerment models currently emphasised in social work education. As Melinda McPherson points out, 'we must engage with migrants and refugees as current and prospective citizens of potential, rather than responding to "our" privileged constitution of them as "problematic"' (2010, p. 565). Women may need support navigating systems with which they are unfamiliar, and assisting women to identify the skills they already possess and to find the tools they need – especially given all the bureaucracy and paperwork – can be an important way of supporting women as they rediscover their agency.

At national and local levels, organisations and policies need to be transformed in order to respond better to the aspirations, needs and skills of refugee women resettling to the US. Resettlement agencies are increasingly asked to provide additional and specialised services without commensurate resources; however affirming women's agency and meeting the needs of diverse refugee communities will require innovative programmes and increased funding. Social workers should be involved in this work as allies, giving priority to and making space for refugee women to speak out for their own rights.

At a more systemic level, there is a need to develop partnerships and alliances with a range of local organisations, for example addressing domestic violence or sexual assault, as well as between all levels of the refugee resettlement infrastructure: federal resettlement governmental agencies, national and international voluntary organisations, local government and community organisations.

Sharing power

Feminist emphases on the importance of sharing power and fostering non-hierarchical relationships and mutuality are critical to social work practice with refugees. Feminisms and other perspectives have provided social work with tools to move beyond the micro or individual understandings of oppression, to highlight and work towards critical consciousness and deconstructing structurally oppressive systems (Sakamoto & Pitner,

2005). Refugee resettlement social workers are powerful and privileged in the service delivery system, and we are thus presented with the need and the responsibility to assess continually how we, and the organisations within which we operate, perpetuate damaging notions of hierarchy at multiple levels (Sakamoto & Pitner, 2005; Sakamoto, 2007).

As a way to monitor and regulate the use of power in social work settings, feminist practice values reflexivity and the effort to reveal and address power inequalities between social worker and client. Reflexive practice obligates social workers to reflect with honesty, depth and vulnerability on the ways in which our understanding and actions are influenced by our social locations (Garcia, 2008; Lum, 2010; Sakamoto & Pitner, 2005). We also need to reflect on how we influence and are influenced by the social worker–client relationship. As a starting point, social workers must engage refugee women as competent individuals with agency, as co-learners, and as allies in a co-constructed process of resettlement (Hölscher & Bozalek, 2012; Sakamoto, 2007). In addition, there may be times when the provider–client boundaries so important in social work (NASW, 2008) are allowed to become a little more porous, flexible and softened by mutuality. Embracing a culturally relevant, respectful and caring communication style with refugee clients oftentimes places the social worker in a position that appears less formal or professional than in other fields of practice. Refugee clients may view the social worker as an extension of their social network, particularly as trust and rapport are established. Furthermore, social workers must be mindful of who is speaking for families, engage refugee women directly in resettlement decisions and ensure communication in the language of their preference (as opposed to only consulting male heads of household or foregoing language interpretation).

Aiming for non-hierarchical relationships and shared power goes well beyond individual (self-reflection) and interpersonal (client–worker relationship) levels. In a field of practice that is intimately interwoven with global structures, social workers need to focus on challenging power inequalities at the level of programme development and policy making. This requires advocacy and attention to macro-level discourse concerning the construction of refugee women within the resettlement system, as well as micro-level clinical interventions. While traditional case management models of service provision are tremendously valuable, rigid notions around the mechanisms through which services are provided may need to be challenged, such as the binary roles of service provider and client (i.e. service provider as 'expert' benefactor and client as passive recipient), the expectations of clients to engage with – and benefit from – prescriptive services with pre-determined and fixed time frames, and assumptions that case management models are the best (or only) ways to respond effectively to refugee women's needs. Embodying a feminist approach, the social work profession can help to carve out much needed space for refugee women to inform modalities for service delivery that is more responsive to their strengths and needs.

Conclusion

Valuing multiple, intersecting and fluid identities, recognising heterogeneity, affirming agency and sharing power are key feminist social work principles, and should become integral to the ways we respond to displaced women. Our call to action, as social workers who operate in multiple realms of practice – micro and macro practice, policy and research – is twofold. First, we need to undertake small acts of resistance in everyday interactions with refugee women. That is, we are mindful of, reflective about and challenge our own power and privilege we bring to our work and possibly perpetuate by failing to allow space for the expertise of refugee women in policy making and programme development. Second, we are called to be intentional and active in challenging the larger structures at play in refugee resettlement – that is, the structures that impede engagement from refugee women themselves and reduce women's experiences and identities to being homogenised, fixed and powerless. We are called to advocate. Ultimately, this entails careful restructuring of our responses to refugees and displaced persons, refugee resettlement programming, training of future resettlement workers and research – and doing so in the spirit of solidarity.

Notes

1 In this chapter, we use the term 'refugee women' because we focus on those termed 'refugees' in the US. We recognise that the broader term 'forced migrant' is used in much of the recent literature.

2 It is important not to speak of '*the* refugee experience', but rather to recognise the diversity among the stories of those who are displaced.

3 In addition to experiencing violence directly, refugee women may witness violence and/or be involved in perpetrating violence associated with war, conflict or displacement.

4 For example, refugee resettlement funding and programmes support placing refugees in jobs *as soon as possible* after arrival, offering English language training *in non-work hours where possible* and providing cash assistance in such a manner *as not to discourage their economic self-sufficiency.*

Further reading

Anzaldúa, G. & Saldívar-Hull, S. (1999) *Borderlands/La Frontera: The New Mestiza.* Aunt Lute Books, San Francisco, CA.

Busch-Armendariz, N.B., Wachter, K., Cook Heffron, L., Nsonwu, M.B. & Snyder, S. (2014) *The Continuity of Risk: A Three City Study of Resettled Congolese Refugee Women.* University of Texas at Austin, Austin, TX.

Chang-Muy, F. & Congress, E. (2008) *Social Work with Immigrants and Refugees.* Springer, New York.

Fiddian-Qasmiyeh, E. (2014) Gender and forced migration. In E. Fiddian-Qasmiyeh, G. Loescher, K. Long & N. Sigona (eds), *The Oxford Handbook of Refugee and Forced Migration Studies.* Oxford University Press, Oxford, pp. 395–408.

Fadiman, A. (2012) *The Spirit Catches You and You Fall Down: A Hmong Child, her American Doctors, and the Collision of Two Cultures.* Macmillan, New York.
Freedman, J. (2007) *Gendering the International Asylum and Refugee Debate.* Palgrave Macmillan, Basingstoke, UK.
Makepeace, A. (producer & director) (2007) *Rain in a Dry Land* [Motion picture]. Anne Makepeace Productions, Lakeville, CT.
Mohanty, C.T. (2003) *Feminism without Borders: Decolonizing Theory, Practicing Solidarity.* Zubaan, New Delhi.

References

Alcoff, L. (1991) The problem of speaking for others. *Cultural Critique*, 20, pp. 5–32.
Anzaldúa, G.E., Ortiz, S.J., Hernández-Avila, I. & Perez, D. (2003) Speaking across the divide. *Studies in American Indian Literatures*, 15(3/4), pp. 7–22.
Balgopal, P.R. (2000) Social work practice with immigrants and refugees: an overview. In P.R. Balgopal (ed.), *Social Work Practice with Immigrants and Refugees.* Columbia University Press, New York, pp. 1–29.
Benson, G.O., Sun, F., Hodge, D.R. & Androff, D.K. (2012) Religious coping and acculturation stress among Hindu Bhutanese: a study of newly-resettled refugees in the United States. *International Social Work*, 55(4), pp. 538–553.
Binder, S. & Tošić, J. (2005) Refugees as a particular form of transnational migrations and social transformations: socioanthropological and gender aspects. *Current Sociology*, 53(4), pp. 607–624.
Busher, D. (2010) Refugee women: twenty years on. *Refugee Survey Quarterly*, 29(2), pp. 4–20.
Castles, S. & Miller, M.J. (2009) *The Age of Migration: International Population Movements in the Modern World.* Palgrave Macmillan, New York.
Chang-Muy, F. & Congress, E. (2008) *Social Work with Immigrants and Refugees.* Springer, New York.
Choi, S., Davis, C., Cummings, S., Van Regenmorter, C. & Barnett, M. (2015) Understanding service needs and service utilization among older Kurdish refugees and immigrants in the USA. *International Social Work*, 58(1), pp. 63–74.
Collins, P.H. (1998) It's all in the family: intersections of gender, race, and nation. *Hypatia*, 13(3), 62–82.
Crawley, H. (1999) Women and refugee status: beyond the public/private dichotomy in UK asylum policy. In D.M. Indra (ed.), *Engendering Forced Migration: Theory and Practice.* Berghahn Books, Oxford, pp. 308–333.
Crenshaw, K. (1991) Mapping the margins: intersectionality, identity politics, and violence against women of color. *Stanford Law Review*, 43(6), pp. 1241–1299.
Deacon, Z. & Sullivan, C. (2009) Responding to the complex and gendered needs of refugee women. *AFFILIA: The Journal of Women and Social Work*, 24(3), pp. 272–284.
Falicov, C.J. (2007) Working with transnational immigrants: expanding meanings of family, community, and culture. *Family Process*, 46(2), pp. 157–171.
Fiddian-Qasmiyeh, E. (2014) Gender and forced migration. In E. Fiddian-Qasmiyeh, G. Loescher, K. Long & N. Sigona (eds), *The Oxford Handbook of Refugee and Forced Migration Studies.* Oxford University Press, Oxford, pp. 395–408.
Fozdar, F. & Hartley, L. (2013) Refugee resettlement in Australia: what we know and need to know. *Refugee Survey Quarterly*, 32(3), pp. 23–51.

Freedman, J. (2007) *Gendering the International Asylum and Refugee Debate*. Palgrave Macmillan, Basingstoke, UK.

Furman, R., Negi, N., Schatz, M.C.S. & Jones, S. (2008) Transnational social work: using a wraparound model. *Global Networks*, 8(4), pp. 496–503.

Garcia, B. (2008). Theory and social work practice with immigrant populations. In F. Chang-Muy & E. Congress (eds), *Social Work with Immigrants and Refugees*. Springer, New York, pp. 79–101.

Gerard, A. & Pickering, S. (2014) Gender, securitization and transit: refugee women and the journey to the EU. *Journal of Refugee Studies*, 27(3), pp. 338–359.

Hajdukowski-Ahmed, M., Khanlou, N. & Moussa, H. (eds) (2008) *Not Born a Refugee Woman: Contesting Identities, Rethinking Practices*. Berghahn, New York.

Hölscher, D. & Bozalek, V.G. (2012) Encountering the other across the divides: re-grounding social justice as a guiding principle for social work with refugees and other vulnerable groups. *British Journal of Social Work*, 42(6), pp. 1093–1112.

Hondagneu-Sotelo, P. & Avila, E. (1997) I'm here, but I'm there. *Gender and Society*, 11(5), pp. 548–571.

hooks, b. (2000) *Feminist Theory: From Margin to Center*. Pluto Press, London.

Horton, S. (2009) A mother's heart is weighed down with stones: a phenomenological approach to the experience of transnational motherhood. *Culture, Medicine, and Psychiatry*, 33(1), pp. 21–40.

Hurtado, A. (1998). Sitios y lenguas: Chicanas theorize feminisms. *Hypatia*, 13(2), 134–161.

Lenette, C. (2015) Mistrust and refugee women who are lone parents in resettlement contexts. *Qualitative Social Work*, 14(1), pp. 119–134.

Loescher, G. (2000) Forced migration in the post-Cold War era: the need for a comprehensive approach. In B. Ghosh (ed.), *Managing Migration: Time for a New International Regime?* Oxford University Press, Oxford, pp. 190–219.

Lum, D. (ed.) (2010) *Culturally Competent Practice: A Framework for Understanding Diverse Groups and Justice Issues*. Cengage Learning, South Melbourne, Vic.

McDowell, L. (1999) *Gender, Identity, and Place: Understanding Feminist Geographies*. University of Minnesota Press, Minneapolis, MN.

McPherson, M. (2010) 'I integrate, therefore I am': contesting the normalizing discourse of integrationism through conversations with refugee women. *Journal of Refugee Studies*, 23(4), pp. 546–570.

Martin, S.F. & Tirman, J. (eds) (2009) *Women, Migration, and Conflict: Breaking a Deadly Cycle*. Springer, Dordrecht.

Mayadas, N.S. & Segal, U.A. (2000) Refugees in the 1990s: a US perspective. In P.R. Balgopal (ed.), *Social Work Practice with Immigrants and Refugees*. Columbia University Press, New York, pp. 198–227.

Mertus, J. (2003) Sovereignty, gender, and displacement. In E. Newman & J. Van Selm (eds), *Refugees and Forced Displacement: International Security, Human Vulnerability and the State*. UN University Press, Tokyo, pp. 250–273.

Miller, K.E. & Rasco, L.M. (eds) (2004) *The Mental Health of Refugees: Ecological Approaches to Healing and Adaptation*. Lawrence Erlbaum Associates, Mahwah, NJ.

Mohanty, C.T. (2003) *Feminism without Borders: Decolonizing Theory, Practicing Solidarity*. Zubaan, New Delhi.

Moraga, C. & Anzaldúa, G. (1981) *This Bridge Called my Back: Writings by Radical Women of Color*. Persephone Press, Watertown, MA.

Moya, P.M.L. (2001) Chicana feminism and postmodernist theory. *Signs*, 26(2), pp. 441–483.

National Association of Social Workers (NASW) (2008) *Code of Ethics*. NASW, Washington, DC.

Nawyn, S.J., Reosti, A. & Gjokaj, L. (2009) Gender in motion: how gender precipitates international migration. *Advances in Gender Research*, 13, pp. 175–202.

Pipher, M.B. (2002) *The Middle of Everywhere: The World's Refugees Come to our Town*. Houghton Mifflin Harcourt, Orlando, FL.

Potocky-Tripodi, M. (2002) *Best Practices for Social Work with Refugees and Immigrants*. Columbia University Press, New York.

Puig, M.E. (2002) The adultification of refugee children: implications for cross-cultural social work practice. *Journal of Human Behavior in the Social Environment*, 5(3–4), 85–95.

Richmond, A.H. (1993) Reactive migration: sociological perspectives on refugee movements. *Journal of Refugee Studies*, 6(1), pp. 7–24.

Sadoway, G. (2008) The gender factor in refugee determination and the effect of 'gender guidelines'. In M. Hajdukowski-Ahmed, N. Khanlou & H. Moussa (eds), *Not Born a Refugee Woman: Contesting Identities, Rethinking Practices*. Berghan, New York, pp. 244–253.

Sakamoto, I. (2007) A critical examination of immigrant acculturation: toward an anti-oppressive social work model with immigrant adults in a pluralistic society. *British Journal of Social Work*, 37(3), pp. 515–535.

Sakamoto, I. & Pitner, R.O. (2005) Use of critical consciousness in anti-oppressive social work practice: disentangling power dynamics at personal and structural levels. *British Journal of Social Work*, 35(4), pp. 435–452.

Schiller, N.G., Basch, L. & Blanc-Szanton, C. (1992) Towards a definition of transnationalism. *Annals of the New York Academy of Sciences*, 645(1), pp. ix–xiv.

Snyder, S. (2012) *Asylum-Seeking, Migration and Church*. Ashgate, Farnham, UK.

UNHCR (2013a) New UNHCR report says global forced displacement at 18-year high. *UNHCR News Stories*, 19 June. www.unhcr.org/51c071816.html (accessed 27 April 2015).

UNHCR (2013b) *Resettlement*. UNHCR. www.unhcr.org/pages/4a16b1676.html (accessed 5 October 2013).

Vervliet, M., De Mol, J., Broekaert, E. & Derluyn, I. (2014) 'That I live, that's because of her': intersectionality as framework for unaccompanied refugee mothers. *British Journal of Social Work*, 44(7), pp. 2023–2024.

Wachter, K., Cook Heffron, L., Snyder, S., Nsownu, M.B. & Busch-Armendariz, N.B. (2015) Unsettled integrations: pre- and post-migration factors in Congolese refugee women's experiences in the United States. *International Social Work*. DOI: 10.1177/0020872815580049.

Walton-Roberts, M. (2004) Transnational migration theory in population geography: gendered practices in networks linking Canada and India. *Population, Space and Place*, 10(5), pp. 361–373.

Westoby, P. & Ingamells, A. (2010) A critically informed perspective on working with resettling refugee groups in Australia. *British Journal of Social Work*, 40(6), pp. 1759–1776.

12 Putting gender in the frame

Feminist social work and mental health

Nicole Moulding

Since second wave feminists drew attention to the connections between mental health and the social conditions of women's lives, feminist social workers have endeavoured to engage with gender in their work with women experiencing mental health problems. This has included developing ways of working that challenge pathologising and paternalistic medical approaches. However, feminist perspectives are in little evidence in mainstream mental health systems, as medical discourses about the biological basis of mental illness and pharmacological treatments continue to dominate, and most social workers therefore practise within highly medicalised settings that are largely gender-blind. In spite of the fact that feminist approaches to women's mental health are marginalised in the mainstream, there has been a burgeoning of feminist research into gender and mental health over the past 30 years, with most of this work originating from outside social work. In this chapter, I explore the contributions of this knowledge for feminist social work, and consider how we might make best use of its insights. I particularly focus on research and practice with women who have histories of gendered violence and abuse because it is increasingly recognised that the heavier burden of poor mental health carried by women is at least in part traceable to this (see Walby, 2004).

The growth of 'gender-blind' perspectives on mental health and illness

Historically, femininity has been closely associated with 'madness' (Ussher, 1991). While women are disproportionately represented among individuals diagnosed with mental health problems, the conflation of femininity and madness is more fundamental than this, and reflects core historical assumptions about femininity and masculinity. Early representations of mental illness often took a female form, and eighteenth and nineteenth century English literature and art are replete with images of 'the mad woman in the attic', reflecting but also reproducing the assumption that women are inherently less psychologically robust than men (Chesler, 2005; Showalter, 1987). During this period, as psychiatry staked its claim over mental illness as a disease rather than a religious or moral affliction, madness became increasingly understood as feminine and was often referred to as 'the female malady' (Showalter, 1987). However, women outnumber men only in the diagnosis of certain conditions. Thus, more women are diagnosed with anxiety and depression (ABS, 2007) and, because these are by far the most common mental health conditions across the population as a whole, the overall numbers of women reporting mental health problems is therefore higher. Women also predominate in relation to eating disorders and the diagnosis of so-called borderline personality disorder (APA, 2013), conditions that are widely recognised as reflecting profoundly gendered and culture-bound discourses and prac- tices in contemporary societies (Bordo, 1988, 1990; Wirth-Cauchon, 2001). Men, on the other hand, outnumber women in drug and alcohol abuse and personality disorders (APA, 2013), while psychotic disorders such as schizophrenia are relatively equal between the genders (ABS, 2007). Thus, women do not outnumber men in the diagnosis of the more severe mental illnesses that are most commonly thought of as 'madness'. The historical conflation of madness with the feminine is therefore somewhat mislead- ing, but it is nonetheless powerful, underpinned as it is by longstanding discourses about the emotional and irrational feminine, and the rational and controlled masculine (Showalter, 1987). More accurately, individual experiences of mental illness can be understood as framed by gender (as well as race, class and other social positionings) in different ways, demon- strated most crudely in the above diagnostic divisions by gender. However, as indicated above, gendered violence and abuse also go at least some way towards explaining the higher burden of poor mental health among women (Walby, 2004), as well as other pressures associated with con- temporary femininities.

As part of the second wave of feminism in western countries in the 1960s and 1970s, critical feminist attention turned to women's experiences of mental illness as a problem borne of gender inequality. Phyllis Chesler's (2005) ground-breaking book *Women and Madness*, first published in 1972, traced the historically higher reports of mental illness among women to patriarchy and misogyny or, in other words, to the complete devaluing of all things feminine. Thus, perhaps for the first time, women's psychologi- cal distress was understood as a function of patriarchal relations and sexism rather than inherent female weakness. As a feminised profession with predominantly female clients and a commitment to social justice, social work had strong and even natural ties with the feminist movement, and many social workers were greatly influenced by these ideas. During this same period, the women's movement was also exposing widespread male-perpetrated sexual assault, child sexual abuse and domestic violence, and gender power relations were also seen as particularly central to these experiences (Breckenridge, 1999). More dedicated feminist attention to the connections between mental health and male-perpetrated violence and abuse came a little later in the 1980s as awareness of the extent of child sexual abuse and adult sexual assault grew (Breckenridge, 1999). Therapeutic work with women who had histories of child sexual abuse became an increasing focus of practice for social workers and other counsellors in feminist women's services in western countries such as Australia, and awareness of sexual abuse as a form of male aggression against women and children remained pivotal to this. I worked as a social worker in women's health centres during this period, and we took an explicitly feminist approach to women's mental health more generally and to working with the effects of male-perpetrated violence in particular.

In spite of feminist efforts to draw attention to the social basis of women's experiences of mental illness, mainstream psychiatry, medicine and psychology have taken an increasingly biological, medical and gender-blind (although not gender-neutral) approach to mental health problems over the past three decades, with genetic explanations and the idea of 'unbalanced' chemicals in the brain pre-eminent (Ussher, 2010). While some conditions that particularly affect women have also been explained through recourse to 'hormones' (Ussher, 1991), most contemporary medical and psychological explanations of mental illness simply fail to account for gender at all. For example, as I mentioned above, eating disorders and borderline personality disorder are far more commonly diagnosed in women yet dominant psychiatric and psychological explanations focus on genes, 'bad' mothering, dysfunctional families and 'personality vulnerabilities' (Moulding, 2003, 2006; Wirth-Cauchon, 2001). In the reductive style of reasoning underpinning positivist science, the social context of women's lives is usually given little explanatory power because not all women experience mental illness: the 'environment' is therefore placed at a distance from the individual and the focus remains on biological, intra-psychic and family factors thought to distinguish 'sick' from 'normal' individuals (Krieger, 1994).

While there continues to be little attention to gender within medicine and mainstream psychology, there has been a burgeoning of interest in the effects of child sexual abuse. When feminists broke the silence on child sexual abuse in the 1980s, the 'child sexual abuse industry' was born (Armstrong, 2000) and now mainly comprises mainstream mental health researchers and clinicians. While the trauma model used to explain the links between abuse and mental health at least gives some credence to the role of environment in mental health problems (Warner, 2009), the child sexual abuse industry has also promulgated the idea of 'victim-illness' (Armstrong, 2000) and the 'harm' story of abuse (O'Dell, 2003), and has largely lost sight of feminist understandings of sexual assault as male aggression based on systems of male privilege (Armstrong, 2000; Warner, 2009). So even in this area, where gender is obviously pivotal, there is virtually no attention to it within medicine and psychology, and health professionals instead focus on determining and treating an array of psychopathologies in victims.

It is against this backdrop of growing medicalisation and individualisation that social work has become increasingly involved in the mental health area as the focus of services has moved from institutional care to care in the community over the past three decades. Most social workers continue to take a broadly social view of mental health and illness (for example, Bland, Renouf & Tullgren, 2015; Tew, 2008), but an explicit feminist perspective is arguably less common now than in the past. The approach to mental health currently dominant in social work is the recovery model. In spite of the fact that most mental health systems around the world remain medically oriented in practice, the past two decades have seen the rise of the recovery approach and, in Australia, this has now been adopted into mental health policy across most jurisdictions as the framework for mental health services (Courtney & Moulding, 2014). The recovery model emerged from the consumer-led mental illness movement in the US and its principles are highly consistent with social work values and ethics (Courtney & Moulding, 2014), emphasising the unique nature of individual lived experience (Deegan, 1996) and the social context of mental illness (Bland et al., 2015). The approach also grew from concern about the treatment of people with more severe mental illness and this orientation usually remains in most versions of the recovery model. However, while the recovery model challenges paternalism and assumptions of chronicity in mental illness, in most of its incarnations it does not particularly trouble medical understandings about the nature and causes of mental illness: indeed, it actively eschews questions of causation and leaves medical definitions and understandings largely intact. Nor does the model particularly engage with the question of gender but instead takes a gender-neutral, humanistic approach that emphasises individual uniqueness. Its focus on the severe end of the mental illness continuum, where the numbers of women and men are relatively equivalent, perhaps also contributes to this gender-neutral perspective. Thus, while more social workers than ever before are involved in the provision of mental health services, most may not particularly relate to feminist ideas and are primarily informed by a relatively gender-neutral recovery model. Over this same period, though, feminist researchers and scholars have built, and continue to build, a substantial body of research and knowledge in gender and mental health. Next, I explore some of this more recent feminist work and consider the implications for feminist-informed mental health practice in social work.

Post-structuralist feminism and mental health

While earlier feminist research into gender and mental health brought important critical insights into the sexism of psychiatry and psychology, and their blindness to the social conditions of women's lives, it also situated women's mental illness quite broadly and universally as a function of patriarchy. As such, feminism could not account very well for why only some women struggled with mental health problems or for differences in women's experiences according to race, class and other social inequalities. More recent feminist research into gender and mental health conducted since the 1990s has been predominantly post-structuralist in orientation, and a characteristic feature of this perspective is that it is not concerned with establishing a particular causal explanation for mental illness, nor does it assume or imply that women's experiences are universal. This body of research has looked instead to the discourses and practices that construct individual experiences, with mental illnesses understood as particular forms of subjectivity rather than as indicative of psychopathology per se. Largely drawing on the ideas of Foucault, post-structuralist feminist approaches have been used to examine historically specific gender and medical discourses applied to women deemed mentally ill, and the intersections and contradictions within them (for example, Bordo, 1988; Malson, 1998; Wirth-Cauchon, 2001). An understanding of power and knowledge as connected and reinforced by the powerful institution of medicine has further enabled deconstruction of psychiatric 'truths' to reveal their basis in gendered social discourses rather than scientific fact.

My own post-structuralist feminist research into eating disorders shows how supposedly gender-neutral psycho-medical theories and treatments are underpinned by gendered discourses about healthy selfhood as masculinised autonomy and control, and unhealthy, deficient selfhood as feminised dependence and lack of control (Moulding, 2003, 2006, 2009). This, I have argued, reproduces the gendered contradictions implicated in producing eating disorders in the first place. For example, Bordo (1990) has demonstrated that women pursue thinness because it symbolises masculinised control over the dangerous, out-of-control female body (Bordo, 1990). I have argued further that reproduction of this tension in traditional psychiatric treatments could help to explain why they have been largely unsuccessful: they rely on women's capitulation to supposed feminine frailty when this is the very positioning that is usually being so strenuously resisted through the eating disorder. In another example, Wirth-Cauchon shows how borderline personality disorder, which is commonly diagnosed in women with sexual abuse histories, has come to replace the Victorian psychiatric condition of hysteria as 'the new female malady' (2001, p. 2). Wirth-Cauchon demonstrates how the conceptualisation of hysteria was focused on a Freudian problematisation of unconscious sexual desire in women in the Victorian era. In contrast, contemporary notions of borderline personality disorder centre the idea of an unstable or even missing 'self' in the context of shifts in women's sexual freedoms and the emergence of 'the regime of the self' in the second half of the twentieth century (Wirth-Cauchon, 2001). Wirth-Cauchon shows how the category of borderline personality disorder therefore reflects contemporary women's social positioning more generally as 'borderline' between 'cultural conceptions of feminine identity and generic selfhood' (p. 6), with this group of women particularly embodying this social violence and paying its costs through their resistance to it.

There is also a robust body of post-structuralist feminist research into the effects of child sexual abuse, mainly from feminist critical psychologists. Reavey (2003) and Warner and Wilkins (2003) show that many of the symptoms identified in women as a result of child sexual abuse are also associated with 'femininity' more generally, that is, irrationality, powerlessness and unreasonableness. However, the assumptions about gender that underlie the identification of these supposed traits are never flagged and remain hidden in mainstream approaches (Reavey, 2003). Warner and Wilkins (2003) point out that the 'symptoms' of borderline personality disorder, such as emotional lability, rage, self-destructiveness, depression and feelings of emptiness, are also commonly associated with 'normative femininity' (p. 172). Thus, they argue that borderline personality disorder can be understood as 'the social embodiment of child sexual abuse, as well as (already pathologised) femininity' (p. 172). O'Dell (2003) shows how a discourse of development enables a positioning of women and children as products of their abusive pasts, with abuse seen as disrupting this developmental pathway so that the abused child becomes 'other' to the non-abused 'normal' child, and women become lifelong, damaged victims. Warner (2009) identifies how the gender discourses in workers' and women's accounts of mental illness and child sexual abuse are often highly contradictory, with women paradoxically both passive and responsible for abuse. She argues that the whole debate must be shifted to asking questions about the worlds women live in rather than making assumptions about 'what's gone wrong in their heads' (p. 139).

Post-structuralist feminist research has therefore demonstrated how women face a double bind in relation to mental health which plays out at two mutually reinforcing discursive levels. Hence, western conceptualisations of healthy and unhealthy selfhood are scaffolded by a derogation of the feminine and a valorisation of the masculine, enabling pathologisation of supposedly 'feminine' traits against a male-defined generic subject. At the same time, many of the mental health problems women face are framed by these self-same cultural contradictions about femininity and generic selfhood. Thus, in relation to child sexual abuse and mental health, feminists have elaborated the ways that gender discourses structure both the explanations of child sexual abuse and the theories used to explain women's subsequent mental health problems. Also common to post-structuralist feminist work on mental health is the elaboration of highly gendered mental illnesses such as eating disorders and borderline personality disorder as forms of resistance to contradictory gender discourses and practices.

Navigating the discursive and the material

Post-structuralist feminism has been criticised for focusing on the symbolic and discursive to the exclusion of the material, lived reality of gender oppression in women's lives (McNay, 2004), as well as for overly romanticising the symptoms of mental illness as protest (Ussher, 2010). However, some contemporary feminist researchers increasingly seek to attend quite explicitly both to the discourses framing women's experiences of mental illness and to the lived, material reality of that experience (for example, Ussher, 2010). In my own work on gendered violence and mental health, I have adopted McNay's (2004) concept of situated intersubjectivity to navigate a path between the discursive and material aspects of women's mental health (Moulding, 2016). Situated intersubjectivity understands the discursive aspects of identity and everyday intersubjective material power relations as inherently intertwined (McNay, 2004). McNay argues that absorbing everything, including society, into language fails to see the 'the complex and uneven ways in which gender inequalities are produced' (p. 174), including underestimating how intractable some forms of oppression are and overestimating how much change can be brought through cultural identity politics. Post-structuralist feminist research into gender and mental health can reflect this problem by remaining only at a discursive level of explanation, and by prioritising individual and conceptual/symbolic change over structural change. As McNay (2004) argues, such an emphasis can become inadvertently complicit with individualism rather than a more radical politics. Moreover, I argue that the need for symbolic and structural change are arguably tied together and both are required simultaneously.

Sometimes post-structuralist feminist work in mental health also approaches knowledge as if all claims are equivalent, and this relativism can play down the identification of dominant discourses and associated gender power relations. On the other hand, materialist feminism can lack a 'hermeneutic notion of self and a coherent account of subjectivity and agency through which the daily experiences of economic, social and cultural oppression might be conceived of as co-extensive rather than crudely determining of each other' (McNay, 2004, p. 175). A notion of the self is important to the study of gender and mental health because without feminist ways of theorising and understanding the thinking, feeling, acting subject and her gendered positioning, we are left with gendered medical notions of psychopathology and damaged selves. Historically, materialist feminism has not particularly applied itself to the field of gender and mental health, or to challenging the dominance of psycho-medical theories and practices: the dominance of this type of feminism in social work might to some extent explain the lack of social work presence in scholarly work on gender and mental health. Thus, as McNay (2004) argues, the concept of situated intersubjectivity is a useful corrective to the individualising tendencies of post-structuralism, because it explicitly embeds the subject in social relations, and also counteracts a materialist tendency to prioritise structures over experience by emphasising intention and agency on the part of the subject.

Gendered violence, abuse and mental health is arguably an area that particularly requires attention to both the discursive and the material:

irrespective of their theoretical persuasion, most feminists would agree that male privilege and unequal gender power relations frame these experiences, and that they have serious material consequences for women's emotional and physical wellbeing. In my own more recent research, I have attempted to navigate the discursive and material dimensions of women's mental health experiences in response to childhood physical, emotional and sexual abuse, and in relation to domestic violence. This research has sought to illuminate women's violence-related emotional distress through deconstruction of the social meanings embedded within the abuse they have experienced and the gender power relations framing this, rather than through recourse to psychological discourses. As such, violence-related emotional distress is located within intersubjective social relationships rather than within individual women (Tew, 2008), including those of race and class in addition to gender.

One of the studies I have undertaken from this perspective involved a narrative-discursive analysis of women's accounts of childhood emotional abuse and later mental health problems. The research focused on childhood emotional abuse because there is evidence that it has the greatest impact on mental health of any single type of childhood abuse (Schneider, Baumrind & Kimerling, 2007; O'Dougherty Wright, Crawford & Del Castillo, 2009). Childhood emotional abuse is also the most common form of abuse (AIHW, 2014; Stoltenborgh et al., 2011). While the negative impact of childhood emotional abuse is now recognised, and there has been some attention to its raced and classed dimensions (May-Chahal, 2006), no existing research considers its gender dimensions in spite of the fact that it is more commonly reported by girls and women (Scher et al., 2004), it often occurs alongside sexual abuse (Briere & Runtz, 1993; Higgins & McCabe, 2001; De Groot & Rodin, 1999; Messman-Moore & Garrigus, 2007) and it seems to have a more negative impact on girls than boys (Itzin, Taket & Barter-Godfrey, 2010), particularly when it is perpetrated by fathers (Downs & Miller, 1998). Both mothers and fathers perpetrate childhood emotional and physical abuse, and in more equivalent proportions than for child sexual abuse, however, examination of gender needs to extend beyond prevalence counts of perpetrators and victims to consider the ways gender discourses, interpersonal gender dynamics and gender power relations frame these experiences (May-Chahal, 2006).

This study demonstrated how childhood emotional abuse can turn up the volume on a host of contradictory gender discourses about women, selfhood, identity and femininity in the context of shifts in contemporary gender relations (Moulding, 2016). In contrast to mainstream research in this area, women were specifically asked what was *done* and *said* to them, by *whom* and in what *context* in order to illuminate the gendered dimensions of their experiences. In response, women described abuse that was highly controlling of their behaviour and often (but not only) concerned with stereotypically feminine domains such as bodily appearance, sexuality and domestic responsibilities. Analysis further demonstrated how this type of abuse reproduces dualistic and moralistic femininity discourses about women as either 'good' or 'bad', or 'for others' versus 'for themselves', which then play out in highly gendered emotions of shame, guilt, ambivalence and worthlessness. While childhood emotional abuse is therefore shown to be a powerful tool of engendering within the family, the study also showed that many women exercise agency in removing themselves from abusive family relationships and in resisting medicalised understandings of their experiences.

I have also been involved with colleagues in a large mixed methods survey and interview study focusing on domestic violence, and this also offered up insights into how specific types of gendered violence and abuse relate to particular forms of emotional distress.[1] Analysis of women's accounts demonstrated how the imposition of domestic, sexual and even financial 'servicing' in violent and controlling relationships is embedded in longstanding sociocultural discourses and practices that position women as sexualised 'objects of exchange' between male subjects rather than as subjects or persons in their own right. The analysis showed how this positioning produces feelings of lost sense of self and agency for many women, which conflict with other contemporary discourses and practices based on notions of gender equality and rights, well as with their own experiences of themselves as agentic selves prior to violent relationships. In common with other forms of gendered abuse, but in its own distinctive way, domestic violence is therefore shown to exaggerate broader contradictions about femininity and generic selfhood in contemporary societies, producing sometimes quite profound feelings of lost identity, shame, guilt, fear (especially of men), ambivalence and worthlessness for many women, but also shock and anger at being stripped of their former status as persons. As in the childhood emotional abuse study, many women also resisted medical understandings of their emotional distress and, in addition to leaving violent relationships, some described feelings of betrayal and a withdrawal from relationships with family and friends because of a perceived lack of understanding and support, and victim blaming.

Both of these studies therefore elaborated the peculiarly *gendered* nature of women's emotional distress in response to specific types of violence and abuse, and showed how the universal psychiatric diagnoses of 'post-traumatic stress disorder', 'anxiety' and 'depression' simply fail to capture this in any meaningful way. Moreover, in the domestic violence study, women's mental health was further compromised by real, ongoing fears about escalating violence, particularly after leaving relationships, as well as significant deterioration in the material conditions of their lives. This included lower incomes, poorer housing, increased child-care responsibilities, reduced work hours, social isolation, the stigma of single parenthood and poverty. Such factors are known to have a compounding negative impact on mental health (Bland et al., 2015), drawing attention in a particularly stark way to the intersections between the discursive, the material and the structural dimensions of women's poor mental health in contexts of gendered violence and abuse.

Feminist-informed approaches to mental health social work

In spite of growing recognition of the connections between gendered violence, abuse and poor mental health, women's symptoms are often detached from the violence and abuse itself in mainstream mental health services, or violence and abuse go unrecognised because practitioners do not enquire into it (Humphreys & Thiara, 2003). While I am not suggesting that mainstream services are incapable of responding appropriately to gendered violence and abuse, I argue that feminist-informed approaches enable a more situated perspective that locates women's distress in the contradictory gender discourses and power relations that frame their lives, thereby avoiding victim blaming and offering greater scope for both individual and social change. Since the second wave women's movement, social workers have endeavoured to develop feminist-informed ways of working with women across multiple levels of practice that are understood to be fundamentally interconnected, including one-to-one therapy and group work, as well as community- and society-wide interventions focused on prevention. Here, I briefly consider feminist approaches at each of these levels of intervention, as well as feminist-informed social work education in mental health, with a specific focus on working with women who are struggling with mental health problems in response to gendered violence and abuse. Before considering these approaches, it is first necessary to point out that, in working with domestic violence in particular, it is important for social workers also to attend to women's and children's safety, and to practical needs for housing, employment and income support, in addition to responding to emotional distress (Itzin et al., 2010).

There are many feminist-informed approaches to therapeutic intervention but I have chosen to briefly discuss Michael White's (2004) narrative therapy approach to working with women who have experienced multiple traumas because it resonates well with many of the insights from the research described earlier. Narrative therapy is not new and is widely known and practised, so I will not outline the approach here (see White & Epston, 1989 for a detailed explanation). In relation to working with women with histories of abuse, White (2004) specifically talks about attending to women's emotional responses, such as feelings of shame, and listening for, encouraging and acknowledging what women have continued to value in life in spite of trauma based on the assumption that abuse has often demeaned their views and realities. As part of this, he describes bringing other trusted individuals into therapeutic conversations as 'outsider witnesses' to acknowledge women's aspirations and values, thereby locating subjectivity in relationships and enabling women to build a stronger sense of themselves that has been eroded by violence and abuse. In line with the research findings outlined earlier, White argues that there is often little continuous 'sense of myself' for women with these experiences, which he suggests is integral to the exercise of personal agency. White's approach therefore strikes a subtle balance between a post-structuralist understanding of the construction of multiple subjectivities in language and intersubjective relationships *and* the material emotional reality of the negative impact of gendered violence and abuse on sense of self over time. As such, this approach eschews a more relativist postmodernist approach to subjectivity as completely fluid and in flux, enabling recognition of the real, highly gendered experience of lost sense of self, agency and shame for women.

The prevention of mental health problems has historically received far less attention than individual therapy and crisis intervention. While there have been efforts in Australia in more recent years to bring a preventive focus to mental health policy and programmes (Commonwealth of Australia, 2009), as with recovery models of mental health, there has been little explicit attention to gender or gendered violence. I argue that one of the most significant ways to reduce the disproportionate burden of poor mental health carried by women is through targeting the prevention of gendered violence and abuse. In line with arguments throughout this chapter, this necessitates attention to both symbolic, attitudinal change but also to structural change in terms of redressing the continuing gender inequalities that frame and enable gendered violence and abuse. There are efforts at both national and international levels by governments across the world focused on the prevention of gendered violence and abuse, for example, through UN Women (2015) and the National Plan to Reduce Violence against Women and their Children 2010–2022 adopted by the Australian federal government in 2013 (National Council to Reduce Violence Against Women and their Children, 2009). Within both these policies, prevention is understood as necessitating both attitudinal change about gender roles, male violence and male privilege, and structural change through the promotion of gender equality across societies. As has been well-established in the public health field, behaviour change is not possible without a coordinated effort that includes both community education and structural social change (Itzin et al., 2010). Feminist social workers can continue to play an important part in bringing a gender perspective to mental health and other relevant social policies that promote the attitudinal and structural changes necessary for the prevention of gendered violence and abuse. However, the women's movement is also galvanising worldwide around the issue of gendered violence and abuse, and there are consequently important opportunities for feminist social workers to be involved in grassroots action, too.

Educating future social workers so that they have an appreciation of the gendered dimensions of mental health problems, and can practise in ways that are sensitive to this, is also critically important. Alongside my teaching team, I coordinate two mental health courses in social work, one at the undergraduate and the other at the postgraduate level. We aim to strike a balance between preparing students to work in mental health systems that continue to be medically oriented in spite of the rhetoric of recovery (Ramon, Healey & Renouf, 2007) and encouraging a critical perspective on mental health and illness. This means ensuring that students are familiar with the diagnostic tools of psychiatry, its language and orientation so that they can work in medical settings but, at the same time, challenging pathologising assumptions and practices by looking to the gender and other social inequalities that frame mental health. The courses also involve extensive use of case studies to illustrate the social dimensions of mental health, and people who have experienced mental health problems facilitate sessions with students to share their experiences, with both of these learning strategies including attention to gendered violence, abuse and mental health. In addition to the development of a critical understanding of mental health and illness, students practise a social approach to recovery in the social work studios where they are encouraged to review their own practice reflexively and receive constructive feedback from staff and peers. The emphasis of this practice-based learning is the development of empathic listening and communication skills to forge partnerships with clients rather than a 'clinical', top-down method of mental health assessment. In line with feminist approaches to practice, students therefore learn a respectful approach to working with clients that situates experience within its social context, and seeks to minimise power relations. The courses also involve attention to the policy context of mental health, and to preventive as well as therapeutic intervention.

Concluding comments

Feminists have offered important critical insights into the gendered dimensions of mental health and illness, with much of this work emanating from a post-structuralist feminist tradition. More recently, some feminist researchers and scholars have sought to move beyond a purely discursive level of explanation to engage also with the material and structural dimensions of women's mental health problems, particularly in response to gendered violence and abuse. Social workers are increasingly involved in the provision of mental health services, and recent feminist scholarly work offers important opportunities for exploring how we might respond to women's distress in ways that engage with its complexity and socially situated nature. There is great scope for social work to build on feminist research into gender and mental health, by continued elaboration of therapeutic models that situate women's distress in its gendered social context, by advocating for symbolic representational and attitudinal changes in relation to gender and through the pursuit of structural social change to reduce gender inequalities and increase women's participation across all sections of society. In particular, reducing the unequal burden of poor mental health experienced by women requires an interconnected, multi-level approach to gendered violence and abuse that pursues social change based on the understanding that the symbolic and the material dimensions of women's lives are fundamentally entwined, and that change in one domain cannot be achieved without corresponding change in the other.

Note

1   These findings are from the following study: Franzway, S., Wendt, S., Moulding, N.T., Zufferey, C. & Chung, D.: 'Gendered violence and citizenship: the complex effects of intimate partner violence on mental health, housing and employment'. The study is funded by the Australian Research Council as a Discovery Project, No.: DP1130104437.

Further reading

Ussher, J. (2010) Are we medicalizing women's misery? A critical review of women's higher rates of reported depression. *Feminism and Psychology*, 20(9), pp. 9–35.

Warner, S. (2009) *Understanding the Effects of Child Sexual Abuse: Feminist Revolutions in Theory, Research and Practice*. Routledge, London.

Wirth-Cauchon, J. (2001) *Borderline Personality Disorder: Symptoms and Stories*. Rutgers University Press, Piscataway, NJ.

References

American Psychiatric Association (APA) (2013) *Diagnostic and Statistical Manual of Mental Disorders (DSM-5)*. APA, Arlington, TX.

Armstrong, L. (2000) What happened when women said 'incest'. In C. Itzin (ed.), *Home Truths About Child Sexual Abuse: Influencing Policy and Practice*. Routledge, London, pp. 27–48.

Australian Bureau of Statistics (ABS) (2007) *National Health Survey*. ABS, Canberra.

Australian Institute of Health and Welfare (AIHW) (2014) *Child Protection Australia 2012–2013*. Australian Government, Canberra. www.aihw.gov.au/publication-detail/?id=60129547965 (accessed 22 April 2015).

Bland, R., Renouf, N. & Tullgren, A. (2015) *Social Work Practice in Mental Health: An Introduction*. Allen & Unwin, Sydney.

Bordo, S. (1988) Anorexia nervosa: psychopathology as the crystallization of culture. In I. Diamond & L. Quinby (eds), *Feminism and Foucault: Reflections on Resistance*. Northeastern University Press, Boston, MA, pp. 46–59.

Bordo, S. (1990) Reading the slender body. In M. Jacobus, E.F. Keller & S. Shuttleworth (eds), *Body/Politics: Women and the Discourses of Science*. Routledge, New York, pp. 83–112.

Breckenridge, J. (1999) Subjugation and silences: the role of the professions in silencing victims of sexual and domestic violence. In J. Breckenridge & L. Laing (eds), *Challenging Silence: Innovative Responses to Sexual and Domestic Violence.* Allen & Unwin, Sydney, pp. 6–30.

Briere, J. & Runtz, M. (1993) Child sexual abuse. *Journal of Interpersonal Violence*, 8(3), pp. 312–330.

Chesler, P. (2005) *Women and Madness.* Palgrave Macmillan, New York.

Commonwealth of Australia (2009) *National Mental Health Policy.* Commonwealth of Australia, Canberra.

Courtney, M. & Moulding, N.T. (2014) Reconciling the irreconcilable? An exploration of how social workers manage tensions between involuntary treatment and the recovery model of mental illness. *Australian Social Work*, 67(2), pp. 1–13.

De Groot, J. & Rodin, G.M. (1999) The relationship between eating disorders and childhood trauma. *Psychiatric Annals*, 29(4), pp. 225–229.

Deegan, P. (1996) Recovery as a journey of the heart. *Psychiatric Rehabilitation Journal*, 19(3), pp. 91–97.

Downs, W.R. & Miller, B.A. (1998) Relationships between experiences of parental violence during childhood and women's psychiatric symptomatology. *Journal of Interpersonal Violence*, 13, pp. 438–457.

Higgins, D.J. & McCabe, M.P. (2001) Multiple forms of child abuse and neglect: adult retrospective reports. *Aggression and Violent Behaviour*, 6, pp. 547–578.

Humphreys, C. & Thiara, R. (2003) Mental health and domestic violence: 'I call it symptoms of abuse'. *British Journal of Social Work*, 33(2), pp. 209–226.

Itzin, C., Taket, A. & Barter-Godfrey, S. (2010) *Domestic and Sexual Violence and Abuse: Tackling the Health and Mental Health Effects.* Routledge, Abingdon.

Krieger, N. (1994) Epidemiology and the web of causation: has anyone seen the spider? *Social Science and Medicine*, 39(7), pp. 887–993.

McNay, L. (2004) Situated intersubjectivity. In B. Marshall & A. Witz (eds), *Engendering the Social: Feminist Encounters with Sociological Theory.* Open University Press, Maidenhead, pp. 171–186.

Malson, H. (1998) *The Thin Woman: Feminism, Post-structuralism and the Social Psychology of Anorexia Nervosa.* Routledge, London.

May-Chahal, C. (2006) Gender and child maltreatment: the evidence base. *Social Work and Society*, 4(1), pp. 53–68.

Messman-Moore, T.L. & Garrigus, A.S. (2007) The association of child abuse and eating disorder symptomatology: the importance of multiple forms of abuse and re-victimization. *Journal of Aggression, Maltreatment and Trauma*, 14(3), pp. 51–72.

Moulding, N.T. (2003) Constructing the self in mental health practice: identity, individualism and the feminisation of deficiency. *Feminist Review*, 75, pp. 57–74.

Moulding, N.T. (2006) Disciplining the feminine: the reproduction of gender contradictions in the mental health care of women with eating disorders. *Social Science and Medicine*, 62(4), pp. 793–804.

Moulding, N.T. (2009) The anorexic as femme fatale: reproducing gender through the father/psychiatrist–daughter/patient relationship. In H. Malson & M. Burns (eds), *Critical Feminist Approaches to Eating Dis/Orders: An International Reader.* Routledge, London, pp. 173–184.

Moulding, N.T. (2016) *Gendered Violence, Mental Health and Recovery in Everyday Lives: Beyond Trauma.* Routledge, London.

National Council to Reduce Violence Against Women and their Children and KPMG Management Consulting (2009) *The Cost of Violence Against Women and their Children*. National Council to Reduce Violence Against Women and their Children, Canberra.

O'Dell, L. (2003) The 'harm' story in child sexual abuse: contested understandings, disputed knowledges. In P. Reavey & S. Warner (eds), *New Feminist Stories of Child Sexual Abuse: Sexual Scripts and Dangerous Dialogues*. Routledge, London, pp. 131–147.

O'Dougherty Wright, M., Crawford, E. & Del Castillo, D. (2009) Childhood emotional maltreatment and later psychological distress among college students: the mediating role of maladaptive schemas. *Child Abuse and Neglect*, 33, pp. 59–68.

Ramon, S., Healy, B. & Renouf, N. (2007) Recovery from mental illness as an emergent concept and practice in Australia and the UK. *International Journal of Social Psychiatry*, 53(2), pp. 108–122.

Reavey, P. (2003) When past meets present. In P. Reavey & S. Warner (eds), *New Feminist Stories of Child Sexual Abuse: Sexual Scripts and Dangerous Dialogues*. Routledge, London, pp. 148–166.

Scher, C.D., Forde, D.R., McQuaid, J.R. & Stein, M.B. (2004) Prevalence and demographic correlates of childhood maltreatment in an adult community sample. *Child Abuse and Neglect*, 28(2), pp. 167–180.

Schneider, R., Baumrind, N. & Kimerling, R. (2007) Exposure to child abuse and risk for mental health problems in women. *Violence and Victims*, 22(5), pp. 620–631.

Showalter, E. (1987) *The Female Malady: Women, Madness and English Culture 1830–1880*. Penguin Books, Harmondsworth.

Stoltenborgh, M., van Ijzendoorn, M.H., Euser, E.M. & Bakermans-Kranenburg, M.J. (2011) A global perspective on child sexual abuse: meta-analysis of prevalence around the world. *Child Maltreatment*, 16, pp. 79–101.

Tew, J. (2008) Social perspectives on mental distress. In T. Stickley & T. Basset (eds), *Learning about Mental Health Practice*. John Wiley & Sons, Chichester, UK, pp. 235–252.

UN Women (2015) *UN Women*. www.unwomen.org/en (accessed 28 May 2015).

Ussher, J. (1991) *Women's Madness: Misogyny or Mental Illness*. Harvester, Hemel Hempstead, UK.

Ussher, J. (2010) Are we medicalizing women's misery? A critical review of women's higher rates of reported depression. *Feminism and Psychology*, 20(9), pp. 9–35.

Walby, S. (2004) *The Cost of Domestic Violence*. Women's Equality Unit, London.

Warner, S. (2009) *Understanding the Effects of Child Sexual Abuse: Feminist Revolutions in Theory, Research and Practice*. Routledge, London.

Warner, S. & Wilkins, T. (2003) Diagnosing distress and reproducing disorder: women, child sexual abuse and 'borderline personality disorder'. In P. Reavey & S. Warner (eds), *New Feminist Stories of Child Sexual Abuse: Sexual Scripts and Dangerous Dialogues*. Routledge, London, pp. 167–186.

White, M. (2004) Working with people who are suffering the consequences of multiple trauma: a narrative perspective. *International Journal of Narrative Therapy and Community Work*, 1, pp. 44–75.

White, M. & Epston, D. (1989) *Literate Means to Therapeutic Ends*. Dulwich Centre Publications, Adelaide.

Wirth-Cauchon, J. (2001) *Borderline Personality Disorder: Symptoms and Stories*. Rutgers University Press, Piscataway, NJ.

13 Child wellbeing, mothering and protection

Fiona Buchanan

In this chapter, I critique current theories that are commonly applied to child wellbeing, mothering and child protection, and I call for social workers to incorporate a radical feminist perspective to address the needs of women and their children. I argue that current applications of attachment and ecological theories do not provide opportunities to discuss children's wellbeing and protection in ways that honour and support women's mothering abilities. I make this argument by drawing on my own research into domestic violence. By taking a radical feminist perspective, I draw on knowledge from the lived experiences of women and children I have worked with in practice and interviewed as a feminist researcher. From this perspective, I propose social work responses that problematise the gendered contexts of women's and children's lives, and support a particular strengths-based approach to work in this area. This chapter promotes feminist understandings of women's knowledge regarding protectiveness and identifies societal challenges to optimal conditions for child wellbeing, mothering and child protection. In doing so, I describe a radical feminist approach that counters gender-blind applied psychological theories that are based on judgements of good or bad mothering, or operate without concern for the gendered contexts of women's and children's lives.

Current approaches to child wellbeing, mothering and child protection

Child wellbeing, based on the ideal of children growing through developmental stages to reach their full potential, is central to the work of many social workers, and all social workers have a specific responsibility to ensure that children are safe (Arney & Scott, 2013). Child safety and child wellbeing have been described as dependent on emotional availability, nurturance, warmth, protection and provision of comfort (Zeanah & Boris, 2000). In most societies, responsibility for the provision of this constellation of optimal child-raising conditions has been placed in the hands of the immediate family (Arney & Scott, 2013). However, when the care of children is questioned, focus is directed towards the primary caregiver rather than the family as a whole. Because of traditional gender roles that continue to operate in all societies, the primary caregiver is most often the child's mother. Thus, from a social work perspective, child wellbeing also concerns mothering, as children's emotional, psychological and physical wellbeing are seen as interconnected with women's mothering capabilities (Krane et al., 2010). Thus, when children are not protected it is most often seen as a failure of the mother (Douglas & Walsh, 2010).

Child wellbeing and protection: looking at attachment

Over 30 years of social work practice, I have seen a focus on the deficits in mothering proliferate as attachment theory, originally conceived of by John Bowlby during the 1950s in the US, has grown in popularity. This has coincided with the growth of neo-liberalism and an increasing dependence on 'evidence-based', individualised, psychological perspectives in relation to a range of health and social problems. Within this context, attachment theory is used to identify patterns of secure or insecure connection by observing interactions between the mother and child to discern whether mothering is sufficient for the child's needs (Prior & Glaser, 2006). Often children's relationships with their mothers are therefore the sole subject of speculation and judgement, with attachment theorists claiming to take the child's perspective (Prior & Glaser, 2006). As the popularity of applied attachment theory has grown, so has evaluation of child wellbeing within narrow dictates that ignore broader societal contexts. In addition, many attachment theorists hold conservative views of societal roles and dated assumptions about social standards and mothering (Jackson & Mannix, 2004). Based on pseudo-scientific experiments, these expert views promote traditional norms through research based on similar values to the middle-class, 1950s world of John Bowlby (1988). Thus, despite the differing reality of many women and children, the stereotypical ideal was one of women as full-time child carers based in the home and supported by a male provider. These parameters are still being applied to mothering in general, regardless of the increasingly diverse and complex contexts of child raising or the varied life experiences of women. Although I see attachment theory as having some merit, I have witnessed many practitioners in community-based services using attachment theory to take an expert position and evaluate women's and children's lives without a critical view of how this narrow, individualised theory fits, or its neo-liberal basis. As a consequence, issues of violence against women, poverty and cultural gendered oppression were often ignored because the focus was solely on the relationship between women and their children.

I am not alone in my concerns. Other feminists, such as Featherstone et al. (2010), have acknowledged that social work practitioners who work with families mostly draw on traditional ideas that children's wellbeing is the prime responsibility of women. Similarly, Franzblau (1999) and Morris (2008) argue this perspective is encouraged by applied attachment theory ideology where the impact of other individuals, groups and systems in the broader community is excluded from responsibility for the wellbeing of children and the prescribed role of women as mothers is not critiqued. Other feminists have taken issue with current applications of theory, describing the attachment field's prescriptive notions of the mothering role as unreasonable, the emphasis on mothering as politically motivated and the rationale for focusing on mothering in isolation from context as patriarchal (Bliwise, 1999; Contratto, 2002). Because of this, attachment theory has been described as part of a continuum of politics that informs policy and 'depoliticizes and removes from historical review the exploita-tive and oppressive conditions under which women reproduce and mother' (Franzblau, 1999, p. 29). Rather than challenging the societal conditions that children are raised in, attachment theory therefore focuses on women as mothers and seeks to alter their behaviour if it is judged that there is any problem with children's wellbeing or safety. This applies wher-ever the threat to child wellbeing originates, and this is particularly prob-lematic in cases of domestic violence where the father may perpetrate the abuse but the mother is held accountable (Humphreys, 2010).

I do not repudiate that the relationship between women and their chil-dren is important, but when women and their children are the sole focus of assessment and treatment, a gendered analysis of broader societal issues impacting on mothering is eclipsed (Lapierre, 2008). Further, as well as having a detrimental effect on women, children's needs are not served when mothers are held responsible for their wellbeing across the lifespan while the impact of gender oppression is ignored. It is disempowering to perceive one's destiny as compromised by an early relationship deemed as deficient through a discourse that negates gender in systems of influence.

Child wellbeing and protection: an ecological systems perspective

Against this backdrop, I argue that a sociological viewpoint is needed to consider how children's wellbeing depends on societal factors such as gender, class, race, discrimination and unequal distribution of wealth. A perspective that is commonly used within social work and human services is the ecological systems perspective based in sociological thought, in which children's wellbeing is affected by the functioning of many multi-layered systems (Bronfenbrenner, 1979). In the following discussion, I explore the possibilities of approaching child wellbeing from this per-spective, but also some of the limitations of the approach.

Ecological systems theory positions children within microsystems of the immediate environment such as family, child care, schools and peers. These microsystems interconnect as mesosystems that are influenced by exosystems such as extended family, neighbourhood and parents' work-places. Macro systems such as governments, culture, economies, mass media and religion also have an impact on children's wellbeing through influences on societal discourses that affect contexts and attitudes to child raising. When social workers take an ecological systems perspective to look at ways to optimise children's development, they consider contexts such as impoverished neighbourhoods, disruption in families and economic systems that support disadvantage (Mattaini, Lowery & Meyer, 2002). Yet, even within an ecosystems perspective it is still women's ability to mother that is commonly under scrutiny because current macrosystems promote the provision of early intervention services staffed by professionals trained in attachment theory. Such services most often target mother–child relationships and apply attachment theory to address perceived deficits (Lapierre, 2010).

As Chodorow (2002) points out, it is also worth noting that, historically, women mothered and children were raised with support from other females in the local community. Practical support allowed women time out from mothering as well as opportunities to gain insights, understanding and expertise from older females within the micro and mesosystems. Also, within this network the challenges of mothering and women's mothering abilities were acknowledged by others who mothered in similar circum-stances. Nowadays the need for supportive contexts is often neglected because, while centring the child, an ecological perspective does not focus on the impact of contemporary systems on the experiences of mothers.

In neo-liberal times, there are also gendered expectations of intensive mothering that promote a view that mothers should be constantly atten-tive and responsible for children's wellbeing. These expectations allow others, including social workers, to hold mothers solely accountable if chil-dren are harmed or at risk of harm. This leads women to feel that they will be judged as bad mothers if they ask others for assistance or question the situation in which they mother. Without awareness of gendered societal factors that impact on mothering, women internalise mother blaming so that they are prevented from achieving a sense of competency and achieve-ment for their successes in child raising. Further, mother blaming deters women from accessing services to help their children and themselves (Jackson & Mannix, 2004).

An ecological systems perspective includes other individuals, groups and systems as significant for children's wellbeing. Recognition that child wellbeing is located in societal connections then leads to a different approach in policy and practice (Eltringham & Aldridge, 2002). However, by centring the child, an ecological systems approach includes mothers as just one element of the microsystem of the family while supporting the use of attachment theory at the mesosystems level. Both attachment theory and ecosystems approaches therefore overlook the impact of multiple gen-dered oppressions that impact on mothering.

Much social work practice is with families and children, and agencies and social work educators often promote the expectation that social workers will hold the needs of children in mind and work with caregivers (usually mothers) to maximise the child's potential (Arney & Scott, 2013). However, women's concern for their children's wellbeing is taken for granted when protection is seen as the prerogative of the state (Humphreys, 2010). Women's protection of their children is only regarded when a woman is perceived as failing to protect or is seen as overprotective. As Mandel states, 'We fail to see how mothers are actively engaged in trying to make their child safer' (2010, p. 531). When assessing child wellbeing from an attachment theory perspective, although the woman's own experience of being mothered may be scrutinised, current experiences of women as mothers are not taken into account (Davies et al., 2007). Instead, expert-driven judgements are applied to many clients who are mothering in impoverished conditions with little support and often while they are enduring gendered violence (Humphreys, 2010). In my practice as a social worker, I noticed that in many situations domestic violence was not even recognised because practitioners' focus was narrowed by an attachment theory approach. Alternatively, social workers can apply an ecological approach and consider the contexts of the child's life. However, within this approach, the link between child wellbeing and mother wellbeing may also be overlooked. As Garbarino (1982) notes, an ecological perspective defines the family as the headquarters of human development. This view does not consider gendered roles within families and the impact of gendered expectations on mothering. Some social workers apply both attachment and ecological systems theories simultaneously, but there is a need to look further and apply a feminist perspective so that women are not relegated to a position where they are either objectified or overlooked.

Feminist ideas about mothering, wellbeing and child protection

As noted earlier, to appraise critically the application of attachment theory and ecosystems approaches to child wellbeing, I take a radical feminist perspective. Radical feminism is based on the belief that 'the personal is political', which is not to say that the personal needs to be politicised, but to recognise that it already is and that politics needs to be redefined to include family life (Bryson, 1999). Radical feminism informs my argument that current theories applied to child wellbeing, child protection and mothering come from a predominantly male view of the world where women have proscribed roles. Taking a radical feminist perspective, Bryson notes: 'Until recently our history, philosophy and public culture has been almost exclusively man made' (2007, p. 38). This does not mean that radical feminism sees men as the enemy: rather radical feminism suggests that awareness of ascribed gendered roles and attitudes can lead to change and better understanding for all. While there is no one radical feminism, for me radical feminism means seeing lived experiences through a lens of patriarchal oppression. Here, patriarchy is defined as 'a social system built on male domination and female subordination' (Browne, 2007, p. 251). With regards to child wellbeing, protection and mothering, countering patriarchy means moving beyond assumptions about women's roles and decentring male perspectives to develop an awareness of women's and children's lived experiences in a gendered context.

Radical feminism has been accused of essentialism and of discounting the experiences of women who have thrived in current systems with supportive male figures in their lives (O'Brien Hallstein, 1999). However, I argue that this misses the point: it is largely good fortune that enables some women to thrive within patriarchy, and we cannot be dismissive about the diversity of systematic oppression of many women in all cultures. The accusation of 'essentialism' is, I believe, a disservice to the many women who are victimised and held culpable within the diverse gender-oppressive systems that are in existence today.

Radical feminist knowledge is created from women's lived experiences with the understanding that women have valuable insights into their needs and the needs of their children. From a radical perspective comes the belief that women, rather than experts, possess ideas for actions needed to help other women in similar situations. This standpoint seeks to empower women and challenges the perspectives of those who hold power through status and institutionalised scientific expertise. To follow Hartsock, 'A standpoint carries with it the contention that there are some perspectives on society from which, however well intentioned one may be, the real relations of humans with each other and with the natural world are not visible' (1998, p. 107).

A radical feminist perspective reveals how many women's experiences conflict with the societal norms that are upheld by men, and this perspective also points out men's positions of power. In contrast, women have much to gain through recognition of the societal norms that constrict their lives and define their view of themselves. With regard to raising children, radical feminism encourages women to see themselves as holding skills and aptitudes that enhance children's wellbeing despite social contexts that oppress them (O'Brien Hallstein, 1999). This includes recognition that, by internalising messages from man-made systems, structures and theories, women hold themselves responsible for any ills that affect their children: for example, many women hold themselves responsible for sexual abuse of their children when it is perpetrated by male relatives. Taking a radical feminist approach means challenging currently applied theories and calling for systemic change.

Child development theorists view human development as an active and flexible process where children adapt and change according to circumstances and societal influences (Eltringham & Aldridge, 2002). However, gender is not included in this equation. As such, child-raising theories ignore gendered life experiences that are produced and reinforced by patriarchy. A radical feminist view frames women as well as children in micro, meso, exo and macrosystems contexts and encourages social workers to perceive women and children as influenced by multiple patriarchal systems of the social world. By taking a radical feminist view, social workers can focus on women's abilities and children's achievements, despite the challenges of gendered discrimination and oppression. Without feminist-informed knowledge garnered from women's lived experiences, social workers risk taking a limited, expert-driven view that distorts the experiences of women and furthers misogynistic discourses of mother blame (Jackson & Mannix, 2004).

In addition, I argue that the wellbeing of children is not served by judgements made with limited knowledge of systems that jeopardise the physical, psychological and emotional safety of their mothers. As Tong notes, 'No person can be expected to remain always cheerful and kind unless that person's own physical and psychological needs are being met' (1998, p. 88). Yet, too often, mothers are expected to be cheerful and kind despite enduring poverty, gendered violence and multiple forms of gendered oppression that underpin challenges to their physical and psychological wellbeing. If an ecological systems approach incorporates consideration of the multiple forms and levels of gender oppression in the micro, exo, meso and macrosystems it becomes clear that systems need to change so that the physical and psychological wellbeing of women, as well as children, is protected.

Applying radical feminist principles in practice

In practice, social workers can engage with mothers to promote awareness of their strengths and resilience, and reduce internalised mother blame. Further, by challenging current unrealistic discourses about mothering, social workers can address the impact of multiple discriminations. In this way, radical feminist ideas can be used to promote a focus on the impact of institutionalised misogyny and encourage change within ecosystems while supporting the strengths that women bring to the mothering role (Davies & Krane, 2006). This is particularly important today when neo-liberal ideology is influencing and shaping contexts of mothering and child wellbeing so that women are expected singlehandedly to ensure that their children's needs are met. With this in mind, I follow with suggestions and ideas for applying radical feminist principles of rights, empowerment, societal change, exposing gender oppression and centring subjective knowledge in practice.

First, with regard to rights in society, there is a need to counter the expectation that 'a woman who has a child is no longer considered as a person but is seen as a mother instead' (Caro & Fox, 2008, p. 148). Too often in social work practice, the idea that women have rights is seen to conflict with the interests of children. When subjected to this view, women find that there is an expectation that their rights are subjugated to the rights of their children. From a radical feminist perspective, women have a right to be regarded, not just in relation to their children, but also as individuals with interests and concerns outside the mothering role. It is understood that, however rewarding the mothering role may be, it is limiting. Most women require adult company, interests outside the home, supportive relationships and acknowledgement of their abilities and strengths to maintain their capacity to mother (Caro & Fox, 2008).

Second, children can be best served in the context of an ecosystems approach that centres women, as well as themselves, at micro, exo, meso and macro levels. By valuing women as more than providers of child care, children benefit from perceiving their mothers as empowered by participation in the social world (Caro & Fox, 2008). Social workers therefore have a role to play in encouraging women to maintain and develop interests beyond mothering. In my own social work practice, I found that encouraging new mothers to seek and sustain interests and relationships outside home was an effective way to address feelings of depression and isolation while simultaneously increasing enjoyment of their children. Using a radical feminist lens to centre women as well as children enables mothers' empowerment and allows children to be raised with an appreciation of the value of women. The child's story relates to the mother's story with attention to the questions of: Who nurtures her? How does society value her? What worth is she granted in the framework of her life? Such self-reflective questions acknowledge that the relationship between mother and child depends on societal conditions (Eltringham & Aldridge, 2002). In recent research conducted with individuals who had been raised in domestic violence, we found that several participants followed society's discourses in blaming their mothers for their father's abusive behaviour (Buchanan, Wendt & Moulding, 2015). In social work practice with clients who share these views, encouraging such individuals to see the pressures that their mothers were under and the discourses about motherhood that encouraged them towards mother blaming could enhance their relationships with their mothers.

Third, within a feminist perspective it is understood that 'mothering is a complex and emotionally challenging relationship and social workers require both theoretical and reflexive knowledge to engage with mothers' (Davies et al., 2007, p. 25). Including gender awareness within an ecological systems perspective fosters acknowledgement of the multiple systems that affect child wellbeing, mothering and child protection. With this awareness, the needs of children, women and society can be appraised. This approach counters the negative impacts of a deficit model applied to women and reinforces the need for changes in societal discourses so that women can enjoy space with, and apart from, their children. From a

radical feminist perspective, when the need for societal change is identified, the focus turns from mother blaming to challenging unjust systems.
For example, when working with women who suffered generalised anxiety
while mothering, I always made a point of asking about their expectations
of motherhood and explored the origins of any unrealistic assumptions.

To address the fourth principle, one way that gendered oppression can
be challenged is by building feminist knowledge to counter received knowledge based on theories that negate gender. Feminism has long influenced
practice through basing theory in research that promotes the voices of
women (Hesse-Biber, 2007). In the arena of child wellbeing, mothering
and child protection, countering individualised, pathologising treatments
through feminist research offers a broader, more holistic view that considers the contexts of lived experiences that can then shape theory. By
undertaking such research, the political as well as the personal is exposed
for critical evaluation (Campbell & Baikie, 2012).

The following example illustrates how feminist research develops theory
by centring subjective experiences to inform practice. This study focused
on the lived experiences of women who had mothered babies in domestic
violence (Buchanan, Power & Verity, 2014). Several of the women who
participated in the research study had been subjected to child protection
investigations. The women's knowledge was acquired through a relational
empowerment methodology where an ethos of mutual support was constructed so that women discussed their experiences in a space where they
were safe to speak openly (VanderPlaat, 1999). Through analysis of the
discussions it became clear that the women formed relationships with their
children within an environment of sustained hostility created by their
abusive partners, isolated from supportive others and with little space for
themselves. In this context, protection of their children was of paramount
importance and the women sought to protect in myriad ways that are not
recognised as motivated by protection in other research and practice contexts. However, in these circumstances, the space to spend time relating to
their children was often constricted because of partners' antagonism
towards the women's focus on children and enforced isolation from
friends and family. All the women saw space to relate as important for
their children and themselves, but all prioritised protection and developed
the relationship with their children from that foundation. They did this in
the context of their partners' hostility, compounded by messages from the
micro, exo, meso and macrosystems that support unrealistic expectations
of intense mothering. In the current context of mother blaming, many of
the women internalised blame, experienced guilt and did not discern that
their role was impacted by the contexts that defined their existence. For
many of the women, despite previous counselling, it was only during their
participation in focus groups with other women that they identified barriers to seeing themselves as able mothers and realised the strengths and
abilities they brought to the mothering role.

This research indicates a need for social workers to reflect on the multiple ways women may protect their children and it illustrates how enquiry into lived experiences can lead to better understanding of child wellbeing, mothering and protection in diverse circumstances. In social work practice that takes a radical feminist perspective, support, sensitivity and attention to gendered oppression can enhance the lives of women and children struggling with issues of wellbeing and safety. Exploring barriers to mothers' protectiveness identifies gendered oppression at all levels of the ecosystem. From there, attention can focus on women's agency and the contributions both mothers and children make to their capacity to thrive.

Feminist research highlights a need to work from a paradigm that utilises a strengths perspective to enquire about gendered contexts, focus on protective feelings, thoughts and actions, and work with ecosystems so that women and children are supported. Deeper insight and further mutual understanding are accessed, and exploring barriers to protection provides opportunities to consider the gendered systems that negatively impact on women as mothers and on the children they are raising. This perspective involves challenging mother-blaming theories, raising awareness of unrealistic expectations placed on women as mothers and confronting systemic barriers to women's and children's wellbeing.

Radical feminist ideas that the personal is political and that theory is built from lived experiences enhance social workers' own awareness levels of women's desires to protect. The relationship between women and their children is important but so is space to relate, and this space can only be obtained if changes are made so that women's rights are acknowledged and each woman's experience in the context of diverse gendered oppressions is identified and examined, and current discourses are challenged. Promoting the wellbeing of both mothers and children depends on recognising the needs of both and working to raise awareness and change the negative discourses that ultimately undermine mothering and child wellbeing.

Conclusion

Radical feminism uses a critical lens to view how patriarchy impacts on the lives of women and children, thus delineating why concerns of child wellbeing, mothering and child protection need to incorporate a gender lens. Through centring women's as well as children's experiences in a sociological framework, radical feminism counters neo-liberal approaches that are shaping child wellbeing, mothering and protection discourses. This framework incorporates an analysis of systemic gender discrimination and highlights the need for changes in the micro, exo, meso and macrosystems. From this perspective social workers are encouraged to increase their awareness of, and resistance to, gender-blind policy and practices and to challenge systems that undermine social justice for women and their children. When it is recognised that knowledge is narrowly constructed by expert views that exclude perspectives from lived experiences, social workers can problematise applied theories that restrict their practice with mothers and children. Incorporating radical feminist principles in social work practice means that women's endeavours to protect are recognised and space for mother–child relationships prioritised. Further, by undertaking research based in diverse lived experiences, social workers can build evidence that will widen the current view of child protection and challenge policies and practices that negate the influences of gendered societal perspectives. Just as radical feminists in second wave feminism challenged proscribed roles for women, social workers can now use radical feminist understandings of rights, empowerment and the need to expose gendered oppression as they centre lived experiences to challenge new orthodoxies that delineate discourses about child wellbeing, mothering and child protection.

Further reading

Benjamin, J. (2013) *The Bonds of Love: Psychoanalysis, Feminism, and the Problem of Domination.* Random House, New York.

Chesler, P. (2011) *Mothers on Trial: The Battle for Children and Custody.* Review Press, Chicago, IL.

Featherstone, B., Hooper, C., Scourfield, J. & Taylor, J. (2010) *Gender and Child Welfare in Society.* Wiley-Blackwell, Chichester, UK.

Porter, M. & Kelso, J. (eds) (2008) *Theorising and Representing Maternal Realities.* Cambridge Scholars, Newcastle.

References

Arney, F. & Scott, D. (2013) *Working with Vulnerable Families: A Partnership Approach,* 2nd edn. Cambridge University Press, Sydney.

Bliwise, N.G. (1999) Securing attachment theory's potential. *Feminism and Psychology,* 9, pp. 43–52.

Bowlby, J. (1988) *A Secure Base: Clinical Applications of Attachment Theory.* Routledge, London.

Bronfenbrenner, U. (1979) *The Ecology of Human Development.* Harvard University Press, Cambridge, MA.

Browne, J. (2007) The principle of equal treatment and gender: theory and practice. In J. Browne (ed.), *The Future of Gender.* Cambridge University Press, Cambridge, pp. 250–280.

Bryson, V. (1999) *Feminist Debates.* Macmillan Press, Houndmills, UK.

Bryson, V. (2007) Perspectives on gender equality: challenging the terms of debate. In J. Browne (ed.), *The Future of Gender.* Cambridge University Press, Cambridge, pp. 35–57.

Buchanan, F., Power, C. & Verity, F. (2014) The effects of domestic violence on the formation of relationships between women and their babies: 'I was too busy protecting my baby to attach'. *Journal of Family Violence,* 29(7), pp. 713–724.

Buchanan, F., Wendt, S. & Moulding, N. (2015) Growing up in domestic violence: what does maternal protectiveness mean? *Qualitative Social Work*, 14(3), pp. 399–415.

Campbell, C. & Baikie, G. (2012) Beginning at the beginning: an exploration of critical social work. *Critical Social Work*, 13(1), pp. 67–81.

Caro, J. & Fox, C. (2008) *The F Word: How we Learned to Swear by Feminism*. University of New South Wales Press, Sydney.

Chodorow, N. (2002) Extract from The reproduction of mothering: psychoanalysis and the sociology of gender. *Feminism and Psychology*, 12(1), pp. 11–17.

Contratto, S. (2002) A feminist critique of attachment theory and evolutionary psychology. In M. Ballou & L.S. Brown (eds), *Rethinking Mental Health and Disorder: Feminist Perspectives*. Guilford Press, New York, pp. 29–47.

Davies, L. & Krane, J. (2006) Collaborate with caution: protecting children, helping mothers. *Critical Social Policy*, 26, pp. 412–425.

Davies, L., Krane, J., Collins, S. & Wexler, S. (2007) Developing mothering narratives in child protection practice. *Journal of Social Work Practice: Psychotherapeutic Approaches in Health, Welfare and the Community*, 21(1), pp. 23–34.

Douglas, H. & Walsh, T. (2010) Mothers, domestic violence, and child protection. *Violence Against Women*, 16, pp. 489–508.

Eltringham, S. & Aldridge, J. (2002) Parenting on shifting sands: the transfer of responsibility for safely managing danger. *Clinical Child Psychology and Psychiatry*, 7(2), pp. 137–145.

Featherstone, B., Hooper, C., Scourfield, J. & Taylor, J. (2010) *Gender and Child Welfare in Society*. Wiley-Blackwell, Chichester, UK.

Franzblau, S.H. (1999) Historicizing attachment theory: binding the ties that bind. *Feminism and Psychology*, 9(1), pp. 22–31.

Garbarino, J. (1982) *Children and Families in the Social Environment*. Transaction Publishers, Piscataway, NJ.

Hartsock, N.C.M. (1998) *The Feminist Standpoint Revisited and other Essays*. Westfield Press, Boulder, CO.

Hesse-Biber, S.N. (2007) Feminist research: exploring the interconnections of epistemology, methodology, and method. In S.N. Hesse-Biber (ed.), *Handbook of Feminist Research: Theory and Praxis*. Sage, Thousand Oaks, CA, pp. 1–28.

Humphreys, C.F. (2010) Crossing the great divide: response to Douglas and Walsh. *Violence Against Women*, 16, pp. 509–515.

Jackson, D. & Mannix, J. (2004) Giving voice to the burden of blame: a feminist study of mothers' experiences of mother blaming. *International Journal of Nursing Practice*, 10, pp. 150–158.

Krane, J., Davies, L., Carlton, R. & Mulcahy, M. (2010) The clock starts now: feminism, mothering and attachment theory in child protection practice. In B. Featherstone, C. Hooper, J. Scourfield & J. Taylor (eds), *Gender and Child Welfare in Society*. Wiley-Blackwell, Chichester, UK, pp. 149–172.

Lapierre, S. (2008) Mothering in the context of domestic violence: the pervasiveness of a deficit model of mothering. *Child and Family Social Work*, 13, pp. 454–463.

Lapierre, S. (2010) Are abused women 'neglectful' mothers? A critical reflection based on women's experiences. In B. Featherstone, C. Hooper, J. Scourfield & J. Taylor (eds), *Gender and Child Welfare in Society*. Wiley-Blackwell, Chichester, UK, pp. 121–148.

Mandel, D. (2010) Child welfare and domestic violence: tackling the themes and thorny questions that stand in the way of collaboration and improvement of child welfare practice. *Violence Against Women*, 16(5), pp. 530–536.

Mattaini, M.A., Lowery, C.T. & Meyer, C.H. (2002) *Foundations of Social Work Practice: A Graduate Text*. NASW, Washington, DC.

Morris, A. (2008) Too attached to attachment theory. In M. Porter & J. Kelso (eds), *Theorising and Representing Maternal Realities*. Cambridge Scholars, Newcastle, pp. 107–117.

O'Brien Hallstein, D.L. (1999) A postmodern caring: feminist standpoint theories, revisioned caring, and communication ethics. *Western Journal of Communication*, 63(1), pp. 32–56.

Prior, V. & Glaser, D. (2006) *Understanding Attachment and Attachment Disorders: Theory, Evidence and Practice*. Jessica Kinsley Publishers, London.

Tong, R. (1998) *Feminist Thought: A More Comprehensive Introduction*. Allen & Unwin, St Leonards, NSW.

VanderPlaat, M. (1999) Locating the feminist scholar: relational empowerment and social activism. *Qualitative Health Research*, 9, pp. 773–785.

Zeanah, C.H. & Boris, N.W. (2000) Disturbances and disorders of attachment in early childhood. In C.H. Zeanah (ed.), *Handbook of Infant Mental Health*. Guilford Press, New York, pp. 353–368.

14 Domestic violence and feminism

Sarah Wendt

Introduction

Feminism was at the cornerstone of making domestic violence visible as a social problem, advocating for shelters/refuges, emotional support for women and children victims, and social change including legal responses to the perpetration of intimate partner abuse (Nichols, 2013). Furthermore, feminism has centralised gender in analyses of domestic violence. In this chapter I outline the debates about gender to explain why men are predominantly perpetrators of domestic violence and women and children victims. I explore how feminism has been instrumental in exposing domestic violence as part of a range of tactics (including physical, sexual, psychological, financial, social and spiritual abuse) used to exercise power and control over women and children. I conclude by arguing that feminism and social work can together lead practice and policy responses to domestic violence so gender continues to remain central.

Throughout the chapter I use the term feminism to speak broadly of a movement across multiple disciplines and professional practices. I acknowledge that feminism is not a single theory or concept; however, I argue it generally advocates for the attainment of rights for women. I also use feminism to reflect a diverse range of scholarship that explores, explains and debates gender (Johnson, 2010). Feminism enables me as a researcher and social worker to look at gender in a critical way. Feminism provides me with a framework to look at social structures, institutions and discourses that impact on and influence women and men. I refer to gender as a social construct, that is, we learn femininity and masculinity through social interactions, but these are bound up with power relations between women and men (Bradley, 2013; Wendt & Zannettino, 2015). Through the contributions of feminism, I will argue domestic violence is an act of gender-based violence, mostly perpetrated by men against women in the context of an intimate relationship, to maintain control over women, a control to which men feel they are entitled (Johnson & Ferraro, 2000).

Understanding the gender debate

There is a long and controversial debate surrounding domestic violence which revolves around the question of whether men's and women's involvement in intimate partner violence is symmetrical or asymmetrical (Johnson, 2006; Krahe, Bieneck & Moller, 2005). The debate generally has two sides. One side argues domestic violence is largely a problem of men assaulting and abusing female intimate partners, while the other side argues that women are at least as violent as men in intimate relationships (Johnson, 2006). These debates will continue because of conceptual and methodological differences in the studies that aim to measure prevalence and incidences of domestic violence (Krahe et al., 2005). However, despite this ongoing debate, I argue that it is feminist analysis that is most compelling and empirically sound for a variety of reasons.

First, feminism has advanced the recognition that domestic violence is a significant social problem. During the second wave feminist movement, activists in Australia, the UK and the US raised awareness of the extent of domestic violence, campaigned and lobbied for social change, and provided practical support through establishing networks of women's shelters/refuges (Buchanan, 2013). Feminist researchers and practitioners have therefore provided the strongest critique of traditional approaches to studying domestic violence. For example, the Conflict Tactics Scale developed by Straus (1979) is a widely used measurement of intimate partner violence. It asks women and men to indicate whether they had ever experienced particular acts of violence (slapped, punched, kicked, forced to have sex). Feminists have exposed that a method that asks about particular acts of violence ignores the essence of abusive relationships. Fear, control and the atmosphere of terror that permeates domestic violence is not captured, as well as the many forms of psychological, social and financial abuse (Laing & Humphreys, 2013). Furthermore, feminists have argued these types of methods in research on domestic violence cannot assess the dynamics of the relationship or the impact and severity of the violence (Boonzaier & Schalkwyk, 2011; Laing & Humphreys, 2013). Feminism has therefore been influential in creating and developing other research instruments to measure the complex dimensions, severity and meaning of domestic violence that have been missing from earlier surveys (Taft, Hegarty & Flood, 2001; Laing & Humphreys, 2013). The Composite Abuse Scale (CAS) is one example, developed by Professor Kelsey Hegarty. This scale is the first validated multidimensional measure of intimate partner violence and has been used extensively globally and is available in ten languages. This measure of partner violence has four dimensions including severe combined abuse, emotional abuse, physical abuse and harassment (Hegarty, Bush & Sheehan, 2005). Feminist researchers are not opposed to large-scale surveys. Feminists understand the importance of revealing the prevalence of domestic violence, but they also argue for the importance of not missing the more nuanced accounts of women's experiences of violence and abuse from an intimate partner. Feminism has highlighted the importance of accounting for individual, interpersonal and sociocultural contexts within which domestic violence occurs (Boonzaier & Schalkwyk, 2011; Wendt & Zannettino, 2015).

Second, feminist scholarship of domestic violence moves beyond 'simply and crudely counting blows' (Krahe et al., 2005, p. 821). Feminist researchers also use qualitative approaches to study domestic violence, which has allowed women to represent their experiences of violence according to their own frames of meaning. Qualitative methods have enabled complexities of intimate partner violence to be explored and for gender to be theorised. In-depth information about the distinctive experiences of abuse in relatively understudied groups of women have therefore emerged (Boonzaier & Schalkwyk, 2011; Wendt & Zannettino, 2015). By engaging in a range of methodologies feminism has provided a concentration of work that explores and examines broader structural and cultural factors that allow so many women to be victimised by their male intimate partners. For example, as DeKeseredy (2011) argues, when sociocultural and structural factors within the institutions of marriage and family as well as law, religion and media are examined, the question of why domestic violence and why gender matters becomes evident. Feminist researchers, scholars and theorists in the past and present have exposed how power and violence are highly gendered and linked to culturally constructed and idealised forms of masculinity and femininity (Hester, 2012; Wendt & Zannettino, 2015); hence feminism has made it possible for domestic violence to be examined within contexts of gender inequality (Hanmer & Itzin, 2000).

Third, feminism has exposed coercive control to highlight the extent, severity and impact of intimate partner violence on women, which has been essential in forming solutions for domestic violence. Stark (2007) explains the gendered nature of coercive control by arguing that men's power (physical, material and social resources) forces women to survive domestic violence by calculating, evaluating and reassessing their own behaviour, including resistance or self-defence. Women become entrapped in domestic violence relationships because of the effect of control on women's health and wellbeing (Stark, 2007). Similarly, Johnson (2006) uses the term intimate terrorism to expose coercive control and to highlight the exertion of power, fear and control as being predominantly perpetrated by men against women. Through his research, he argues men's violence produces more physical injuries, more negative psychological consequences and more fear (Johnson, 2010).

Feminism has not ignored women's use of violence and abuse in intimate partner relationships. Hester (2012) outlined key studies which have found that women are rarely the initiators of violence and those who are violent to their male partners are more likely to be using 'violent resistance' for self-defence and retaliation against violent male partners. Studies have also shown that those with a long history of victimisation from previous male partners and in childhood use violence to decrease their own chance of further victimisation. In summary, feminist scholarship, research and practice has contributed much to understanding the complexities of domestic violence and gender differences. From decades of feminist-informed research, theorising and advocacy, the evidence is strong that domestic violence involves more death, injury, fear and psychological damage when perpetrated by men rather than women (Johnson, 2010).

Feminism has successfully led and presented compelling empirical evidence that domestic violence is largely perpetrated by men (Johnson, 2006). While the debates about the extent and nature of domestic violence will continue and the question of gender will remain, I argue that feminism is vital in this space for two reasons. First, feminism keeps gender central in explanations and understandings of domestic violence. Second, feminism exposes and challenges the dominance of masculinities and heteronormative power within these debates. Feminism stresses that gender is relational and ever-present; hence these debates about domestic violence happen within a context of challenging gender power relations.

Understanding the gendered nature of domestic violence

Domestic violence did not even exist as a concept or phenomenon before feminist activism, research and scholarship (Wendt & Zannettino, 2015). It was feminism that exposed and named domestic violence and documented the gendered nature of such abuse. Feminist-informed definitions of domestic violence have included coercive control and a range of abusive behaviours such as physical, sexual, psychological, social, economic and spiritual abuse (Laing & Humphreys, 2013; DeKeseredy, 2011). To demonstrate the importance and value of this work, I cite examples from research, mainly my own, to show the range of abusive behaviour that is perpetrated against women. These examples show how men engage with constructions of gender in domestic violence in sophisticated ways to create fear for women (Yodanis, 2004). The examples also show that women are rarely only victimised by one type of assault.

Feminist researchers and practitioners have long argued that physical abuse includes not only any act of physical violence but the threat of it. The threat of male violence is enough to create fear and control. For example, Boonzaier and Schalkwyk (2011) explored women's narratives of domestic violence in South Africa. They quote a woman talking about physical abuse:

> I'm like this, I can't keep quiet. I must talk back. And he does not want that! If I talk back or say something back, then it seems like he

can give me one hell of smack. I decided, one day I decided, it is better if I keep my mouth shut. Because if I stay quiet it seems like he will also be quiet.

(p. 275)

This quotation shows many practices of gender such as women being blamed for provoking abuse and the many ways women try to understand and please their partner to stop abuse. Similar to physical abuse, feminists have also argued that sexual abuse is not only unwanted physical invasion or penetration of a woman's body that is sexual in nature, but includes a range of insidious coercive practices that control women. Sexual abuse is also humiliation, degradation and violation of women's sexual integrity (Hlavka, 2014; Kelly, 1990). For example, a woman I interviewed about her experiences of domestic violence wanted to talk about rape and asked me many times if rape can occur in marriage. She shared examples of feeling uncomfortable and compelled to have sex with her husband.

I thought 'I have to be the submissive wife, I must give in even if I don't want it and even if my period's not quite finished yet, even if you're not comfortable with it'.... Anyway so I just put up with it. I've gotten to the point that my skin crawls if my husband touches me.

(Wendt & Zannettino, 2015, p. 100)

Feminism has exposed and critiqued the heteronormative discourses that consistently link female sexuality with passivity, vulnerability and submissiveness, and male sexuality with dominance, aggression and desire (Hlavka, 2014). Liz Kelly has long argued that sexual violence needs to be understood to occur along a continuum of coercive behaviours, gender inequality and sexism (Kelly, 1990).Within the context of domestic violence, many women experience difficulties in naming sexual abuse because it incorporates shame and humiliation for women, fear of retaliation from a partner and ideas of male entitlement to sex (Boonzaier & Schalkwyk, 2011; Hlavka, 2014).

Sexual and physical abuse are also emotional abuse. No one strand of abuse can be isolated and viewed on its own as each receives support from the others (DeKeseredy, 2011). Emotional abuse can sometimes be referred to as psychological abuse or verbal abuse and it is diverse; however, feminists have documented many stories from women including engendering fear or humiliation, enforcement of social isolation (social abuse) and taking or withholding finances (financial abuse) as examples of emotional abuse. Emotional abuse generates anxiety, and impoverishes and undermines self-esteem (Jewkes, 2010). Feminist scholarship has pointed out that these strands of emotional abuse together with socio-cultural constructions of gender explain coercion, control and fear in domestic violence (DeKeseredy, 2011). The quotations below from my own research demonstrate gender power relations along the continuum of emotional abuse.

> At the dinner table he would treat me like a child. I never used to eat many vegetables and he was, well, how can you expect the kids to eat vegetables, and just look at me, like you better eat those vegetables. And the kids never said a word and as soon as dinner was finished they would get up and one had to do the dishes, even my daughter who was 4 years old. And I when I think about it, why didn't I stop it? It was because I was too scared, scared of the wrath, the ranting and the raving and glaring ... that could go on all night and escalate with his drinking.
>
> (Wendt, Buchanan & Moulding, 2015, p. 8)

Financial abuse is tied up with emotional abuse. It includes a perpetrator controlling or withholding finances, spending finances for his use only causing inadequate finance for essential living costs, as well as perpetrators sabotaging victims' access to employment and income (Chung & Wendt, 2015).

> I feel like a hopeless mother because I couldn't protect them [her children], because I was living in such absolute terror all the time and desperation all the time. We never had enough to eat, we weren't well, we were unhealthy.
>
> (Wendt & Zannettino, 2015, p. 53)

> I'm sure the power imbalance that it caused [she is talking about her employment] contributed to his actions or his attitudes. He was quite happy for me to work and to spend my money but he didn't like me to talk about my work at all ... he didn't want to hear about anything that I did, he made it quite clear.[1]

These two quotations show gendered expectations that women can and should navigate and meet both partners' and children's needs all the time, even in dangerous contexts. Perpetrators of abuse can draw on such discourses to make women feel guilt, doubt and blame in domestic violence.

Social abuse is often referred to as controlling the victim through forms of surveillance and monitoring, for example, of where she goes, who she sees and what she wears. It also includes perpetrators isolating victims from family and friends by convincing them they do not need anyone else or sabotaging contact with them (Chung & Wendt, 2015). 'He always wanted me to dress a particular way, like wearing trousers and pants was just wrong, short hair was sinful' (Wendt & Zannettino, 2015, p. 95).

> I was doing a course and having a lot of fun and actually making friends for the first time and he was getting jealous of that and kept

on threatening and getting aggressive and threatening that he was going to kill himself if I didn't stay with him and trying to disconnect me from all the friends there. Later on, I think throughout the relationship, every time that I made friends he kept on putting those friends against me or putting them down in front of me and making sure that I never had any connection with them. It got to the stage where you couldn't have anyone even around the house.[2]

These two quotations show a sense of male entitlement and expectations of women serving and meeting the needs of men. Women are positioned as the property of men.

There is also emerging literature that has focused on religion and domestic violence and hence spiritual abuse has also been named. Spiritual abuse is evident when the perpetrator uses the realm of a woman's spiritual experiences and connectedness to hurt her as well as the misuse of religious beliefs or practices to justify physical and other forms of abuse (Wendt & Zannettino, 2015, p. 87). For example, I interviewed a Christian woman about her experiences of domestic violence and she showed me her Bible numerous times, referring to biblical texts that her partner used to force her to stay with him.

> He defiled my Bible. In Genesis, Chapter 2 and Verse 16 when after Adam and Eve had eaten the forbidden fruit, God said, 'Your desire will be for your husband and he will rule over you…'. He underlined and with exclamation marks 'he will rule over you'. My husband circled 'your desire will be for your husband and he will rule over you'.
>
> (Wendt & Zannettino, 2015, p. 90)

In this example, masculine authority and feminine submission is constructed as divinely ordained and this reinforcement of gender can diminish women's beliefs in their right to, or their sense of, equality (Allen & Devitt, 2012).

The qualitative responses above show that men use countless and complex highly gendered abuse tactics to establish coercive control in domestic violence. Domestic violence cannot be understood as a list of isolated incidences, or violent acts. Domestic violence encompasses patterns of coercive control that result from everyday unequal gender power relations. Men who use violence in intimate relationships draw on discourses of gender systematically to degrade and belittle women, eroding self-worth and consequently creating entrapment. Gender positioning and how power is played out in the contexts of intimate relationships is central to understanding domestic violence, its continuation and justification across time (Wendt & Zannettino, 2015). In short, feminism has exposed the gendered nature of domestic violence, which reflects patterns of male domination in most societies (Taft et al., 2001).

What happens when gender disappears: what does this mean for social work?

By centralising gender, feminism has shaped policy and practice responses to domestic violence. Domestic violence responses are largely and appropriately targeted to women victims and their children (Taft et al., 2001). Intervention therefore focuses on enhancing women's safety, providing psychological and emotional support, and increasing access to resources such as housing, income and child care. Gender analysis in policy and practice is most obvious in the work of women's shelters/refuges. Women's shelters/refuges provide protection and serve as a hiding place for women and their children when leaving domestic violence. They provide a range of services including information and understanding about domestic violence and offer a supportive social atmosphere in which women can think about and plan for their future (Jonker et al., 2014). Women's shelters/refuges also help women understand and overcome the fear and anxiety that are a consequence of coercive control, violence and abuse. Through close contact with other women who have endured domestic violence women begin to see the patterns of abuse that denote domestic violence as a societal issue not of their making and thus they can let go of shame and self-blame. In addition shelters/refuges provide advocacy services, legal counselling and referrals to other services. Principles of empowerment underpin the work of shelters/refuges in order to enable women to regain confidence and skills to function on their own (Haj-Yahia & Cohen, 2009; Jonker et al., 2014). In summary, feminist-informed responses to domestic violence aim to raise women's collective consciousness and social awareness that domestic violence is not related to women's personal failure in marriage or intimate partners' idiosyncratic behaviours or pathology, but are the result of broader social gender inequality (Mason, 2007).

Feminism is essential in domestic violence research, and policy and practice responses, because advances in the domestic violence field are continually met with counterattack or undermining of the gains made (DeKeseredy & Schwartz, 2013). De-gendering of domestic violence happens in multiple ways with perhaps the most aggressive coming from organised anti-feminist groups in western capitalist countries (Flood, 2004). It also happens in more subtle ways by social and legal policy adopting gender-neutral language when naming domestic violence. Furthermore, de-gendering domestic violence work can also be the result of funding pressures, competitive tendering processes and domestic violence work being absorbed or morphed into generic services such as homelessness and family counselling. These pressures are always present and can be seen across the western world. For example, in both Australia and the UK in the previous 12 months specialised domestic violence services that respond to women and children have been defunded, closed or at minimum received funding on yearly contracts (see Bullen, 2015; Laville, 2014; Neate, 2014). I argue social work is well positioned to engage with and utilise feminist scholarship so gender remains central in domestic violence analysis, policy and practice. Social work is a profession that strives to raise awareness of structural and systemic inequities, which fits with the broader goals of feminism to explore and expose oppression and disadvantage in the lives of diverse groups of women. Feminism enables social workers to see how women and men are affected by broader societal structures and discourses (Teater, 2010). As Dominelli (2002) argues, feminist theories provide a platform for anti-oppressive practice, a critical component for social workers to work against marginalisation and disadvantage. Without gender analysis, I argue, domestic violence becomes an issue of individual pathology that is reflective of women's so-called poor choices and victimisation and something only men with particular psychological problems perpetrate. Domestic violence is therefore positioned as a problem for particular individuals, which diminishes the broad-scale harmful effects on women and children. De-gendering thereby eliminates collective action and hence ignores the importance of social change that is required to stop domestic violence (DeKeseredy & Schwartz, 2013).

Conclusion

For social work, continuous reflections are required to ensure that policy and practice responses to domestic violence do not separate the experiences of individual women from their social contexts (Laing & Humphreys, 2013). It is through the recognition of social contexts that feminism has exposed the gendered nature of domestic violence. Without its gendered social context, the social and historical causes of male violence disappear. A contextual and political understanding is fundamental to action and needed to reduce or eliminate domestic violence. Feminism enables social work not to forget the social context of gender power relations and hence be part of the solution to end domestic violence.

Notes

1 This interview was conducted as part of an Australian Research Council Grant titled Project ID: DP130104437, Gendered violence and citizenship: the complex effects of intimate partner violence on mental health, housing and employment.
2 The interview was conducted as part of the study reported in Wendt, Buchanan and Moulding (2015).

Further reading

Johnson, M. (2006) Conflict and control: gender symmetry and asymmetry in domestic violence. *Violence Against Women*, 12(11), pp. 1003–1018.

Laing, L. & Humphreys, C. (2013) *Social Work and Domestic Violence: Developing Critical and Reflective Practice.* Sage, London.
Wendt, S. & Zannettino, L. (2015) *Domestic Violence in Diverse Contexts: A Re-Examination of Gender.* Routledge, London.

References

Allen, M. & Devitt, C. (2012) Intimate partner violence and belief systems in Liberia. *Journal of Interpersonal Violence*, 27(17), pp. 3514–3531.
Boonzaier, F. & van Schalkwyk, S. (2011) Narrative possibilities: poor women of color and the complexities of intimate partner violence. *Violence Against Women*, 17(2), pp. 267–286.
Bradley, H. (2013) *Gender*, 2nd edn. Polity, Cambridge, UK.
Buchanan, F. (2013) A critical analysis of the use of attachment theory in cases of domestic violence. *Critical Social Work*, 14(2). www1.uwindsor.ca/criticalsocial work/critical_analysis_attachment_theory (accessed 15 July 2015).
Bullen, J. (2015) The evidence supports specialist refuges for domestic violence. *Conversation*, 18 February. https://theconversation.com/the-evidence-supports-specialist-refuges-for-domestic-violence-37066 (accessed 15 July 2015).
Chung, D. & Wendt, S. (2015) Domestic violence against women: policy, practice and solutions in the Australian context. In A. Day & E. Fernandez (eds), *Preventing Violence in Australia: Policy, Practice and Solutions*. Federation Press, Annandale, NSW, pp. 202–215.
DeKeseredy, W. (2011) *Violence against Women: Myths, Facts, Controversies*. University of Toronto Press, Ontario, Canada.
DeKeseredy, W. & Schwartz, M. (2013) *Male Peer Support and Violence Against Women: The History and Verification of a Theory*. Northeastern University Press, Boston, MA.
Dominelli, L. (2002) *Feminist Social Work Theory and Practice*. Palgrave, Basingstoke, UK.
Flood, M. (2004) Backlash: angry men's movements. In E.E. Rossi (ed.), *The Battle and Backlash Rage On: Why Feminism Cannot be Obsolete*. Xlibris Corporation, New York, pp. 261–278.
Haj-Yahia, M. & Cohen, H. (2009) On the lived experience of battered women residing in shelters. *Journal of Family Violence*, 24(2), pp. 95–109.
Hanmer, J. & Itzin, C. (eds) (2000) *Home Truths about Domestic Violence: Feminist Influences on Policy and Practice, a Reader*. Routledge, London.
Hegarty, K., Bush, R. & Sheehan, M. (2005) The Composite Abuse Scale: further development and assessment of reliability and validity of a multi-dimensional partner abuse measure in clinical settings. *Violence and Victims*, 20(5), pp. 529–547.
Hester, M. (2012) Portrayal of women as intimate partner domestic violence perpetrators. *Violence Against Women*, 18(9), pp. 1067–1082.
Hlavka, H. (2014) Normalising sexual violence: young women account for harassment and abuse. *Gender and Society*, 28(3), pp. 337–358.
Jewkes, R. (2010) Emotional abuse: a neglected dimension of partner violence. *Lancet*, 376(9744), pp. 851–852.
Johnson, M. (2006) Conflict and control: gender symmetry and asymmetry in domestic violence. *Violence Against Women*, 12(11), pp. 1003–1018.

Johnson, M. (2010) Langhinrichsen-Rolling's confirmation of the feminist analysis of intimate partner violence: comment on 'Controversies involving gender and intimate partner violence in the United States'. *Sex Roles*, 62, pp. 212–219.

Johnson, M. & Ferraro, K. (2000) Research on domestic violence in the 1990s: making distinctions. *Journal of Marriage and the Family*, 62, pp. 948–963.

Jonker, I., Jansen, C., Christians, M. & Wolf, J. (2014) Appropriate care for shelter-based abused women: concept mapping with Dutch clients and professionals. *Violence Against Women*, 20(4), pp. 465–480.

Kelly, L. (1990) How women define their experiences of violence. In K. Yllo & M. Bograd (eds), *Feminist Perspectives on Wife Abuse*. Sage, Newbury Park, CA, pp. 114–132.

Krahe, B., Bieneck, S. & Moller, I. (2005) Understanding gender and intimate partner violence from an international perspective. *Sex Roles*, 52(11/12), pp. 807–827.

Laing, L. & Humphreys, C. (2013) *Social Work and Domestic Violence: Developing Critical and Reflective Practice*. Sage, London.

Laville, S. (2014) Domestic violence refuge provision at crisis point, warn charities. *Guardian*, 4 August. www.theguardian.com/society/2014/aug/03/domestic-violence-refuge-crisis-women-closure-safe-houses (accessed 15 July 2015).

Mason, R. (2007) Building women's social citizenship: a five-point framework to conceptualise the work of women-specific services in rural Australia. *Women's Studies International Forum*, 30(4), pp. 299–312.

Neate, P. (2014) Closing domestic violence refuges is the most dangerous thing of all for women. *Telegraph*, 5 August. www.telegraph.co.uk/women/womens-life/11013739/UK-domestic-violence-refuge-closures-the-most-dangerous-thing-of-all-for-women.html (accessed 15 July 2015).

Nichols, A. (2013) Meaning-making and domestic violence victim advocacy: an examination of feminist identities, ideologies, and practice. *Feminist Criminology*, 8(3), pp. 177–201.

Stark, E. (2007) *Coercive Control: How Men Entrap Women in Personal Life*. Oxford University Press, New York.

Straus, M. (1979) Measuring intrafamily conflict and violence: the Conflict Tactics (CT) scales. *Journal of Marriage and the Family*, 41(1), pp. 75–88.

Taft, A., Hegarty, K. & Flood, M. (2001) Are men and women equally violent to intimate partners? *Australian and New Zealand Journal of Public Health*, 25(6), pp. 498–500.

Teater, B. (2010) *An Introduction to Applying Social Work Theories and Methods*. McGraw Hill and Open University Press, Maidenhead, UK.

Wendt, S. & Zannettino, L. (2015) *Domestic Violence in Diverse Contexts: A Re-Examination of Gender*. Routledge, London.

Wendt, S., Buchanan, F. & Moulding, N. (2015) Mothering and domestic violence: understanding maternal protectiveness within gender power relations. *AFFILIA: The Journal of Women and Social Work*, 30(4), pp. 533–545.

Yodanis, C. (2004) Gender inequality, violence against women, and fear: a cross-national test of the feminist theory of violence against women. *Journal of Interpersonal Violence*, 19(6), pp. 655–675.

15 Rape and sexual assault

Using an intersectional feminist lens

Fiona Buchanan and Lynn Jamieson

In this chapter, we examine the feminist idea of 'intersectionality' in order to elaborate its potential as a theoretical perspective that social workers can draw on in their efforts to divest rape and sexual assault of their power to demean women. Before moving into discussion of feminist understandings of rape and sexual assault, and the more recent contribution of an intersectional feminist lens, we will first set some parameters around our discussion by examining understandings of rape and sexual assault in the contemporary context.

Defining the parameters of rape and sexual assault

Rape and sexual assault are global issues affecting the health and well-being of people in all communities. Understandings of the contexts and incidence of rape and sexual abuse are arbitrated by different cultures and rape is defined differently in diverse legal jurisdictions. A definition of rape with international recognition, although not universal incorporation into national jurisdictions, is that adopted by the World Health Organization (WHO) on behalf of the United Nations. The WHO defines rape as 'physically forced or otherwise coerced penetration – even if slight – of the vulva or anus, using a penis, other body parts or an object' (WHO, 2002). Oral rape is missing from this definition but is included in many legal definitions in various jurisdictions throughout the world (Cook et al., 2011).

WHO (2002) broadly describes sexual abuse as

> any sexual act, attempt to obtain a sexual act, unwanted sexual comments or advances, or acts to traffic, or otherwise directed, against a person's sexuality using coercion, by any person regardless of their relationship to the victim, in any setting, including but not limited to home and work.

The World Health Organization (2002) identifies difficulties of collecting rape data in multi-country comparisons and cites the unreliability of police statistics. Despite these difficulties survey reports indicate unacceptable levels of rape and sexual abuse perpetrated against women in all cultures.

Legal and health sector definitions of sexual assault and rape generally specify the nature of the sexual act and sometimes provide a description of what constitutes non-consent and coercive tactics used to compel (Cook et al., 2011). How to establish absence of consent or presence of coercion is a contested issue in many sexual offence cases. Legal jurisdictions place more or less emphasis on the use of physical force, psychological intimidation, threats or blackmail. Whatever the circumstances, rape and sexual assault negatively affect the physical, mental and social health of survivors and can cause sexual and reproductive health problems both in the short and long term (WHO, 2002).

Whether rape is committed against women, transgendered people or men, the control exercised by the perpetrator is widely understood as an attack on the agency and self-worth of the survivor. However, rape and sexual abuse is most often perpetrated by men against women (WHO, 2002). Female sex offending makes up a very small percentage of all sexual assaults and Australian research has found that half of all convicted female sex offenders co-offended with a male perpetrator, suggesting that when women abuse they are often coerced by a male partner (Stathopoulos, 2014). While sexual violence is not infrequently directed against men, this is usually by men who seek power over other men. Men's sexual violence against men is becoming more visible and increasingly a subject of enquiry (Davies, Gilston & Rogers, 2012; Peterson et al., 2011; Sleath & Bull, 2010), but rape and sexual assault of women continues to represent a major social problem. For example, in a telephone survey of 3,000 randomly selected American women, the researchers concluded that 18 per cent had been raped and only 16 per cent of those raped had reported it to the police (Kilpatrick et al., 2007).

In times of peace, most rapes and sexual assaults are perpetrated by persons known to the victim, whether they are a partner, family member, friend, work colleague or acquaintance. For example, in a review of research in the United States, the authors note that being raped by their partner is an aspect of the experience of 40–50 per cent of women enduring domestic violence (Martin, Taft & Resick, 2007). In specifying that rape and sexual assault are violations, regardless of the perpetrator's relationship with the victim, the WHO is mindful of the high prevalence of sexual victimisation within marriage where, as one facet of domestic violence, rape and sexual assault are used to subjugate women. This is borne out by the prevalence of rape shown in large-scale studies and evidence gathered across countries and cultures throughout the world although, given taboos about talking about rape in some cultures, rape is likely to be significantly underreported (WHO, 2002).

Rape and sexual assault are still systematically used as acts of warfare (Brownmiller, 2013; Kelly, 2000; Zurbriggen, 2010). To this day, armed men 'rape and pillage', with women's bodies used as spoils of war. In 'peace times', acts of rape and sexual assault are also used to subjugate minority groups, whether racialised (Crenshaw, 1991) or marginalised because of sexual or transgender orientation (Lombardi et al., 2002; McNeil et al., 2012; Stotzer, 2009). Acts of sexual assault are often directed at the most vulnerable in society, including people with disabilities (Hollomotz, 2012; Lin et al., 2009), aged people and those with mental impairment, all of which are groups likely to be referred to social workers (McMahon & Schwartz, 2011).

Feminist understandings of rape and sexual assault

In the 1970s radical feminists pioneered a critical analysis of rape, locating it in patriarchal systems of male privilege, power and control over women and their bodies. By listening to the voices of rape and sexual assault survivors, second wave feminists conceptualised rape as a manifestation of male abuse of power. Susanne Brownmiller was one of a number of early feminists who argued that all men benefit from women's fear of rape, as this fear causes women to censor their own movements and to seek male protection (Brownmiller, 2013). From a radical feminist perspective male abuse of power results from and is sustained by patriarchal systems – including economic, political and cultural institutions – that allocate most of the control and resources, status and power to men, sustaining a view of gender inequality as a legitimate outcome of presumably natural male superiority over women. Feminist work also specifically uncovered social attitudes about gender and sexuality that enable and sustain male-perpetrated rape and sexual abuse. For example, feminists showed how victim blaming for rape was based on categorising women into those deserving of men's protection and those who are culpable for the sexual abuse perpetrated against them. Such victim-blaming discourses were shown to be based on ideas of women as 'temptresses' and men as naturally unable to hold back their 'sex drive'.

Many feminists also adopted Liz Kelly's (1988) idea of a continuum of sexual violence: she argued that the small ways in which men intrude into women's spaces and bodies to harass and demean them are at one end of the continuum, with rape and murder at the other. Kelly (1988) therefore used the idea of a continuum to capture both the common underlying coercive exercise of power by men and their continuity with women's experiences of harassment and abuse. Minor forms of misogyny and sexual harassment are not typically counted in official statistics or research despite the understanding that they are part of the context that makes rape possible. Feminists have also shown that women themselves do not always define their experiences of rape and sexual assault in the same way as legal categories (Koss, 2005). In addition to her concept of a continuum of sexual violence, Kelly (1988) also coined the terms 'pressurised sex' and 'coercive sex' to capture how women talk about unwanted sex when reluctant to use the concept of rape. These practices continue: in a recent large survey of 13–17 year olds in the UK, 10 per cent of girls reported being pressured into having sexual intercourse when they did not want to (Barter & McCarry, 2012). In her research on the trafficking of women, Kelly (2000) also notes that reluctance to name abuse and exploitation is because some elements of coercion are normalised, and because of creeping gradations of entrapment.

While the concept of 'patriarchy' has become less fashionable, contemporary feminists nonetheless continue to document the reproduction of gender inequalities. This includes critical attention to persistent binary cultural ideals of masculinity that valorise 'being a man' as the antithesis of femininity. The essence of this hegemonic masculinity is power over others and, while this includes other men, it particularly rests on an assumption of power and control over women (Connell & Messerschmidt, 2005). While not all men seek to live up to this cultural ideal of hegemonic masculinity, the image of the conquering hero who gains women's sexual favours by heroic acts of physical conquest is as much an expression of women's subordination as the rapist who presumes he can take women for his use and abuse.

Historically, women have been treated as men's property and many jurisdictions defined rape in terms of a crime committed by one man against another's property; it has taken decades of feminist struggle to enable the human rights focus of current United Nations definitions (Bourke, 2008). However, criminal justice systems still typically fail many women. Adversarial systems enable patriarchal perspectives to influence the application of the law of rape, distorting understandings of consensual sex and undermining the credibility of women as witnesses. Through such processes women can be further humiliated and objectified in court procedures in which legal representatives of the accused seek to suggest that they are fabricating or somehow to blame for the events. Thus, issues of the woman's lifestyle choices, appearance, behaviours, location and honesty are brought into question, often despite attempts to exclude irrelevant sexual history and character evidence (Adler, 1987; Brown, Burman & Jamieson, 1993, Daly & Bouhours, 2010; Edwards et al., 2011; Naffine, 2014; Temkin, 2002). In no other field of law is the character of a victim attacked to this extent. By evoking stereotypes of 'authentic' rape and sexual assault as deviant acts perpetrated by a stranger and occurring only within a narrow set of circumstances – outside the home and invoking physical resistance from the person under attack – women who are raped in other circumstances are exposed to disbelief and critical appraisal (Edwards et al., 2011). Lack of understanding about various forms of coercion also allows victim blaming and disavows that women refrain from physical resistance because of fear, intimidation and threats to self or others, such as children. Myths about women's propensity to lie are played on to reframe acts of rape and sexual assault as spurious attempts to vilify the abuser. Such tactics deny justice to women and deter women who have been raped and sexually assaulted from seeking legal retribution.

Advancing feminist understandings of rape and sexual assault: intersectional feminism

Patriarchal views and practices are still present in most if not all social systems around the world, including many legal systems, although now they are sometimes more subtly expressed. In particular, victim blaming continues to be supported by myths about rape despite feminist ideas supposedly becoming more mainstream (Bohner et al., 2013; Bernhardsson & Bogren, 2012; Edwards et al., 2011; Gavey, 2013; Horvarth & Brown, 2009). At the same time, academic theorisation of gender and power has become increasingly sophisticated, and the concept of 'intersectionality' now informs much feminist discussion. Intersectional feminism grew from the work of African-American feminists who first theorised the interrelationships of gender with racism and class inequalities (Crenshaw, 1991; Dill, McLaughlin & Nieves, 2007). Intersectional feminists also worked to counter what has been described as 'hegemonic feminisms' that privilege the perspective of middle-class white women (Martinez, 2011, p. 148). However, we argue that intersectional feminism builds on the work of radical feminists by expanding our vision rather than replacing it with a different premise. Intersectional feminism furthers our understanding by drawing out the diverse ways that oppression and discrimination intersect to disadvantage women. An intersectional perspective pays attention to how social circumstances and cultural norms promote and proscribe particular ways of being, identifying as and displaying being a woman. Focusing on women's identities as affected by how they are treated enables understanding from disenfranchised groups of how multifaceted oppression exacerbates distress and distrust of systems which should protect the human rights of all people (Dill et al., 2007).

In situations of rape and sexual assault, the lens of intersectional feminism makes more visible women's experiences across diverse ages, abilities, cultures, socioeconomic classes and sex/gender identities, such as lesbian and transsexual women. For example, issues of poverty, discrimination and racism differentiate the experiences of many women from that of white, middle-class women. The perspective can also work against simply individualising difference as a matter of unique psychology or reducing difference to simplistic one-factor explanations such as 'culture'. For example, studies of the prevalence of rape and sexual assault show differences in prevalence between ethnic groups and by social class but such differences are produced by interacting social processes. They are not adequately explained by 'culture' or 'identity' without both remembering that men's violence against women is a problem in all cultures and looking for the interlocking systems of inequality that frame its specific forms (Gavey, 2013; Gill, 2013). Circumstances of poverty create stresses that exacerbate levels of violence, and findings of different rates of sexual violence between ethnic groups sometimes disappear when controlling for socioeconomic circumstances (Sokoloff & Dupont, 2005).

In the case of African-American women and Indigenous women in white settler societies, the interaction of poverty with the constant incursion of racism alongside legacies of subjugation through colonisation or slavery have more explanatory power than a simplistic use of 'culture' or 'identity'. The idea that particular marginalised or multiply disadvantaged groups have 'rape cultures' also enhances prejudice and stigma that cause further harm to women who are raped. The vulnerability of Indigenous women is demonstrated through the finding that they are twice as likely to experience rape as other women in the population (Nixon & Humphreys, 2010). In Australia, McCalman et al. (2014) note that an inordinately high incidence of rape against Aboriginal women is exacerbated by fear of disclosure. Racist discourse denigrating Aboriginal people, the terrible history of colonisation, and negative experiences of government agencies and services amplify the risks of rape and disclosure of rape. This backdrop means that the incidence of abuse feeds racist discourses about Aboriginal people and it fractures trust in help-giving services. This makes rape more possible and promotes questioning and condemnation of disclosure within Aboriginal communities that may result in family retaliation, community condemnation and blame (McCalman et al., 2014).

Absence of legal redress or appropriate assistance from support services is particularly common in the experience of disadvantaged groups. The reasons for this failure are entwined with the systems of inequality underpinning their disadvantage. Women with physical and intellectual disabilities are particularly vulnerable to rape but the disadvantages of gender and disability mean they are often disbelieved or disregarded (Lin et al., 2009; Hollomotz, 2012). The failure of agencies to deliver appropriate support is also documented as a commonplace experience of the transgender community (Namaste, 2000; McNeil et al., 2012; Whittle et al., 2008). Research suggests very high rates of sexual assault as part of a pattern of hate crime and prejudice against transgender people (Stotzer, 2009), particularly against male to female and female to male transsexual people (Lombardi et al., 2002). In many jurisdictions, definitions of rape remain gendered in ways that create insurmountable difficulties when transgender people seek legal redress as rape victims; at the same time transgender people have been convicted of sexual assault for failing to disclose their gender history prior to consensual sex (Sharpe, 1994, 2014). It takes a particular awareness among service providers to recognise and resist the interplay between misogyny, discrimination and intolerance of difference that leads to rape as a method for further targeting and demoralising disenfranchised groups.

The concept of 'intersectionality' therefore draws attention to the fluid and supporting ways in which systems of inequality and social division generate hybrid forms of social disadvantage (Anthias, 2014). The term signals a theoretical approach that goes beyond treating gender inequality as the only relevant story in understanding gender and sexual violence. The 'intersection' metaphor is one of social position rather than individual attributes (Sokoloff & Dupont, 2005). It is important not to reduce individuals to carriers of disadvantage but rather to understand how the joint operations of social worlds create exposure to sexual abuse, and reduce both recognition and opportunities to seek redress. For example, it is the ways in which social worlds privilege men, white ethnicities and able-bodied people that diminish the room for manoeuvre of many women, not the attributes of gender, skin colour or bodily disabilities in themselves.

As the earlier examples show, systems of inequality other than gender can increase victimisation of women, reduce protection against rape and sexual assault, increase the silencing of victims and create barriers to assistance with recovery. Equality policies and protections against discrimination, as well as legal redress for sexual assault, are often insensitive to multiple disadvantages in ways which marginalise and exclude women who should have access to legal redress. Unacknowledged legacies of cultural stereotyping as an aspect of treating subordinate groups as 'others' can discourage clients from disclosing to service providers and contribute to service providers failing to recognise sexual assault, thus inadvertently discouraging reporting and missing opportunities to enquire about needs for support. Colonial histories of subordination and ideologies denigrating others, such as racism, homophobia and bigotry, deny members of the subordinated group the authority to speak, sometimes producing self-censoring because of fear of stigma and defeat (Collins, 2004). If social workers are to show that they are part of the solution and not part of the problem they may have to build a history of protecting the community from the abuse of racism or other histories of discrimination before being able to protect individuals from the abuse of assault (Sokoloff & Dupont, 2005).

Rape and sexual assault as a social work issue: an intersectional lens

The persistence of men's sexual assaults on women, children and other men, and the potential depth of the consequent harm, gives all social workers cause to address rape and sexual assault as human rights and social justice issues across the whole range of social work practices. An appropriate social work response requires understanding of how the production, incidence, experience and harm of men's violence against women intersects with inequalities and disadvantages other than gender.

The experience of women who stand at the intersections of disadvantage, for example, poor women from racially abused ethnic minorities or lesbian women within stigmatised religious groups, remind us that men's gendered control over women is not the only dimension of power shaping the harms of sexual assault.

Social workers have a mandate to advocate for human rights within the ideal of a just society; rape and sexual assault represent a denial of both. However, as McMahon and Schwartz (2011) have documented in their research, attention to this topic within social work is limited. Yet from a feminist and human rights perspective, social workers should be at the vanguard of rape prevention and addressing the needs of rape survivors (McMahon & Schwartz, 2011).

It is, therefore, essential that social workers are able to ask about rape and sexual assault sensitively during assessments and have the skills and knowledge to address any disclosures. In particular, social workers in mental health services, homeless accommodation, community-based programmes, migrant and refugee services, and disability services will be working with women who have been raped or sexually assaulted, including women from diverse social backgrounds. In some instances, the difficulties clients are experiencing will have been caused or exacerbated by undeclared rape and sexual assault in the recent or more distant past. If rape and sexual assault are not identified as a cause or contributing factor, distressing thoughts, feelings and circumstances related to the assault cannot be resolved. Without appropriate responses women may be re-victimised by service providers, including social workers, and societal myths that intensify shame and self-blame may be reinforced (McMahon & Schwartz, 2011). Social workers who lack knowledge in this area therefore may not only silence women but can also exacerbate harm.

An intersectional feminist lens can particularly offer social work practitioners and policy makers a perspective from which to view disparities in the incidence of rape and a means to address the impact of myths which compound the effects of rape and sexual assault. Social work intervention can be understood as sitting along a continuum from social activism to support of individuals. This continuum includes advocacy, policy development, political lobbying, work in communities, counselling, therapy and working with disadvantaged and vulnerable people in all sectors of society. Social workers in specialist rape and sexual assault services are adept at using their social work knowledge and skills to have a positive impact along this continuum. Likewise, there are social workers within services who incorporate anti-rape practice in their work. However, all social workers have a mandate to promote social justice. Given that social work is concerned with the needs of vulnerable communities all social workers need to be conversant with and skilled in using feminist knowledge, based in diverse lived experiences of survivors, to address rape and sexual abuse. An important element of this knowledge base is an understanding of rape myths, including how their operation misrecognises and exacerbates multiple disadvantages, and feeds on and perpetuates not only misogyny but other forms of prejudice.

Rape myths have long histories and permeate religious, legal and media institutions. Edwards et al. (2011) offer a review of how each myth has come about and is being sustained. The myth that women frequently tell lies about rape co-exists comfortably with legal systems which demand proof of physical resistance in rape cases and conclude that the absence of such proof indicates telling lies. Women's social position at the intersections of disadvantage further affects the ways they are subjected to the charge of lying in rape cases. For example, working-class women may be faced with defence tactics that appeal to class-based prejudices of supposed unreliability and poor self-control. Defence lawyers may draw the attention of the court to any circumstances reflecting disadvantage, such as living in stigmatised housing areas, growing up in state care or a history of glue sniffing (Brown et al., 1993; Phipps 2009). Such details can become part of a general strategy of undermining a woman's credibility (Jordan, 2011; Temkin, 2002; Temkin & Krahé, 2008) because in many cultures ideas about 'good' and 'bad' character are deeply infused with prejudices about social class and ethnicity as well as gender. Skeggs (2004) has documented how feminine 'respectability' has been culturally aligned with images of white, middle-class women in the UK, making it difficult for working-class and ethnic minority women to claim this for themselves. The perception that women lie about rape supports and draws on a more general misogyny, portraying women as dishonest and unreliable, or motivated by revenge. Similarly, tactics drawing on prejudices about ethnicity, religion, able-bodiedness or sexuality buy into racism, bigotry, denigration of disability and homophobia. Edwards et al. (2011) trace the suggestion that women lie about rape back to biblical texts and point to contemporary echoes in criminal justice systems. In some jurisdictions, efforts to improve the experience of women have focused on changing the attitudes and practices of the police and legal practitioners, with mixed success (Burman, Jamieson & Nicholson, 2007; Daly & Bouhours, 2010; Jordan, 2011; Naffine, 2014; McMillan & Thomas, 2013). The tactics of defence lawyers are not typically the focus of such efforts at changing professional cultures, and research into mock juries suggests defence tactics are effective (Ellison & Munro, 2009). Some sociolegal scholars advocate bringing expert witnesses into the courts explicitly to counteract the repertoire of rape myths that defence lawyers play on (Temkin & Krahé, 2008; Krahé & Temkin, 2009).

Media biases also lend support to rape myths. Ideas about ethnicity, 'race' and social class are often implicit in media accounts of rape with the ideal-typical victim being white and middle-class (Berrington & Jones 2002; Dowler, 2006; Kitzinger 2013; Soothill & Walby, 1991; Gill, 2007). There is a long and well-documented history of racist assumptions about black men and rape of white women which still surface in popular discourse (Collins, 2004).

There is now a very significant body of feminist research documenting the prevalence of rape myths across diverse populations. Much of it documents higher rates of acceptance of sceptical victim-blaming myths among men than women (Edwards et al., 2011; Foster & Kidd, 2014; Grubb & Turner, 2012). Edwards et al. (2011) cite many studies which find that 'the invitation to rape' myth is pervasive in diverse communities, nurturing and supported by the misplaced belief that women who confine themselves to stereotypical roles avoid rape. This view may be reinforced when public announcements made by the police, following publicised rape cases, ask women to restrict their movements. The message reinforces the idea that if women are in the public domain they are putting themselves at risk and that women who stay indoors will be safe. Such a message may weigh particularly heavily on women who are defying local cultural conventions by travelling alone and those who lack the economic resources to avoid forms of transport and places associated with risk. In contradiction to this message, surveys of victimisation show that there are high numbers of women, including women from diverse ethnic backgrounds, abilities and sexualities, who are sexually assaulted at home, often by males that they know as partners, relatives or friends. Abuse of women and children who are frail or vulnerable residents in care homes is also known to be perpetrated primarily by carers in positions of trust (Daly & Bouhours, 2010; Edwards et al., 2011). The suggestion that home is safe and public space is a place of danger for women is an insidious myth that partially continues the effect of more explicit patriarchal questioning of women's right to participate in public life, whether or not there is social acceptance for such views.

In many jurisdictions legislation was, and in some cases still is, in place so that men cannot be charged with raping their wives. Some interpretations of religious doctrines support this idea of a husband's access to his wife's body which allows men to rape their wives with impunity (Edwards et al., 2011). In addition to some jurisdictions denying women the right to seek justice, many women either do not know that they have the right or have lost belief in their rights. Women who are segregated and isolated may not have access to information that contradicts their husband's beliefs about his entitlement to sex. Research has documented the debilitating, confidence-destroying impact of the coercive control of an abusive partner (Stark, 2007). An abuser exercising coercive control engineers a woman's social isolation but women who are already isolated, for example, distanced from friends and family by migration and facing language barriers in making new ties, are especially vulnerable. Myths about rape add to the smokescreen obscuring possibilities of exit for women who are being raped by a partner exercising coercive control. An intersectional lens encourages further consideration of how some social situations offer fewer routes of exit than others. Women who believe their legal right to citizen-ship or means of economic support depend on their relationships with their abusers are particularly cut off from means of redress.

Intersectional feminist principles for social work

If the role of social work is to promote positive social change, then it is highly appropriate to make the values of social justice and human rights explicit when addressing rape and sexual assault. Further, social work is distinguished by using a strengths approach to enable empowerment of clients and client groups. Following an intersectional feminist approach recognising multiple identities (Damant et al., 2008), a focus on women's diverse strengths and identities can help to ensure that survivors of rape and sexual abuse are not solely defined by the trauma that they have endured. By integrating feminist-informed knowledge into practice, alternative messages can be used to refute internalised prejudices. With knowledge of myths, and practice at their rebuttal, social workers can chal-lenge clients' experiences of shame and self-blame and influence how rape and sexual assault survivors see themselves.

Working directly with rape and sexual assault survivors begins with established social work skills of taking a non-judgemental attitude, and showing empathy and acceptance (Chenoweth & McAuliffe, 2015). Through building respectful relationships with clients combined with awareness of barriers they are likely to face, truly listening and enabling women to tell their story in their own time, questions about possible rape and sexual assault can be asked sensitively. Using social work skills with survivors of rape and sexual assault should create openings for disclosure, following the clients' leads, and acknowledging their right to make their own decisions. When working with survivors from a strengths perspective, there is scope to recognise and reinforce individual women's agency by seeking to understand and acknowledge each woman's survival strategies. From an intersectional feminist perspective, honouring individual women's strengths, despite multiple oppressions, means that women are not defined by the act of rape and the strengths gained from varied identi-ties can be valued.

Good social work practice is already sensitive to cultural stereotyp-ing. An intersectional perspective reinforces the importance of resist-ing ethnocentric assumptions dressed up as if they reflect 'universal civilisation', by listening to and honouring knowledge rooted in the experiences of women in circumstances of disadvantage and minority cultures (Ono 2013; Sokoloff & Dupont, 2005). Appropriate assistance to rape victims may mean acknowledging sources of expertise outside the social work community and being aware of the range of community supports available to particular groups. For example an Australian Aboriginal woman may draw strength from being encouraged to speak with a trusted woman who is an elder in her community and better positioned to understand the impacts of multigenerational discrimination and abuse suffered by her people and by Aboriginal women in general.

Social workers working in policy have an important role to play in ensuring that the voices of women from minority groups are included. Analysis of policy documents shows that, even when the diversity of women's circumstances is acknowledged, along with recognition that women with particular disadvantages may have particular needs, the voices of disadvantaged minorities are seldom heard, despite being the obvious experts on their own needs (Strid, Walby & Armstrong, 2013). Researchers and campaigners working to reduce violence against women can point to policies and practices formed with good intentions but which, without consulting ethnic minority women, have caused them harm. For example, absolute confidentiality is much more important for women's safety and wellbeing in some communities than others and practices of sharing information across professional groups can be experienced as a serious breach of trust (Kelly, 2010).

Research, including practitioner research, which draws on intersectional feminist perspectives can add to the knowledge base supporting practice and activism to promote change at individual, policy and societal levels. Social work researchers can inform practice through a social work evidence base which delineates incidence, issues, prevention programmes and effective practice strategies with diverse client groups. When researching participants' experiences of rape and sexual assault, social work skills fit with feminist methods of qualitative research and are particularly helpful in research with diverse vulnerable groups because they simultaneously uncover deep and rich meaning while helping participants to feel valued and empowered (Liamputtong, 2007).

Although there is sparse coverage of rape and sexual assault in the social work literature, feminist researchers have developed a knowledge base that social workers can use to counter societal views which disempower women who have endured rape and sexual assault (Edwards et al. 2011; Fisher & Cullen, 2000; Littleton, 2011; Macy et al., 2010; Martin et al., 2007; McMahon & Schwartz, 2011). Knowledge about rape myths and openness to understanding effects of multiple layers of discrimination are tools that social workers can bring to address rape and sexual abuse. In addition, social workers who are conversant with the systems and legislation in their jurisdiction can help women to make choices about seeking justice.

Social workers can contribute to combating the climate in which rape flourishes through promoting discourses on gender, sexism, racism, homophobia and other forms of oppression, for example, by supporting school and community prevention programmes which promote tolerance of differences and respectful relationships (Edwards et al., 2011; Horvarth

& Brown, 2009; Jones, 2012; Littleton, 2011). Social workers who have made it their business to understand the specific barriers to justice for women at intersections of multiple disadvantage are well placed to interact with criminal justice systems on their behalf, as advocate or witness, and they have an opportunity to educate police, lawyers and court officials (Sokoloff & Dupont, 2005).

Visible involvement in anti-violence activities such as Reclaim the Night Marches and online campaigns which inclusively acknowledge gendered injustices adds a social work voice to resistance to violence against women in diverse communities. Through advocating, lobbying, policy work and educating, systems can be influenced from inside and out.

Social workers can similarly build a knowledge base that will help to make the case for including women at intersections of disadvantage in policy consultation. By conducting qualitative and quantitative research into the instance, effects and interventions for women in diverse populations using intersectional feminist approaches, social workers can promote recognition of the varied ways in which discrimination oppresses women. Feminist research on rape and sexual assault can expose how racism and other prejudices may lead to higher rates of assault, increased adverse effects, particular assaults on identities and reduced access to justice for women across a range of disadvantaged groups.

Conclusion

In this chapter we have outlined the definition and incidence of rape and sexual assault, and considered the contribution that radical and intersectional feminisms bring to our understanding of these problems. Social workers, no matter in which sector of service provision or policy writing, will be working with women who have survived rape, yet this is an area of social work that is insufficiently recognised. There is little research and evidence of reflection on practice. All social workers can raise awareness of societal myths and how they sustain victim blaming, which allows systemic discrimination against vulnerable individuals and groups to persist. There is much to be done to combat rape and sexual abuse but social work skills and values combined with knowledge based in feminist perspectives puts social workers in a position to support clients and promote social change. Working across the continuum of social work practice can promote knowledgeable, just societies which refute patriarchal belief systems and help to empower survivors of rape and sexual abuse to speak out and have their voices heard. Moreover, social workers can work with survivors to use their agency in collective efforts for social change. Since the 1970s feminists have dreamed of a world free from rape, and we believe that social workers continue to have an important role to play in helping to realise that dream.

Further reading and websites

Bourke, J. (2008) *Rape: A History from 1860 to the Present Day.* Virago, London.

Lombard, N. & McMillan, L (eds) (2013) *Violence against Women: Current Theory and Practice in Domestic Abuse, Sexual Violence and Exploitation.* Jessica Kingsley Publishers, London.

Ullman, S.E. (2010) *Talking about Sexual Assault: Society's Response to Survivors.* American Psychological Association, Washington, DC.

International websites

End Violence Against Women International includes information about best practice in a range of service provision settings: www.evawintl.org/.

Sexual Violence Research Initiative is a South African-based programme with a very useful website offering news about conferences and research papers. This site also has information about availability of funding for new research: www.svri.org/.

Australian websites

Sexual Violence Research, Australian Institute of Family Studies: www.aifs.gov.au/acssa/.

National Association of Services Against Sexual Violence: www.nasasv.org.au/index.htm.

References

Adler, Z. (1987) *Rape on Trial.* Routledge, London.

Anthias, F. (2014) The intersections of class, gender, sexuality and 'race': the political economy of gendered violence. *International Journal of Politics, Culture, and Society,* 27(2), pp. 153–171.

Barter, C. & McCarry, M. (2012) Love, power and control: girls' experiences of relationship exploitation and violence. In N. Lombard & L. McMillan (eds), *Violence Against Women: Current Theory and Practice in Domestic Abuse, Sexual Violence and Exploitation.* Jessica Kingsley Publishers, London, pp. 103–124.

Bernhardsson, J. & Bogren, A. (2012) Drink sluts, brats and immigrants as others: an analysis of Swedish media discourse on gender, alcohol and rape. *Feminist Media Studies,* 12, pp. 1–16.

Berrington, E. & Jones, H. (2002) Reality vs. myth: constructions of women's insecurity. *Feminist Media Studies,* 2, pp. 307–323.

Bohner, G., Eyssel, F., Pina, A., Siebler, F. & Viki, G.T. (2013) Rape myth acceptance: cognitive, affective and behavioural effects of beliefs that blame the victim and exonerate the perpetrator. In M. Horvath & J. Brown (eds), *Rape: Challenging Contemporary Thinking.* Routledge, Abingdon, pp. 17–45.

Bourke, J. (2008) *Rape: A History from 1860 to the Present Day.* Virago, London.

Brown, B., Burman, M. & Jamieson, L. (1993) *Sex Crimes on Trial: The Use of Sexual Evidence in Scottish Courts.* Edinburgh University Press, Edinburgh.

Brownmiller, S. (2013) *Against our Will: Men, Women and Rape.* Open Road Media, New York.

Burman, M., Jamieson, L. & Nicholson, J. (2007) *Impact of Aspects of the Law of Evidence in Sexual Offence Trials: An Evaluation Study.* Scottish Government, Edinburgh. www.scotland.gov.uk/Publications/2007/09/12093403/1 (accessed 24 June 2015).

Chenoweth, L. & McAuliffe, D. (2015) *The Road to Social Work and Human Service Practice*, 4th edn. Cengage, South Melbourne.

Collins, P.H. (2004) *Black Sexual Politics: African Americans, Gender and the New Racism.* Routledge, New York.

Connell, R.W. & Messerschmidt, J.W. (2005) Hegemonic masculinity: rethinking the concept. *Gender and Society*, 19, pp. 829–859.

Cook, S.L., Gidycz, C.A., Koss, M.P. & Murphy, M. (2011) Emerging issues in the measurement of rape victimization. *Violence Against Women*, 17(2), pp. 201–218.

Crenshaw, K. (1991) Mapping the margins: intersectionality, identity politics, and violence against women of color. *Stanford Law Review*, 43(6), pp. 1241–1299.

Daly, K. & Bouhours, B. (2010) Rape and attrition in the legal process: a comparative analysis of five countries. *Crime and Justice*, 39(1), pp. 565–650.

Damant, D., Lapierre, D., Kouraga, A., Fortin, A., Hamelin-Brabant, L., Lavergne, C. & Lessard, G. (2008) Taking child abuse and mothering into account: intersectional feminism as an alternative for the study of domestic violence. *AFFILIA: The Journal of Women and Social Work*, 23(2), pp. 123–133.

Davies, M., Gilston, J. & Rogers, P. (2012) Examining the relationship between male rape myth acceptance, female rape myth acceptance, victim blame, homophobia, gender roles, and ambivalent sexism. *Journal of Interpersonal Violence*, 27(14), pp. 2807–2823.

Dill, B.T., McLaughlin, A.E. & Nieves, A.D. (2007) Future directions of feminist research: intersectionality. In S.N. Hesse-Biber (ed.), *Handbook of Feminist Research: Theory and Praxis.* Sage, Thousand Oaks, CA, pp. 629–637.

Dowler, K. (2006) Sex, lies, and videotape: the presentation of sex crime in local television news. *Journal of Criminal Justice*, 34, pp. 383–392.

Edwards, K.M., Turchik, J.A., Christina, M., Dardis, C.M., Reynolds, N. & Gidycz, C.A. (2011) Rape myths: history, individual and institutional-level presence, and implications for change. *Sex Roles*, 65, pp. 761–773.

Ellison, L. & Munro, V.E. (2009) Reacting to rape exploring mock jurors' assessments of complainant credibility. *British Journal of Criminology*, 49(2), pp. 202–219.

Fisher, B.S. & Cullen, F.T. (2000) Measuring the sexual victimization of women: evolution, current controversies, and future research. *Criminal Justice*, 4, pp. 317–390.

Foster, C. & Kidd, G.J. (2014) Acquaintance rape: associations between rape myths, blame, and attitudes towards women. *Asian Journal of Humanities and Social Studies*, 2(3). www.ajouronline.com/index.php?journal=AJHSS&page=article&op=view&path%5B%5D=1356 (accessed 24 June 2015).

Gavey, N. (2013) *Just Sex? The Cultural Scaffolding of Rape.* Routledge, New York.

Gill, A. (2013) Intersecting inequalities: implications for addressing violence against black and minority ethnic women in the United Kingdom. In N. Lombard & L. McMillan (eds), *Violence against Women: Current Theory and Practice in Domestic Abuse, Sexual Violence and Exploitation*, Jessica Kingsley Publishers, London, pp. 141–158.

Gill, R. (2007) *Gender and the Media.* Polity, Oxford.

Grubb, A. & Turner, E. (2012) Attribution of blame in rape cases: a review of the impact of rape myth acceptance, gender role conformity and substance use on victim blaming. *Aggression and Violent Behavior*, 17, pp. 443–452.

Hollomotz, A. (2012) Disability, oppression and violence: towards a sociological explanation. *Sociology*, 47(3), pp. 477–493.

Horvath, M. & Brown, J. (2009) Setting the scene: introduction to understanding rape. In M. Horvath & J. Brown (eds), *Rape: Challenging Contemporary Thinking*. Routledge, Abingdon, pp. 1–14.

Jones, H. (2012) On sociological perspectives. In J.M. Brown & S.L. Walklate (eds), *Handbook on Sexual Violence*. Routledge, Abingdon, pp. 181–202.

Jordan, J. (2011) Silencing rape, silencing women. In J. Brown & S. Walklate (eds), *Handbook on Sexual Violence*. Routledge, London, pp. 253–287.

Kelly, L. (1988) *Surviving Sexual Violence*. Polity Press, Cambridge.

Kelly, L. (2000) Wars against women: sexual violence, sexual politics and the militarised state. In S. Jacobs, R. Jacobson & J. Marchbank (eds), *States of Conflict: Gender, Violence and Resistance*. Zed Books, London, pp. 45–65.

Kelly, L. (2010) Foreword. In R.K. Thiara & A.K. Gill (eds), *Violence against Women in South Asian Communities: Issues for Policy and Practice*. Jessica Kingsley Publishers, London, pp. 9–13.

Kilpatrick, D.G., Resnick, H.S., Ruggiero, K.J., Conoscenti, L.M. & McCauley, J. (2007) *Drug-Facilitated, Incapacitated, and Forcible Rape: A National Study*. National Crime Victims Research and Treatment Center, Medical University of South Carolina, Charleston, SC.

Kitzinger, J. (2013) Rape in the media. In M. Horvath & J. Brown (eds), *Rape: Challenging Contemporary Thinking*. Routledge, Abingdon, pp. 74–99.

Koss, M.P. (2005) Empirically enhanced reflections on 20 years of rape research. *Journal of Interpersonal Violence*, 20(1), pp. 100–107.

Krahé, B. & Temkin, J. (2009) Addressing the attitude problem in rape trials: some proposals and methodological considerations. In M. Horvarth & J. Brown (eds), *Rape: Challenging Contemporary Thinking*. Routledge, London, pp. 301–321.

Liamputtong, P. (2007) *Researching the Vulnerable*. Sage, London.

Lin, L., Yen, C., Kuo, F., Wu, J. & Lin, J. (2009) Sexual assault of people with disabilities: results of 2002–2007 national report in Taiwan. *Research in Development Disabilities*, 30, pp. 969–975.

Littleton, H. (2011) Rape myths and beyond: a commentary on Edwards and colleagues. *Sex Roles*, 65, pp. 792–797.

Lombardi, E.L., Wilchins, R.A., Priesing, D. & Malouf, D. (2002) Gender violence: transgender experiences with violence and discrimination. *Journal of Homosexuality*, 42(1), pp. 89–101.

McCalman, J., Tsey, K., Bainbridge, R., Rowley, K., Percival, N., Lynette, O. & Judd, J. (2014) The characteristics, implementation and effects of Aboriginal and Torres Strait Islander health promotion tools: a systematic literature search. *BMC Public Health*, 14(1), pp. 1–12.

McMahon, S. & Schwartz, R. (2011) A review of rape in the social work literature: a call to action. *AFFILIA: The Journal of Women and Social Work*, 26(3), pp. 250–263.

McMillan, L. & Thomas, M. (2013) Police interviews of rape victims: tensions and contradictions. In M. Horvath & J. Brown (eds), *Rape: Challenging Contemporary Thinking*. Routledge, London, pp. 255–280.

McNeil, J., Bailey, L., Ellis, S., Morton, J. & Regan, M. (2012) *Trans Mental Health and Emotional Wellbeing Study*, Scottish Transgender Alliance and Sheffield Hallam University, Sheffield, UK.

Macy, R.J., Giattina, M.C., Parish, S.L. & Crosby, C. (2010) Domestic violence and sexual assault services: historical concerns and contemporary challenges. *Journal of Interpersonal Violence*, 25(1), pp. 3–32.

Martin, E.K., Taft, C.T. & Resick, P.A. (2007) A review of marital rape. *Aggression and Violent Behaviour*, 12, pp. 329–347.

Martinez, P.R. (2011) Feminism and violence: the hegemonic second wave's encounter with rape and domestic abuse in USA (1970–1985). *Cultural Dynamics*, 23(3), pp. 147–172.

Naffine, N. (2014) *Feminism and Criminology*. John Wiley & Sons, New York.

Namaste, V. (2000) *Invisible Lives: The Erasure of Transsexual and Transgendered People*. University of Chicago Press, Chicago, IL.

Nixon, J. & Humphreys, C. (2010) Marshalling the evidence: using intersectionality in the domestic violence frame. *Social Politics*, 17(2), pp. 137–158.

Ono, E. (2013) Violence against racially minoritized women: implications for social work. *AFFILIA: The Journal of Women and Social Work*, 28(4), pp. 458–467.

Peterson, Z.D., Voller, E.K., Polusny, M.A. & Murdoch, M. (2011) Prevalence and consequences of adult sexual assault of men: review of empirical findings and state of the literature. *Clinical Psychology Review*, 31(1), pp. 1–24.

Phipps, A. (2009) Rape and respectability: ideas about sexual violence and social class. *Sociology*, 43(4), pp. 667–683.

Sharpe, A. (2014) Criminalising sexual intimacy: transgender defendants and the legal construction of non-consent. *Criminal Law Review*, 3, pp. 207–223.

Sharpe, A.N. (1994) The precarious position of the transsexual rape victim. *Current Issues in Criminal Justice*, 6(2), 303–307.

Skeggs, B. (2004) *Class, Self, Culture*. Routledge, London.

Sleath, E. & Bull, R. (2010) Male rape victim and perpetrator blaming. *Journal of Interpersonal Violence*, 25(6), pp. 969–988.

Sokoloff, N.J. & Dupont, I. (2005) Domestic violence at the intersections of race, class, and gender challenges and contributions to understanding violence against marginalized women in diverse communities. *Violence Against Women*, 11(1), pp. 38–64.

Soothill, K. & Walby, S. (1991) *Sex Crime in the News*. Routledge, London.

Stark, E. (2007) *Coercive Control: How Men Entrap Women in Personal Life*. Oxford University Press, Oxford.

Stathopoulos, M. (2014) *The Exception that Proves the Rule: Female Sex Offending and the Gendered Nature of Sexual Violence*. ACSSA Research Summary No. 5. Australian Institute of Family Studies, Melbourne. www3.aifs.gov.au/acssa/pubs/research-summary/ressum5/index.html (accessed 4 April 2014).

Stotzer, R.L. (2009) Violence against transgender people: a review of United States data. *Aggression and Violent Behavior*, 14(3), pp. 170–179.

Strid, S., Walby, S. & Armstrong, J. (2013) Intersectionality and multiple inequalities: visibility in British policy on violence against women. *Social Politics: International Studies in Gender, State and Society*, 20(4), pp. 558–581.

Temkin, J. (2002) *Rape and the Legal Process*. Oxford University Press, Oxford.

Temkin, J. & Krahé, B. (2008) *Sexual Assault and the Justice Gap: A Question of Attitude*. Bloomsbury Publishing, London.

Whittle, S., Turner, L., Coombs, R. & Rhodes, S. (2008) *Transgender Eurostudy: Legal Survey and Focus on the Transgender Experience of Health Care*. ILGA Europe, Brussels.

World Health Organization (2002) *Violence against Women.* Fact Sheet No. 239. WHO, Geneva. www.who.int/mediacentre/factsheets/fs239/en/ (accessed 2 March 2014).

Zurbriggen, E.L. (2010) Rape, war, and the socialization of masculinity: why our refusal to give up war ensures that rape cannot be eradicated. *Psychology of Women Quarterly*, 34, pp. 538–549.

16 Homelessness and intersectional feminist practice

Carole Zufferey

Homelessness is a gendered and multidimensional human rights issue. The United Nations General Assembly adopted the Universal Declaration of Human Rights in 1948, which states that every person has the right to a standard of living that is adequate for their health and wellbeing, including access to food, clothing, housing and medical care (Article 25). Global definitions of homelessness tend to focus on literal homelessness, which is living without shelter and with few possessions, 'sleeping in the streets, in doorways or on piers, or in any other space, on a more or less random basis' (United Nations, 1998, para. 1.328). Western policy definitions of homelessness concentrating on literal, primary or visible homelessness (such as 'rough sleeping' in Britain and 'street people' in America) also tend to focus on men, who are more likely to experience and remain in this type of homelessness (Passaro, 1996). In western countries, these literal definitions of homelessness are contested, and dominant definitions of homelessness have been criticised for being gender-neutral. Gender-neutral perspectives on homelessness can obscure gendered experiences, rendering invisible the types of homelessness experienced by women and their children. This is because housing-based definitions of homelessness assume that housing is the solution and that homelessness is the problem (Tomas & Dittmar, 1995), yet women tend to be victims of gendered violence in their own homes.

Broader definitions of homelessness imply a continuum of homelessness and housing that extend beyond primary (or literal) homelessness. Australian researcher Chris Chamberlain (1999) outlines an approach to primary, secondary, tertiary and marginal levels of homelessness, with primary homelessness capturing literal homelessness. Secondary homelessness includes people with no place of usual residence (such as 'couch surfing' or living in temporary shelters). Tertiary homelessness includes people who are inappropriately or insecurely housed, living in culturally defined substandard accommodation. Marginal housing refers to people who are 'at risk' of homelessness (such as people living in boarding houses, financial housing crisis or overcrowded conditions). Similarly, the European Typology of Homelessness and Housing Exclusion (Amore,

Baker & Howden-Chapman, 2011) also defines homelessness as a continuum: roofless, which is people sleeping rough and living in public spaces; houseless, which includes people living in homeless services, women's shelters, hospitals and prisons; insecure housing, which includes a lack of security of tenure and living with the threat of violence; and inadequate housing, which relates to overcrowding, houses unfit for habitation and temporary housing such as mobile homes.

Worldwide, there are over 100 million people without shelter, and the majority are women and children (UNCHS, 1996). The Australian Bureau of Statistics (ABS) Census (2011) collates demographic data and estimates the prevalence of homelessness using six predefined operational groups: persons in improvised dwellings, tents or sleeping out; in supported accommodation for the homeless; staying temporarily with other households; in boarding houses; in other temporary lodgings; and living in severely crowded dwellings. However, despite widening understandings of homelessness, housing-based definitions do not consider the embodied and gendered lived experiences of homelessness. In contrast, feminist theorising of homeless experiences draws on diverse and inclusive feminist ethics and principles, and acknowledges how lived experiences of home and homelessness are embodied and gendered. As an example, feminist theorising centres the observation that the main cause of women's homelessness is gendered violence in the context of unequal gender and other social power relations.

Homelessness is therefore multidimensional and complex, influenced by changing historical, gender, cultural, discursive and structural contexts (Somerville, 1992). Homelessness also involves 'physiological (lack of bodily comfort or warmth), emotional (lack of love or joy), territorial (lack of privacy), ontological (lack of rootedness in the world, anomie) and spiritual (lack of hope, lack of purpose)' dimensions (Somerville, 2013, p. 384).

Australian researchers such as Robinson (2009, 2011) and Farrugia (2010) have studied how homelessness is embodied, felt and lived, noting that power relationships and emotions are central to the embodied subjectivities of (young) people experiencing homelessness. These authors focus on intersubjectivities, identity, belonging, the sociology of the body, social geographies of place, embodiment and emotions, drawing on critical and reflexive ethnographic methodologies to engage with the 'lived experiences' of homelessness. However, feminism has largely not been central to contemporary sociological theorising about homelessness.

Feminism has much to contribute to expanding knowledge and challenging social work practice in the field of homelessness (Watson & Austerberry, 1986). Feminist researchers in this field, including myself, have examined subjective definitions and experiences of identity, home and homelessness (Wardhaugh, 1999), 'everyday' lived experiences of homelessness (Zufferey & Kerr, 2004) and feminist social work responses to domestic violence and homelessness (Seymour, 2012; Zufferey, 2009; Johnson & Richards, 1995). However, feminist researchers have tended to focus on home as gendered, rather than homelessness.

Feminists have focused on the public–private divide of women's lived experiences in their physical spaces and places of home (Smith, 2012). Home has been related to identity, 'place(s), space(s), feeling(s), practices, and/or an active state of state of being in the world' (Mallett, 2004, p. 62). Western interpretations of the meaning of home may include a sense of security, stability, privacy, safety and the ability to control a living space (Gurney, 1999). Home is variously conflated with the private domain: a house, the family, a haven or refuge, as well as a prison for those who experience violence and abuse in their 'home' (Mallett, 2004, p. 71). Home can be related to feelings of 'being at home', creating or making home and the 'ideal' home (Mallett, 2004, p. 62). Home can be an 'ideal' and a 'reality', both an 'actual' and 'remembered' journey, which occurs across time and in diverse places and spaces (Mallett, 2004, p. 69). Therefore, women's experiences of home and homelessness relate to feelings of 'belonging' that evolve throughout our lives and in our relationships with others (Jackson & Scott, 2010). While home, like homelessness, involves subjective feelings, not feeling 'at home' does not mean that people identify as 'homeless' (Mallett, 2004). Feeling 'at home' relates to feeling a sense of belonging, while feeling 'homeless' relates to experiences and feelings of exclusion and displacement (Yuval-Davis, 2011). As such, some women express feeling 'homeless' in their own homes due to experiencing domestic violence but this is not the experience of all women.

Feminism and homelessness

There are many different forms of feminism that can be taken up by social workers working in the field of homelessness. In this chapter, I particularly draw on intersectional feminism to explore understandings of homelessness. Similar to feminism, a central aim of social work is to influence social change and redress inequalities (Allen, Pease & Briskman, 2003). Feminism and social work have a long and intertwined history, with compatible commitments to activism and the betterment of society (Kemp & Brandwein, 2010). However, feminism and social work have been criticised for promoting white, western, middle-class women's experiences and neglecting to acknowledge diversity (hooks, 2000; Crenshaw, 1990). In responding to such criticisms, authors such as Jackson argue that 'the ways in which gender intersects with other forms of inequality, especially those founded on racism and colonialism, has been under-theorised' (1998, p. 24). Intersectional feminism has now become a powerful and useful political tool to frame social work advocacy efforts (Yuval-Davis, 2006).

There has been a considerable amount of literature published on intersectionality. As Carbin and Edenheim argue, intersectionality is now 'presented as *the* feminist theory' (2013, p. 245) in gender research and practice. The social work and intersectionality literature is diverse and includes advocating for teaching intersectionality to students of diverse disciplines at undergraduate and postgraduate levels (Carbin & Edenheim, 2013), using it as a human rights policy frame (Yuval-Davis, 2006), incorporating it in social work practice, research, policy and education (Murphy et al., 2009) and using it as a tool for critical reflection in social work for analysing a critical incident (Mattsson, 2014).

Intersectional theorising in the 1980s and 1990s criticised the essentialism of white identity-based politics by highlighting the inseparability of racial and gender oppressions and the socio-political location and standpoint of black feminists (Mehrotra, 2010, p. 420). Unlike the experience of 'home' feeling like a 'prison' for some women who experience violence, black feminist scholars have argued that, for black women, home is a 'haven' from a racist society and a site of resistance to 'white supremacist capitalist patriarchy' (hooks, 1990, 2000). However, research studies nonetheless consistently find that the majority of women who experience homelessness were once victims of domestic violence. The most severe and lethal domestic violence disproportionately occurs among low-income women of ethnic minority backgrounds, challenging the mainstream feminist contention that domestic violence affects all women equally (Sokoloff & Dupont, 2005). For example, African-American women and Aboriginal Australian women are more likely to have children in their care, be poor, experience violence, be discriminated against in employment and have fewer accommodation options, all of which occur in the gendered context of the increasing feminisation of poverty (Richards et al., 2010).

An intersectional framework broadens feminist activism in the area of homelessness and domestic violence, which includes focusing on social categories, such as gender, race, ethnicity, culture, sexuality, class, ability, age, mobility, wealth and religion, as well as geographical locations, such as urban/rural regions, nation-states and a country's social and economic developmental context (Yuval-Davis, 2006; Nixon & Humphreys, 2010). For example, in Australia it is important to acknowledge the colonisation and dispossession of Indigenous Australians and that 'the sense of belonging, home and place enjoyed by the non-Indigenous subject', whether that be the colonisers, migrants or refugees, is 'based on the dispossession of the original owners of the land' and the denial of Indigenous Australians' rights under 'international customary law' (Moreton-Robinson, 2003, p. 23).

In my own research, I have reflected on the value of intersectional feminism to contribute further to understandings of homelessness. Specifically focusing on social work, I have examined how social workers' bodies and identities are gendered when working in diverse fields of homelessness, including gendered violence (Zufferey, 2009). I found that social work is experienced and constructed as 'women's work', that unspoken gender relations are experienced by female workers in client–worker relationships with the opposite sex, that being a man or a woman can function as an invisible form of oppression, that a woman's physical appearance plays an important symbolic role in cultural constructions of, and responses to, gender and that social workers feel that feminist approaches are preferable when working with women who are homeless due to domestic violence (Zufferey, 2009, p. 386). In this feminist analysis of social work responses to homelessness, I centralise gender and power relations, emphasising the importance of embracing feminism in social work practice in the field of homelessness and gendered violence (see Zufferey, 2014).

Feminist social work responses to homelessness

Feminist-informed social work practice is particularly relevant to the field of domestic violence and homelessness. Drawing on my research and practice experiences in the field of homelessness, I have found that feminist approaches to homelessness enable a critical examination of how homelessness is responded to by social workers when shaping policy and practising in the field of homelessness. Twelve out of 39 participants in my PhD research on social work responses to homelessness advocated for a feminist approach to practice, especially when working with women in gendered violence (Zufferey, 2008). The feminist approach assists social workers to analyse power differentials from a human rights perspective, which can combine macro and micro practice to 'reframe' client circumstances. As one social worker said:

> Contextualising their [clients'] experience within the larger sociopolitical structures ... which sounds quite sort of intellectual and basic but ... in the everyday practice of our work it is kind of that feminist consciousness raising that happened in the 70s and 60s and you can still see the way that that really gets women to feel that they are not isolated nor are they pathologised, once they are there and they start recollecting their experience to us, a group or a body of women, and that recognises that we are quite different, there is not one kind of women but we do share similar kinds of oppressions.
>
> (Female, aged 21–30, government worker)

This collective feminist approach akin to 'making the personal political' (Kemp & Brandwein, 2010) merges individual and collective approaches to women's homelessness, where feminist community activism can complement individualist case management approaches. Intersectional feminist practice can also include a macro-political analysis of the structural positioning of social groupings and provide a multilayered analysis of social structures, constructions of identities and symbolic representations of social issues (Winker & Degele, 2011) such as homelessness. This involves socially locating and positioning social work and homelessness within organisational contexts and social institutions that are unequal, multilayered, dynamic and complex. For example, in both media representations of homelessness and social work organisational contexts, client–worker relationships are constructed as dichotomous, based on powerless/powerful identities where homelessness is a social problem to be 'fixed' by the service provider (Winker & Degele, 2011; Zufferey, 2008).

A key consideration for social work practitioners, policy makers and educators in the fields of social work is to be well-informed about the intersectional inequalities and discrimination affecting their client group(s). Yuval-Davis (2011) calls for a dialogue between people from different positionings and, in the field of homelessness, this could involve frontline social workers engaging in a dialogue with diverse groups of service users and policy makers. I argue that social workers play an important role in advocating for service users' voices to be heard and incorporated into policy responses, as well as making visible gaps in policy that prevent better outcomes for people who experience homelessness (Zufferey, 2011). This challenges 'one size fits all' policies and practices often criticised by people who experience homelessness and by frontline social workers too (Zufferey, 2008, 2009, 2011; Zufferey & Kerr, 2004). However, in my research and practice I have found that social workers are involved in resisting as well as supporting dominant social institutions and inequalities, which can be critiqued using an intersectional feminist lens.

Reflections on intersectional feminism and social work

Intersectional feminist approaches to homelessness enable social workers to deconstruct how unequal power relations (related to, for example, gender, class, race, ethnicity and sexual orientation) intersect to constitute embodied experiences of homelessness and social work. Embracing intersectionality in social work practice with people who are homeless involves examining how homelessness and social work are constituted through unequal and intersecting power relations. This requires a critical exploration of how social identity categories (such as Indigeneity, race, ethnicity, gender, class, age, sexuality, ability and other markers of identity) shape the embodied identities and experiences of men and women who are defined as homeless. This includes acknowledging how diverse and intersecting social identity categories and social locations structurally increase vulnerability and risk of homelessness. For example, women living in poverty of ethnic minority backgrounds are structurally disadvantaged and discriminated against, increasing their vulnerability to and risk of homelessness. Intersectionality also involves reflecting on social workers' social locations (for example white race privilege, race relations, ethnicity, gender, class, age, sexuality, ability, religious and social orientation, and other markers of social location) and how these social locations are experienced differently by different service users. Social work practitioners drawing on intersectional feminism can emphasise the importance of responding to diverse, embodied and interrelated inequalities, by giving due accord to the agency of service users, without losing sight of the structural inequalities that impact on people who experience homelessness.

In the context of social work practice responses to homelessness, intersectional feminism allows for a more complex, flexible, multilayered analysis of diverse social identities and power locations. It also enables a level of theoretical complexity in terms of incorporating research strategies that are anti-categorical, intra-categorical and inter-categorical (McCall, 2005; Christensen & Jensen, 2012). An anti-categorical approach examines how concepts, terms and categories are constructed, problematising the process of categorisation, which aligns with post-structuralist feminist understandings. For example, in practice, this approach may assist to deconstruct problematic categorisations and the fixing of homed–homeless identities in the context of gender inequalities, racial differences, class disadvantage, age stereotypes and sexuality. At the policy level, the anti-categorical approach may be useful to deconstruct dominant policy terminology and definitions of home and homelessness, using the perspectives of diverse people who have experienced homelessness. Intra-categorical approaches take identity categories into account but acknowledge that identities are fluid and multiple, tending to focus on 'neglected points of intersection' and on individuals at the micro level (McCall, 2005; Winker & Degele, 2011). This approach enables social workers to examine neglected and multiple identity categories and different stakeholders in the field of homelessness in more depth. For example, focusing on the neglected area of social work responses to homelessness, I have explored the personal and professional identities of individual social workers and how they embodied power, gender, class and cultural relations (Zufferey, 2009). As well, given that sexuality is often neglected in social work practice, a colleague and I have explored how sexuality and notions of home and homelessness are embodied and imagined (see Zufferey & Rowntree, 2014). We found that for a small group of lesbian women in Adelaide, South Australia, home involved the embodiment (and imagining) of physical spaces and locality (houses and landscapes) and the identification with communities of shared interest (lesbian communities and environmental movements). This study challenged heteronormative assumptions that currently influence how home, homelessness and sexuality are understood (Zufferey & Rowntree, 2014). Inter-categorical approaches focus on the relationships between categories where existing categorical differences are predefined. This can be used to document and measure inequality across multiple dimensions and how categories and inequalities change over time. For example, our recent research on how intimate partner violence (IPV) negatively affects women's mental health, housing stability and employment demonstrates that women's citizenship is eroded over time, across each of these predefined dimensions. The online survey with 658 Australian women showed that the majority of respondents reported they did not regain the levels of mental health, the quality of housing or the employment status which they had achieved before their experiences of IPV.[1] Therefore, the complexities of intersectional categories, including anti-categorical, intra-categorical and inter-categorical, make intersectionality a useful tool for constructing inclusive and multiple approaches to social work policy, practice and research in the field of homelessness and specifically gendered violence (McCall, 2005; Christensen & Jensen, 2012; Gressgård, 2008; Damant et al., 2008).

Conclusion

Intersectional social work practice involves embracing the complexities of the lived experiences of homelessness and positioning homelessness within a complex gendered frame that also incorporates other social axes of difference. The challenge for feminist social work practitioners is how to respond collectively to the intersecting inequalities experienced by their clients within organisational contexts that focus on individual issues, such as drug and alcohol, or mental health or other disabilities. The challenge for feminist social work policy makers relates to constructing categories from which to collect homelessness data that are unambiguous and mutually exclusive, whilst also acknowledging the intersections between categories of social identity and the social locations of policy makers. The challenge for feminist social work academics is to maintain a focus in their teaching on how gender intersects with other forms of disadvantage to constitute social problems such as homelessness, as well as social work responses to them. My vision as a social work educator is to graduate social work students who appreciate that homelessness and social work responses to it are complex and gendering. My hope for the future is that intersectional feminism can increasingly be used in social work policy, practice, research and education to advance practice responses to homelessness that are inclusive and respectful of diversity.

Note

1 This preliminary finding comes from an Australian Research Council Discovery Grant No. DP130104437, titled, *Gendered Violence and Citizenship: The Complex Effects of Intimate Partner Violence on Mental Health, Housing and Employment* (S. Franzway, S. Wendt, N. Moulding, C. Zufferey & D. Chung).

Further reading

Naples, N., Hoogland, R., Wickramasinghe, M. & Wong, A. (eds) (2015) *The Wiley-Blackwell Encyclopedia of Gender and Sexuality Studies*. Wiley-Blackwell, Malden, MA.

Smith, S.J. (ed.) (2012) *International Encyclopedia of Housing and Home.* Elsevier Science, Burlington, VT.

Wahab, S., Anderson-Nathe, B. & Gringeri, C. (eds) (2015) *Feminisms in Social Work Research.* Routledge. New York.

References

Allen, J., Pease, B. & Briskman, L. (eds) (2003) *Critical Social Work.* Allen & Unwin, Sydney.

Amore, K., Baker, M. & Howden-Chapman, P. (2011) The ETHOS definition and classification of homelessness: an analysis. *European Journal of Homelessness,* 5(2), pp. 19–37.

Australian Bureau of Statistics (ABS) (2011) *2049.0, Census of Population and Housing: Estimating Homelessness, 2011.* ABS, Canberra. www.abs.gov.au/AUSSTATS/abs@.nsf/Lookup/2049.0Explanatory%20Notes12011 (accessed 8 March 2014).

Carbin, M. & Edenheim, S. (2013) The intersectional turn in feminist theory: a dream of a common language? *European Journal of Women's Studies,* 20(3), pp. 233–248.

Chamberlain, C. (1999) *Counting the Homeless: Implications for Policy Development.* Australian Bureau of Statistics, Canberra.

Christensen, A. & Jensen, S. (2012) Doing intersectional analysis: methodological implications for qualitative research. *Nordic Journal of Feminist and Gender Research,* 20(2), pp. 109–125.

Crenshaw, K. (1990) Mapping the margins: intersectionality, identity politics, and violence against women of color. *Stanford Law Review,* 43, pp. 1241–1299.

Damant, D., Lapierre, S., Kouraga, A., Fortin, A., Hamelin-Brabant, L., Lavergne, C., et al. (2008) Taking child abuse and mothering into account: intersectional feminism as an alternative for the study of domestic violence. *AFFILIA: The Journal of Women and Social Work,* 23, pp. 123–133.

Farrugia, D. (2010) Youth, homelessness and embodiment: moralised aesthetics and affective suffering. Paper presented at the Australian Sociological Association Conference, Sydney, 6–9 December.

Gressgård, R. (2008) Mind the gap: intersectionality, complexity and 'the event'. *Theory and Science,* 10, pp. 1–16.

Gurney, C. (1999) Pride and prejudice: discourses of normalization in public and private accounts of home ownership. *Housing Studies,* 14(2), pp. 163–183.

hooks, b. (1990) *Yearning: Race, Gender and Cultural Politics.* South End Press, Boston, MA.

hooks, b. (2000) *Feminist Theory: From Margins to Center.* South End Press, Boston, MA.

Jackson, S. (1998). Feminist social theory. In S. Jackson & J. Jones (eds), *Contemporary Feminist Theories.* Edinburgh University Press, Edinburgh, pp. 12–33.

Jackson, S. & Scott, S. (2010) *Theorising Sexuality.* McGraw-Hill Education, Maidenhead, UK.

Johnson, A.K. & Richards, R.N. (1995) Homeless women and feminist social work practice. In N. Van Den Berg (ed.), *Feminist Practice in the 21st Century.* NASW Press, Washington, DC, pp. 232–257.

Kemp, S. & Brandwein, R. (2010) Feminisms and social work in the United States: an intertwined history. *AFFILIA: The Journal of Women and Social Work*, 25(4), pp. 341–364.

McCall, L. (2005) The complexity of intersectionality. *Signs: Journal of Women in Culture and Society*, 30(3), pp. 1771–1800.

Mallett, S. (2004) Understanding home: a critical review of the literature. *Sociological Review*, 52, pp. 62–89.

Mattsson, T. (2014) Intersectionality as a useful tool: anti-oppressive social work and critical reflection. *AFFILIA: The Journal of Women and Social Work*, 29(1), pp. 8–17.

Mehrotra, G. (2010) Toward a continuum of intersectionality theorizing for feminist social work scholarship. *AFFILIA: The Journal of Women and Social Work*, 25(4), pp. 417–430.

Moreton-Robinson, A. (2003) I still call Australia home: Indigenous belonging and place in a white postcolonizing society. In S. Ahmed, C. Castaneda, A. Fortier & M. Sheller (eds), *Uprootings/Regroundings: Questions of Home and Migration*. Berg, Oxford, pp. 23–40.

Murphy, Y., Hunt, V., Zajicek, A.M., Norris, A.N. & Hamilton, L. (2009) *Incorporating Intersectionality in Social Work Practice, Research, Policy, and Education*. NASW Press, Washington, DC.

Nixon, J. & Humphreys, C. (2010) Marshalling the evidence: using intersectionality in the domestic violence frame. *Social Politics*, 17(2), pp. 137–158.

Passaro, J. (1996, Reprint 2014) *The Unequal Homeless Men on the Streets, Women in their Place*. Routledge, London.

Richards, T.N., Garland, T., Bumphus, V.W. & Thompson, R. (2010) Personal and political? Exploring the feminization of the American homeless population. *Journal of Poverty*, 14(1), pp. 97–115.

Robinson, C. (2009) Homelessness felt. *Cultural Studies Review*, 15, pp. 167–172.

Robinson, C. (2011) *Beside One's Self: Homelessness Felt and Lived*. Syracuse University Press, New York.

Seymour, K. (2012) Feminist practice: who I am or what I do? *Australian Social Work*, 65(1), pp. 21–38.

Smith, S.J. (ed.) (2012) *International Encyclopedia of Housing and Home*. Elsevier Science, Burlington, VT.

Sokoloff, N. & Dupont, I. (2005) Domestic violence at the intersections of race, class and gender: challenges and contributions to understanding violence against marginalized women in diverse communities. *Violence Against Women*, 11(1), pp. 38–64.

Somerville, P. (1992) Homelessness and the meaning of home: rooflessness or rootlessness? *International Journal of Urban and Regional Research*, 16(4), pp. 529–539.

Somerville, P. (2013) Understanding homelessness. *Housing, Theory and Society*, 30(4), pp. 384–415.

Tomas, A. & Dittmar, H. (1995) The experience of homeless women: an exploration of housing histories and the meaning of home. *Housing Studies*, 10(4), pp. 493–513.

UNCHS (1996) *An Urbanising World: Global Report on Human Settlements*. Oxford University Press, Oxford.

United Nations (1998) *Principles and Recommendations for Population and Housing Censuses*. United Nations, New York.

Wardhaugh, J. (1999) The unaccommodated woman: home, homelessness and identity. *Sociological Review*, 47(1), pp. 91–110.

Watson, S. & Austerberry, H. (1986) *Housing and Homelessness: A Feminist Perspective.* Routledge, London.

Winker, G. & Degele, N. (2011) Intersectionality as multi-level analysis: dealing with social inequality. *European Journal of Women's Studies*, 18(1), pp. 51–66.

Yuval-Davis, N. (2006) Intersectionality and feminist politics. *European Journal of Women's Studies*, 13(3), pp. 193–209.

Yuval-Davis, N. (2011) *The Politics of Belonging.* Sage, London.

Zufferey, C. (2008) Responses to homelessness in Australian cities: social worker perspectives. *Australian Social Work*, 61(4), pp. 357–371.

Zufferey, C. (2009) Making gender visible: social work responses to homelessness. *AFFILIA: The Journal of Women and Social Work*, 24(4), pp. 382–393.

Zufferey, C. (2011) Homelessness, social policy, and social work: a way forward. *Australian Social Work*, 64(3), pp. 241–244.

Zufferey, C. (2014) Intersectional feminism and social work responses to homelessness. In S. Wahab, B. Anderson-Nathe & C. Gringeri (eds), *Feminisms in Social Work Research.* Routledge, New York, pp. 90–102.

Zufferey, C. & Kerr, L. (2004) Identity and everyday experiences of homelessness: some implications for social work. *Australian Social Work*, 57(4), pp. 343–353.

Zufferey, C. & Rowntree, M. (2014) Finding your community wherever you go? Exploring how a group of women who identify as lesbian embody and imagine 'home'. Paper presented at the Australian Sociological Association Conference, Adelaide, 24–27 November.

17 Sexuality, social work and the feminist imaginary

Margaret Rowntree

Traditionally, the social work discipline has not given sexuality the same level of attention as class, gender, ethnicity, age or health. When or if sexuality has been considered, the term is mostly used to mean sexual orientation, with social workers' mandate largely derived from addressing inequities arising from the lesser status of minority sexual communities. However, the ways in which sexuality is spoken about are broadening as its place on the western social work agenda finally gains impetus. In this chapter I add to this nascent but growing body of knowledge by advocating for social work to attend to sexuality through a perspective that privileges the role of the imaginary in feminist projects, in this case the feminist sexual project. Quite simply, the feminist sexual project seeks liberating forms of sexual relations for women, and men. In doing so, I principally draw upon the work of feminist philosopher Rosi Braidotti (2002, 2003, 2005, 2011), and in particular her materialist theory of becoming. Rather than promoting social conditions that enable rights and freedoms to express who we are, or what sexual orientation we are, the focus here is on who, what and how we want to become (sexually) in the world. This venture is surely in line with social work's mission of promoting the empowerment and liberation of people to enhance wellbeing (AASW, 2010). Rather than seeing sexuality as a social category or social identity, in this chapter I conceptualise sexuality as an axis of social analysis, and follow Stevi Jackson's understanding that it encompasses wide-ranging aspects of erotic life, namely 'desires, practices, relationships and identities' (2006, p. 106).

Feminist engagement with sexuality

While historically sexuality may not have been a leading item on the social work agenda, it has been a noteworthy and sustained item on the western feminist agenda. Here I briefly review some notable historical highlights in feminism's engagement with sexuality, particularly although not exclusively women's sexuality. In doing so, I lay the groundwork for my argument for social work's contemporary engagement with sexuality from a materialist feminist perspective, which I later elaborate upon. First, feminists during the second wave of the women's movement in the 1960s and 1970s rallied around concerns about the double standard of sexual conduct between men and women, identifying it as a marker of gender inequality and patriarchal oppression (Firestone, 1971; Morgan, 1970; Oakley, 1972). Other feminists at the time were keen to use the momentum of the movement to imagine alternative sexual paradigms and challenge existing status quo arrangements (Cixous, 1996; Greer, 1971). It is widely recognised, though, that these feminist aspirations were largely unrealised in comparison to the movement's other achievements for women (hooks, 1984). Here bell hooks describes the challenge of feminism's sexual project:

> It has been a simple task for women to describe and criticize negative aspects of sexuality as it has been socially constructed in sexist society; to expose male objectification and dehumanization of women, to denounce rape, pornography, sexualized violence, incest etc. It has been a far more difficult task for women to envision new sexual paradigms, to change the norms of sexuality.
>
> (1984, p. 148)

By the early 1980s feminists had become deeply embroiled in conflict over sexuality, leading to the eventual fracturing of the women's movement. What has since become known as the 'sex wars' involved polemical disputes between one faction of feminists who championed sexual freedom and highlighted sexual pleasure, and another faction that championed freedom from sexism and highlighted sexual dangers (Chancer, 1998).

It was not until the 1990s that women's sexual expression came into the spotlight again – this time taken up by women describing themselves as a third wave of the feminist movement. Keen to distinguish themselves from what they saw as the inflexibility of politically correct second wave feminists, these women sought to do feminism in their own way (Bail, 1996). Recuperating the word 'girl' from one of personal insult to one of fun-loving self-avowal, they incorporated traditional feminine accessories into their dress codes, pairing femininity and feminism together in sympathy rather than at odds. The so-called 'New Girl Order' called for women to use their right to express their sexuality in any and as many ways as they wanted (Karp & Stoller, 1999). According to Debbie Stoller, a prominent advocate in this movement, the employment gap for women was temporarily 'set aside' to address 'the orgasm gap' (Karp & Stoller, 1999, p. 76). 'Sexuality, in all its disguises, has become a kind of lightning rod for this generation's hopes and discontents' write Nan Bauer Maglin and Donna Perry (1996, p. xvi) in their description of the times. While Deborah Siegel in her later reflections upon this period recalls that women's 'demand for sexual freedom was vintage radical feminist. But their hallmark call for multiplicity was third wave' (2007, p. 147).

The 1990s also saw feminists engaging with queer theory, spearheaded by the landmark works of Judith Butler (1990) in *Gender Trouble: Feminism and the Subversion of Identity* and Eve Kosofsky Sedgwick (1990) in *Epistemology of the Closet.* Sedgwick's book draws attention to the hysterical social fear of the 'closet', or that which is the underside of assumed normative sexuality, while Butler's book puts forward the radical idea that it is not just gender that is discursively constructed but also sex. She elaborates:

> When the constructed status of gender is theorized as radically independent of sex, gender itself becomes a free-floating artifice, with the consequence that *man* and *masculine* might just as easily signify a female body as a male one, and *woman* and *feminine* a male body as easily as a female one.
>
> (p. 6)

For Butler, gender is a process, involving the resignification of speech and bodily acts through reiterative performativity – like a parade or masquerade. There is, however, no doer behind Butler's performer but rather the performance itself that constitutes the self (Butler, 1990). Queer theorists have, subsequently, lifted ideas from Butler's theory of performativity to argue for more artful and fluid gender and sexuality parodies. Arguably, queer theory's contribution to feminism has been about assaulting normative and dichotomous identity configurations of gender and sexuality.

The last highlight I refer to is feminism's current attention to 'post-feminist' culture. Post-feminism is a term that captures ideas about the redundancy of feminism and the achievement of gender equality (McRobbie, 2004) – ideas that many feminists claim to be flawed. In relation to sexuality, post-feminism often manifests in representations of women exhibiting highly sexualised behaviour. For Rosalind Gill (2003), this development is no sign of feminist progress but rather the latest form of sexual governance for women:

> The figure of the autonomous, active, desiring subject has become – I suggest – the dominant figure for representing young women, part of the construction of the neo-liberal feminine subject. But sexual subjectification, I would argue, has turned out to be objectification in new and even more pernicious guise.
>
> (p. 105)

On the same page is journalist Ariel Levy (2005) who lambasts the highly public display of women's sexuality, a phenomenon that she calls 'raunch culture', as nothing more than women becoming 'female chauvinist pigs', and doing the sexually objectifying work of the old patriarchy. Feona Attwood (2006) worries, though, that equating post-feminism with repressive sexist views closes down discussions on how to materialise active sexual subjectivities for women. She asks for great consideration of the extent to which 'new forms of post-feminist representation and practice ... embody transgressive female sexualities' (p. 83). In this vein, Stéphanie Genz and Benjamin Brabon (2009) argue that post-feminism offers new potentially productive territory for feminist engagement. Uncannily, these highly contested debates about whether a hypersexualised post-feminist culture is progressive or regressive in feminist terms is reminiscent of those fought out during the 1980s 'sex wars'.

So far I have pointed out the importance of sexuality, especially but not solely women's sexuality, to a range of feminists over the last 50 years. For women, it has been about invigorating, even liberating, their sexuality, but it has also been about envisaging what they want in terms of sexual expression, a project that is arguably still ongoing. The feminist sexual project is, thus, about vision – trying to imagine how gender and sexual relations could become and what they might look like.

Social work's engagement with sexuality

The examination of matters to do with sexuality is, for the most part, a latecomer in the discipline of social work. Recently, however, sexuality has been receiving long overdue attention, particularly in the UK (Bywater & Jones, 2007; Charnley & Langley, 2007; Dunk, 2007; Dunk-West, 2012; Dunk-West & Hafford-Letchfield, 2011; Fish, 2008; Hicks, 2008a, 2008b; Jeyasingham, 2008; Myers & Milner, 2007), and to a lesser extent in Canada and the US (Crisp, 2006; Crisp & McCave, 2007; Fredriksen-Goldsen et al., 2011; Hylton, 2005; Van den Bergh & Crisp, 2004; Walls et al., 2009) and in Australia (Furlong & Mansel-Lee, 2006; Hughes, 2003, 2007, 2009; Rowntree, 2014c; Willis, 2007). Based on its mandate to address social injustices and inequities, social work has responded primarily by supporting the rights and concerns of people who identify with minority sexual communities. However, different understandings of sexuality, and the ways they then shape social work, are emerging. At this time there are two main, somewhat polarised, social work approaches to sexuality reflecting what can be described as the modernist–postmodernist paradigmatic divide.

One school, espousing more modernist thinking, encourages social workers to practise in gay-affirmative ways (Crisp, 2006; Crisp & McCave, 2007; Hughes, 2003, 2007, 2009; Van den Bergh & Crisp, 2004). According to Nan Van Den Bergh and Catherine Crisp (2004), gay-affirmative practice is akin to culturally competent practice, whereby social workers are required to acquire particular knowledge, attitudes and skills in order to work affirmatively and competently with specific client groups and their concerns. This affirmative social work effort also aims to promote anti-homophobic attitudes and redress unjust exclusionary policies and practices, such as access to the institution of marriage on the basis of sexual identity or status. The gay-affirmative approach appreciates the power that collective identity politics can wield in raising and promoting the concerns and rights of minority sexual communities, and the part social work has traditionally taken or still takes in supporting this endeavour. This approach is consistent with the discipline's modernist mandate of address-ing social inequities between groups and communities disadvantaged by their particular location in society.

Departing radically from the above ideas and the practices they inform, the other school reflects more postmodernist thinking, preferring to disturb all settled ideas about sexual identities and boundaries. This second school of thought belongs to a vein of growing interest by social work educators in studies of sexuality influenced by post-structuralist and queer ideas (Hicks, 2008a, 2008b; Jeyasingham, 2008; Martinez, Barsky & Singleton, 2011; Rowntree, 2014c; Willis, 2007). These educators' main quarrel with the competency model for gay-affirmative practice is its impli-cation of a universal reality and its failure to recognise the different ways that people express and describe their sexuality. Indeed, Paul Willis (2007) argues that social work has adopted, quite uncritically, taken-for-granted truths about sexualities based on an essentialist framework for understanding the different needs of same-sex-attracted people. Instead he appeals for a social work pedagogy that draws from queer ideas in order to destabilise dominant understandings of sexual divisions and to open up the possibility for refashioning the expression of sexual desires.

Referring to the gay-affirmative approach as the 'ethnic identity' model, Stephen Hicks (2008a, p. 68) is particularly critical of the way it constructs sexual identities into sexual types such that those who do not identify with the dominant category of heterosexuality are set apart as different or infe-rior. As the other, social workers are then required to understand and cater for the assumed special needs of minority sexual groups. Hicks calls for an educational approach that reveals how heterosexuality works, how social work has been and is still implicated in a heteronormative view of sexuality, and how a focus on sexual diversity also renders heterosexuality invisible to interrogation. In order to reduce the risk of stereotyping people from sexual minority groups, Mark Furlong and Virginia Mansel-Lee (2006, p. 43) advocate for social workers to take 'a stance of informed not-knowing' to understanding people's experiences of discrimination. This educational approach takes as its starting point a particular stance that does not assume competence but rather conveys the desire by the social worker to learn about people's particular and different lived experi-ences of homophobia.

In my own past work I have sought to reveal the valorisation of heter-onormative processes within social work. I have argued that, by default, affirmative social work efforts that seek to redress unjust exclusionary pol-icies, such as access to the institution of marriage, then constitute hetero-sexual and other sexual categories as inherent. Whilst social work has clearly taken on board social constructionist and postmodernist under-standings in relation to gender and ethnicity, this has clearly not been the case in relation to sexuality. By and large, sexuality in social work refers to and means a fixed sexual orientation. In contrast, drawing on the work of Alfred Kinsey, Wardell Pomeroy and Clyde Martin (1949) and more recent queer theory, I join with other academics (Epstein et al., 2012; Garnets & Peptau, 2000) to conceptualise sexuality as ranging and moving along a continuum bookended by the dichotomous and exclusive positions of het-erosexuality and homosexuality (Rowntree, 2014b). Based on their sex studies, Kinsey and his colleagues calculated that approximately 46 per cent of the population has both homosexual and heterosexual experi-ences over the life span (1949, p. 656). They declared that 'the living world is a continuum in each and every one of its aspects. The sooner we learn this concerning human sexual behavior the sooner we shall reach a sound understanding of the realities of sex' (p. 639).

Further, I have argued that by exploring the social construction of het-erosexuality and the processes by which boundaries are made between sexual identities that then regulate access to a range of social institutions, including marriage, social work is less likely unintentionally to fall in line with the dominant tenets of institutional heterosexuality. Here heterosex-uality is more than a marker of sexual identity; it is also a primary organ-ising principle in society that extends beyond the dimension of sexuality. This is where, as Jackson argues, the term heteronormativity has purchase as 'shorthand for the numerous ways in which heterosexual privilege is woven into the fabric of social life, pervasively and insidiously, ordering everyday existence' (2006, p. 108). Arguably, the exploration of institu-tional heterosexuality may raise social workers' awareness of their part in the invisible social architecture that orders heteronormative life, such as the condoning of alternative sexual expression only when it follows in the image of heterosexual marriage and family patterns. This exposé follows in the footsteps of the discipline's recent interrogation of the workings of white middle-class privilege in subordinating the different lived experi-ences of people who are not Anglo-Celtic and middle class.

Those of us that are more affiliated with the second school of thought want social work to expand its orthodox mandate beyond gay-affirmative practice. The intention is not to ignore the place that identity politics has and does play for people who identify with minority sexual communities, or the part social work has traditionally taken or still takes in supporting the sexual rights and concerns of such marginalised groups. Rather, a per-spective influenced by post-structuralist and queer ideas aims to provide different insights about people's sexuality to those of social work's rights-based approach to social injustices and inequities. It offers the possibility of considering sexuality as a more fluid and changeable concept than normative sexual identities, and thus requires a more nuanced social work response.

My feminism

Given the many forms contemporary feminisms can and do take, I now particularise mine. Like Caroline Ramazanoğlu and Janet Holland who describe feminism as concerned with 'gendered lives, experiences, relationships and inequalities' (2002, p. 5), my understandings focus on the transformation and promotion of non-exploitative gender and sexual relations. This contemporary feminist political commitment is, thus, wider than matters pertaining to 'the woman' or 'the feminine'. Nevertheless, the impetus for non-exploitative and transformative gender and sexual relations is more likely to emerge from the experiences, subjugated knowledge and imaginings of women because of their history of oppression and exclusion. This position follows the work of a number of feminists who recognise the imaginary as salient to the changing face of feminism and its projects (Braidotti, 2002, 2003; de Lauretis, 1987; Rose, 1995). According to Gillian Rose the feminist project is a political endeavour motivated by that which is not yet realisable and which is concerned with 'an escape from the limits of phallocentrism' (1995, p. 334). Similarly Teresa de Lauretis describes this feminist project as 'the space off, the elsewhere' (1987, p. 26) – that which is left out of masculine-defined representations and discourses.

It is to Rosi Braidotti and her affirmative politics, though, that I turn most for my feminist inspiration. Rather than separating reason from imagination, Braidotti (2002, 2003, 2005, 2011) conjoins them in her materialist theory of becoming, questioning who we want to become. The imaginary in this contemporary feminism is definitely no fanciful, self-referential reverie. Her feminist project involves mapping these transformations, or what she calls figurations. For Braidotti a figuration is 'a transformative account of the self – it's no metaphor' (2003, p. 54). These 'living maps' are 'highly specific geopolitical and historical locations: it's history tattooed on your body' (p. 54). Increasingly complex in today's world, the subjects of these living maps are like nomads, Braidotti (2005) suggests, in the sense that they often criss-cross over different identity borders while still anchored to historical locations. For example, while the intersection of gender with other social locations means that there are many different subject positions taken amongst women and even within a woman, women are still connected at some level through gender. Braidotti vehemently argues that the process of becoming new subjects emerges from the materialism of people's lives, particularly from those with 'memories of the non-dominant kind' (2002, p. 8). For example, women's embodied experiences highlight the confines of masculine-located patterns of thinking, while black women's embodied experiences reveal the limitations of white women's located knowledge. Previously invisible, these embodied accounts of power relations can become catalysts for new figurations of subjectivity – for new ways of becoming.

The feminist imaginary is, thus, very much part of, and born out of, the everyday embodied and socially embedded experiences – 'enfleshed materialism' (2002, p. 15). Yet embodied ways of being are embedded and not easily discarded and, as Braidotti acknowledges, redefinitions in subjectivity require conscious reiterative mimesis to subvert established codes. She also concedes that in the present post-postmodern moment nomadic figurations may express complicated, contradictory and contested subject positions (2005), such as the coexistence of gay tolerance and homophobia, or multiculturalism and xenophobia. While politically these nomadic figurations may zigzag in conflicting ways in the early part of the trimillennium, she argues that the feminist quest is about seeking out those that are transforming ways of becoming woman. Here woman is not the *Other* of man but, as Braidotti (2002, 2003) puts it, 'the other of the *Other*' (emphasis added). She elaborates further:

> In other words, the subject of feminism is not Woman as the complementary and specular other of man but rather a complex and multi-layered embodied subject who has taken her distance from the institution of femininity. 'She' no longer coincides with the disempowered reflection of a dominant subject who casts his masculinity in a universalistic posture. She, in fact, may no longer be a she, but the subject of quite another story: a subject in process, a mutant, the other of the Other, a post-Woman embodied subject cast in female morphology.
>
> (2003, p. 45)

In terms of sexuality, my feminism is in keeping with Braidotti's affirmative materialist feminism; it is strategic, looking for fissures to release new ways of becoming that involve fluid, multiple and nomadic subjectivities that underscore 'passions, empathy and desire' (2002, p. 266). Social work, I suggest, with its mission of promoting social wellbeing and its mandate of embracing social diversity, is one such apt opening.

Social work's engagement with sexuality underpinned by a feminist materialist theory of becoming

The ability to empathise with people from diverse social locations and their alternative viewpoints and experiences is one of the key tools in the social work kitbag. Crucially, the development of empathy as a social work skill is underpinned by a capacity to imagine – to envisage what life might be like from another subject position. However, the imaginary is largely under-acknowledged as a skill in social work projects, with the discipline preferring to use words such as creativity and innovation to describe this important visionary function. Yet, social change is not possible without vision. On the other hand, feminists have long recognised the imaginary as vital to its political projects – to envisage what life might be like if it were not cast predominantly in masculine definition. This visionary imperative for a more socially just and equitable future provides the suture between feminism and social work.

As a feminist social worker concerned about sexuality, I am not claiming that all existing sexual relations are oppressive for women, or that all people who identify with or practise non-normative sexualities face discrimination. In line with post-structuralist and queer theory, I believe that there is diversity within sexual practices and relations and in ways of doing sexual desire. What Braidotti's (2002, 2003) work on the imaginary brings to the sexual project is its value and potential in giving rise to transformations that are not necessarily in the heteronormative and phallogocentric mould.

How can the ideas within this feminist conceptual framework – a materialist theory of becoming – inform social work education and practice on the topic of sexuality? First, these ideas urge social work researchers, educators, students and practitioners to embrace sexuality as a matter for social change attention, similar to other axes of social location, injustice and analysis. As social change agents, social workers are charged with the task of promoting the value of diversity not just in relation to the social locations of gender, class, race, ethnicity, ability, age and their intersections, but also of sexuality. This mandate, therefore, requires the discipline to acknowledge the heteronormativity of past and present practices and to take responsibility not to repeat more of the same. By taking up this mantle social work practitioners are invited to reflect on their practice for heterosexual bias – no mean feat given the difficulties of seeing from within. Another way of learning more about our implication in heterosexual privilege is to heed Braidotti's (2002) advice about the insights that can be gleaned from those at the margins of the dominant mode. Here social workers would inquire sensitively about sexuality, particularly from those who have non-dominant memories. This line of inquiry does not advocate for competence but for curiosity (Rowntree, 2014c). Taking a stance of curiosity is a humbling experience; it involves listening, hearing and learning about a range of socially embedded and embodied experiences of women and men in relation to sexuality, and the effects of their intersections with other socially embedded locations

Another application of the feminist ideas in Braidotti's materialist theory of becoming is for social work researchers, educators and practitioners to ask themselves and the people they work with to imagine how they would like to express their sexuality, or how they would like sexuality represented in media and popular culture. While this might seem a particularly bold and socially risky venture to undertake, it has been my experience that women and men are eager, by and large, to discuss a topic that oftentimes is considered private and somewhat taboo (Rowntree, 2014a). For example, in advertising for interviewees in a study of the influence of ageing on baby boomers' sexualities, an internet survey had to be set up to meet the high numbers of people keen to participate. The data in this study revealed that it is important for many women and men of the baby boomer generation to dispel existing widespread ideas that they are asexual. Indeed, this study found a strong trend towards baby boomers becoming more confident and comfortable with their sexuality as they aged.

My audience study on post-feminist representations of feminine sexuality in popular culture is also noteworthy in showing a distinct level of discontent amongst women across age groupings towards what they perceive as heterosexist and overly narrow conventional heterosexual imagery (Rowntree, 2014b). Indeed, few participants read these post-feminist images as reflecting gender equality. In the main, study participants expressed a strong preference for a broader and more diverse range of feminine sexual representations, and for women to be depicted with more active sexual subjectivities. These findings suggest that women in contemporary times may not be as anti-feminist or post-feminist in their views as some feminist critics in academia fear, but rather may hold aspirations that align with feminist politics.

Closely following the ideas of the feminist imaginary, my research on sexual daydreams has been illuminating, not just in terms of revealing the shifts in sexual relations and representations that women would like to see occur, but also the insights into women's current sexual lives (Rowntree, 2011). For example, the data revealed that a number of women imagine expressing their sexuality in safe, emotionally intimate and flexible relationships, ones that are often absent or impoverished in their present lives. Thus, the data provides insight into a contrasting link between women's imagined and everyday lived sexual experiences, with the imaginary vicariously providing for absences in their lives. Moreover, the study provides evidence of the very real constraints of heteronormativity on women's everyday lives and their impatience with its regulation over their sexual conduct. The findings demonstrate that there are contemporary women who are keen to challenge dominant sexual paradigms with alternative figurations to compulsory heterosexual monogamy (Rowntree, 2011, 2013). These figurations thus fill in some of the details omitted in contemporary hegemonic representations of women and their sexuality. Nonetheless, the inspiration for these new ways of becoming, such as those within the sexual daydreams of the women in this research project, is born from the 'trauma of gender' (de Lauretis, 1987, p. 21), the pain of embodied sexual experiences embedded in social structures of gender asymmetry and sexual injustice.

These few examples illustrate what can be learnt and what transformations can emerge when people are asked about cultural representations, lives and imaginings of sexuality. The mapping and valorisation of these different erotic figurations is in keeping with Braidotti's vision for an affirmative feminist politics, and her materialist theory of becoming.

Conclusion

In this chapter I have made the case that the feminist sexual project of seeking out non-exploitative transformative sexual relations for women and men aligns closely with social work's mission of promoting the empowerment and liberation of people to enhance wellbeing, its mandate for addressing social injustices and inequities, and its social change remit. Following this logic, I have called for social workers to give sexuality the attention shown to other social axes of analyses and their intersections. Doubtless, some social workers will take more of a lead in facilitating transformations of sexual relations and practices than others, but to overlook the topic is, arguably, unethical for those people we work with whose sexuality and sexual experiences are repressed, suppressed or oppressed. In taking on board this sexual project, it is worthwhile looking both backwards and forwards. Looking backwards provides the opportunity for social work researchers, educators, practitioners and students to take stock of heteronormative underpinnings within the discipline's thinking and the practices it informs, and to vow to chart a more inclusive course. In looking forwards to chart this broader course, I have suggested the value of appropriating feminist ideas about the imaginary. These imaginings, though, are born from the experiences of 'enfleshed subjects' (Braidotti, 2002, p. 60). Building upon ideas associated with a feminist materialist theory of becoming, I have provided examples of how social workers can learn humbly from the people we work with and for, particularly from those at the margins, about their sexual lives and aspirations.

Further reading

Braidotti, R. (2002) *Metamorphoses: Towards a Materialist Theory of Becoming.* Polity, Cambridge.

Braidotti, R. (2011) *Nomadic Subjects: Embodiment and Sexual Difference in Contemporary Feminist Theory,* 2nd edn. Columbia University Press, New York.

Dunk-West, P. & Hafford-Letchfield, T. (2011) *Sexual Identities and Sexuality in Social Work: Research and Reflections from Women in the Field, Contemporary Social Work Studies.* Ashgate, Farnham, UK.

Hicks, S. (2008a) Thinking through sexuality. *Journal of Social Work,* 8(1), pp. 65–82.

Hicks, S. (2008b) What does social work desire? *Social Work Education,* 27(2), pp. 131–137.

References

Attwood, F. (2006) Sexed up: theorizing the sexualization of culture. *Sexualities,* 9(1), pp. 77–94.

Australian Association of Social Workers (2010) *Code of Ethics.* AASW, Canberra.

Bail, K. (1996) *DIY Feminism.* Allen & Unwin, St Leonards, NSW.

Bauer Maglin, N. & Perry, D. (1996) Introduction. In N. Bauer Maglin & D. Perry (eds), *'Bad Girls'/'Good Girls': Women, Sex, and Power in the Nineties.* Rutgers University Press, New Brunswick, NJ, pp. xiii–xxvi.

Braidotti, R. (2002) *Metamorphoses: Towards a Materialist Theory of Becoming*. Polity, Cambridge.

Braidotti, R. (2003) Becoming woman: or sexual difference revisited. *Theory, Culture and Society*, 20(3), pp. 43–64.

Braidotti, R. (2005) A critical cartography of feminist post-postmodernism. *Australian Feminist Studies*, 20(47), pp. 169–180.

Braidotti, R. (2011) *Nomadic Subjects: Embodiment and Sexual Difference in Contemporary Feminist Theory*, 2nd edn. Columbia University Press, New York.

Butler, J. (1990) *Gender Trouble: Feminism and the Subversion of Identity*. Routledge, New York.

Bywater, J. & Jones, R. (2007) *Sexuality and Social Work: Transforming Social Work Practice*. Learning Matters, Exeter, UK.

Chancer, L.S. (1998) *Reconcilable Differences: Confronting Beauty, Pornography, and the Future of Feminism*. University of California Press, Berkeley, CA.

Charnley, H.M. & Langley, J. (2007) Developing cultural competence as a framework for anti-heterosexist social work practice: reflections from the UK. *Journal of Social Work*, 7(3), pp. 307–321.

Cixous, H. (1996 [1975]) *The Newly Born Woman*, ed. C. Clement. I.B. Tauris, London.

Crisp, C. (2006) The Gay Affirmative Practice Scale (GAP): a new measure for assessing cultural competence with gay and lesbian clients. *Social Work*, 51(2), pp. 115–126.

Crisp, C. & McCave, E. (2007) Gay affirmative practice: a model for social work practice with gay, lesbian, and bisexual youth. *Child and Adolescent Social Work Journal*, 24(4), pp. 403–421.

de Lauretis, T. (1987) *Technologies of Gender: Essays on Theory, Film, and Fiction*. Indiana University Press, Bloomington, IN.

Dunk, P. (2007) Everyday sexuality and social work: locating sexuality in professional practice and education. *Social Work and Society*, 5(2), pp. 135–142.

Dunk-West, P. (2012) The sexual self and social work and policy, or, why teenage pregnancy prevention programmes miss the point. *Social Work and Society: International Online Journal*, 10(2). www.socwork.net/sws/article/view/338/675 (accessed 27 May 2015).

Dunk-West, P. & Hafford-Letchfield, T. (2011) *Sexual Identities and Sexuality in Social Work: Research and Reflections from Women in the Field*. Ashgate, Farnham, UK.

Epstein, R., McKinney, P., Fox, S. & Garcia, C. (2012) Support for a fluid-continuum model of sexual orientation: a large-scale internet study. *Journal of Homosexuality*, 59(10), pp. 1356–1381.

Firestone, S. (1971) *The Dialectic of Sex: The Case for Feminist Revolution*. Cape, London.

Fish, J. (2008) Far from mundane: theorising heterosexism for social work education. *Social Work Education*, 27(2), pp. 182–193.

Fredriksen-Goldsen, K.I., Woodford, M.R., Luke, K.P. & Gutiérrez, L. (2011) Support for sexual orientation and gender identity content in social work education: results from national surveys of US and anglophone Canadian faculty. *Journal of Social Work Education*, 47(1), pp. 19–35.

Furlong, M. & Mansel-Lee, V. (2006) Not one of us is without bias: identifying and challenging racism and homophobia. *Advances in Social Work and Welfare Education*, 8(1), pp. 38–54.

Garnets, L.D. & Peptau, L.A. (2000) Understanding women's sexualities and sexual orientations: an introduction. *Journal of Social Issues*, 56(2), p. 181.

Genz, S. & Brabon, B.A. (2009) *Postfeminism: Cultural Texts and Theories*. Edinburgh University Press, Edinburgh.

Gill, R. (2003) From sexual objectification to sexual subjectification: the resexualisation of women's bodies in the media. *Feminist Media Studies*, 3(1), pp. 100–106.

Greer, G. (1971) *The Female Eunuch*. McGraw-Hill, New York.

Hicks, S. (2008a) Thinking through sexuality. *Journal of Social Work*, 8(1), pp. 65–82.

Hicks, S. (2008b) What does social work desire? *Social Work Education*, 27(2), pp. 131–137.

hooks, b. (1984) *Feminist Theory: From Margin to Center*. South End Press, Boston, MA.

Hughes, M. (2003) Talking about sexual identity with older men. *Australian Social Work*, 56(3), pp. 258–266.

Hughes, M. (2007) Older lesbians and gays accessing health and aged-care services. *Australian Social Work*, 60(2), pp. 197–209.

Hughes, M. (2009) Lesbian and gay people's concerns about ageing and accessing services. *Australian Social Work*, 62(2), pp. 186–201.

Hylton, M.E. (2005) Heteronormativity and the experiences of lesbian and bisexual women as social work students. *Journal of Social Work Education*, 41(1), pp. 67–82.

Jackson, S. (2006) Interchanges: gender, sexuality and heterosexuality: the complexity (and limits) of heteronormativity. *Feminist Theory*, 7(1), pp. 105–121.

Jeyasingham, D. (2008) Knowledge/ignorance and the construction of sexuality in social work education. *Social Work Education*, 27(2), pp. 138–151.

Karp, M. & Stoller, D. (eds) (1999) *The Bust Guide to the New Girl Order: The Magazine for Women with Something to get off Their Chests*. Penguin, London.

Kinsey, A.C., Pomeroy, W.B. & Martin, C.E. (1949) Sexual behavior in the human male. *Journal of Nervous and Mental Disease*, 109(3), p. 283.

Kosofsky Sedgwick, E. (1990) *Epistemology of the Closet*. University of California Press, Berkeley, CA.

Levy, A. (2005) *Female Chauvinist Pigs: Women and the Rise of Raunch Culture*. Free Press, New York.

McRobbie, A. (2004) Postfeminism and popular culture. *Feminist Media Studies*, 4(3), pp. 255–264.

Martinez, P., Barsky, A. & Singleton, S. (2011) Exploring queer consciousness among social workers. *Journal of Gay and Lesbian Social Services*, 23(2), pp. 296–315.

Morgan, R. (ed.) (1970) *Sisterhood is Powerful: An Anthology of Writings from the Women's Liberation Movement*. Random House, New York.

Myers, S. & Milner, J. (2007) *Sexual Issues in Social Work*. Polity Press, Bristol.

Oakley, A. (1972) *Sex, Gender and Society*. Maurice Temple Smith, London.

Ramazanoğlu, C. & Holland, J. (2002) *Feminist Methodology: Challenges and Choices*. Sage, London.

Rose, G. (1995) Making space for the female subject of feminism: the spacial subversions of Holzer, Kruger and Sherman. In S. Pile & N. Thrift (eds), *Mapping the Subject: Geographies of Cultural Transformation*. Routledge, London, pp. 332–354.

Rowntree, M.R. (2011) Women's sexual lives in the new millennium: insights from their daydreams. Paper presented at the Cultural Studies of Australasia Association Conference: Cultural ReOrientations and Comparative Colonialities, Adelaide, 22–24 November.

Rowntree, M.R. (2013) New millennium's feminine subject of feminism. *Feminist Review*, 105(3), pp. 65–82.

Rowntree, M.R. (2014a) 'Comfortable in my own skin': a new form of sexual freedom for ageing baby boomers. *Journal of Ageing Studies*, 31, pp. 158–153.

Rowntree, M.R. (2014b) Feminine sexualities in the chick genre: women's readings and preferred readings. *Feminist Media Studies*, 15(3), pp. 508–521.

Rowntree, M.R. (2014c) Making sexuality visible in Australian social work education. *Social Work Education*, 33(3), pp. 353–364.

Siegel, D. (2007) *Sisterhood, Interrupted: From Radical Women to Grrls Gone Wild*. Palgrave Macmillan, New York.

Van den Bergh, N. & Crisp, C. (2004) Defining culturally competent practice with sexual minorities: implications for social work education and practice. *Journal of Social Work Education*, 40(2), pp. 221–238.

Walls, N.E., Griffin, R., Arnold-Renicker, H., Burson, M., Johnston, C., Moorman, N., Nelson, J. & Schutte, E.C. (2009) Mapping graduate social work student learning journeys about heterosexual privilege. *Journal of Social Work Education*, 45(2), pp. 289–307.

Willis, P. (2007) 'Queer eye' for social work: rethinking pedagogy and practice with same-sex attracted young people. *Australian Social Work*, 60(2), pp. 181–196.

18 Constructing gender

Feminist gerontology and social work practice

Jill Chonody and Barbra Teater

Introduction

Ageing is a normal biological process and is typified by physical changes, both internal and external, and along with gender and race it is among the first thing that we notice about other people. These physical indicators then in turn influence the way others are treated. Nonetheless, ageing (along with gender and race) is socially constructed. Decline in the body is overemphasised; old age is designated as a time for loss (Cruikshank, 2009). This reductive definition of ageing is reinforced by ageist beliefs and contributes to the marginalisation of older people.

Ageism perpetuates the myth that older people are of little social value and therefore can legitimately be devalued within the social system (Nelson, 2011). For example, research indicates that young people tend to infantilise older people in a number of ways, including speaking to them as if they are children ('elderspeak') or saying paternalistic things like, 'aren't you so cute?' These encounters can lower the self-esteem of older people and cause them to question their ability. Much like other forms of oppression, it can be challenging to recognise the salience and importance of age, especially when we are in a position of privilege, namely youth; even if one experiences oppression or disadvantage due to other social conditions (e.g. race), the effects of ageism can still be difficult to see (Calasanti, Slevin & King, 2006). Moreover, the intentionality of ageist attitudes and behaviours are difficult to determine (Chonody & Teater, forthcoming) and may be born out of a desire to help.

Ageism is often equated with other types of 'isms' such as sexism or racism; however, it is qualitatively different in that an individual lives with her/his gender or race across the lifespan, whereas ageism is only associated with later years and unique to that developmental period (Cruikshank, 2009). Ageism is also something that may be faced by everyone, and thus is an issue that has broad social and interpersonal implications – from employment to sexuality. The concepts of ageing and ageism are important within the context of feminist social work as they encompass the norms that dictate beliefs about and attitudes towards this period of the life course and how such beliefs and attitudes differ based on gender.

To frame our discussion of women, ageing and social work, we draw from feminist gerontology, which we use to examine age, gender, power and the intersection of oppression throughout the life span. This perspective provides a basis from which to critique the response from the state and society on women as they age, acknowledge diversity among women and target inequality, and promote diversity through micro, mezzo and macro practices (Hooyman et al., 2002). This theoretical perspective is useful for understanding issues such as social relationships, care giving, work, income and retirement, health care, social and personal issues, and abuse.

Through this chapter, we define and explain feminist gerontology and what it has to offer social work practice. We will look at the ways in which ageing can have an impact on women, particularly due to social and economic structures, and will address the intersectionality of oppression. We will examine how social work practice, based on feminist gerontology, can be used to tackle ageing-related oppression and discrimination and facilitate an ageing process that is meaningful and psychologically, physically and socially healthy for women. Finally, we will consider ways in which feminist gerontology can be applied to social work practice at the micro, mezzo and macro levels.

The gendered construction of ageing and its impact on women

Gendered relations are part of our everyday lives and the maintenance of differential power is sustained across the life course. These differences impact on the experience of women and lead to less opportunity, including in education, work and economic power. However, ageing has traditionally been the domain of gerontology, while women's issues have been examined from various feminist perspectives that typically ignored ageing women by focusing on younger/middle-aged women and issues such as child care or reproductive rights (Calasanti & Slevin, 2006). At this intersection of gerontology and feminism we can achieve a greater understanding of how women experience ageing in a culture that worships youth and production within the marketplace, and sees maleness as the ideal. Feminist gerontology helps bridge the gap between these two theories to address aspects of ageing as they relate to socially constructed gender dynamics and how this relates to the intersectionality of oppression.

Feminist theory and critical gerontology are the foundation for feminist gerontology. Broadly speaking, feminist approaches attempt to raise social consciousness with regard to the oppressive social structures that privilege men (Garner, 1999), and critical gerontology attempts to deconstruct the social interpretation of ageing (Moody, 1988). Age stratification within society creates differential rewards, including power and status, associated with particular periods in the life course; this allows certain groups to benefit from ageism (Calasanti, 2005). 'Old age does not just exacerbate other inequalities but is a social location in its own right, conferring a loss of power for all those designated "old" regardless of their advantages in other hierarchies' (Calasanti et al., 2006, p. 17). Moreover, these disadvantages and inequalities associated with older age are viewed as 'natural, and thus beyond dispute' (Calasanti et al., 2006, p. 18). But feminist gerontology offers a theoretical standpoint to critique the social and cultural construction of ageing (Hooyman et al., 2002) and promotes an empowerment approach to practice.

Women's experiences of growing older are not homogeneous, but rather differ based on gender, class and ethnicity. Therefore, exploring the potential differences in ageing for women is a crucial first step when working with older women in social work practice. The following section examines some specific aspects of ageing that are particularly relevant for women but, as we will discuss later in the section on intersectionality, the experiences described below will differ among older women based on class, ethnicity and sexual orientation.

Gender inequality and gender roles

Gender inequality is particularly evident among older adults in terms of income and pensions in later life and the need to access social services. Women have traditionally been, and still are, paid less than men for similar work and have accumulated smaller pensions (Arber & Ginn, 2005). The differences in terms of income and pensions in later life results in a gender difference in standard of living, with women more likely to live in poverty (Arber & Ginn, 2005) and having increased dependence on the state as they age (Estes, 2005). Estes argues that this phenomenon pertains to the division of labour and power between men and women, their roles and related institutional structures.

Gender differences in terms of economic and social relationships among older adults are argued to be the result of a state, economy and social institutions that have been developed and maintained by men (Acker, 1988). Such a patriarchal state has historically defined and supported men's roles in the capitalist marketplace, whereas women's roles have been defined and encouraged to create and foster family and social relationships (Estes, 2005). A man's worth and status comes from his position within the marketplace and economic standing whereas a woman is expected to provide and participate in family roles and social relationships, which are not valued or compensated (Estes, 2005). Estes argues that this discrepancy in historic gender expectations is a central dynamic concerning old age. For example, Estes suggests that the gendered state is 'the contradiction between the *needs* of women throughout the lifecourse and the organization of work, and the modes of *distribution* based on the recognition (and compensation) and non-recognition (and non-compensation) of "work"' (2005, p. 554).

When considering social services for older women we need to acknowledge that gender differences are a result of a patriarchal state and social system. In particular, as women live longer than men they are more likely to need support from the state as they age. Moreover, given that they are more likely to live in poverty than men, they will likely need more assistance in meeting their basic needs due to income/pension constraints (Estes, 2005). Older women are also more likely to provide long-term care to family members or friends and are more likely to require care themselves. As women live longer, it is becoming more a reality that ageing parents will need care well into the middle/late ages of adult children. That is, it will become a more common scenario for a woman in her 60s or 70s to be caring for her mother who is in her 80s or 90s. This not only has additional economic consequences for older women, but additional repercussions for women's health and wellbeing.

Women and relationships

As women age, there is a greater likelihood that they will become widowed, particularly in heterosexual relationships (Arber & Ginn, 2005). Nearly half of women over 65 years old are widowed, and this increases to nearly 80 per cent of women who are widowed at age 85 or over, in contrast to 60 per cent of men who are still married at age 80 and over (Arber & Ginn, 2005). Based on the patriarchal state as described above, becoming divorced, separated or widowed changes not only the living arrangements for older women but their living standards, social supports/relationships, income and access to a caretaker if a woman becomes frail or ill.

Women can experience a loss or change in relationship differently from men. First, older women are more likely to have better social relationships with friends and family when compared to men (Arber & Ginn, 2005), and women who are widowed can experience a new sense of autonomy (Davidson, 2001). Although women may experience a loss of a spouse or partner, they may also gain social and emotional supports from other widows. Social connections and relationships are linked to physical and mental health (Umberson & Montez, 2011), and women who report having more contact with friends and family report lower levels of loneliness (De Jong Gierveld, 2003). Therefore, the extent to which an older woman experiences social isolation and loneliness, and has access to social relationships should be assessed when providing social services.

Women and their bodies

Gender inequality is also evident in societal expectations of the physical aspects of ageing. The ageing body is often held in contempt for its loss of youthful appearance and its failure to behave in ways that we have grown to expect. For the ageing woman, significant status loss may occur due to these outward changes. For example, a woman's age is intertwined with her sexuality and women are largely seen to be at the height of their 'sexual value' in their youth. With each passing year, this gradually diminishes (Sontag, 1997). By menopause, some women may feel their sexual attractiveness is lost forever. These anti-ageing norms are socially constructed and expressed through and reinforced by an anti-ageing movement that includes both outward appearance and physicality. The idea that youth can – and should – be maintained throughout life, particularly for women, is expressed in terms like 'successful ageing' or 'active ageing', which implies failure if certain benchmarks cannot be met. The 'active older woman' is inherently a middle-class ideal in that, to achieve some 'success', she must be youthful, physically fit and socially engaged. All of these characteristics assume access to resources, and even then many women cannot maintain this standard over time. Women's experience with their ageing body and changing sexuality are important considerations for practice and will have varying degrees of impact on women's lived experiences.

Feminist gerontology and the intersectionality of oppression

The intersectionality of multiple forms of oppression (e.g. class, gender, race, sexual orientation, gender identity) is related to a patriarchal social system that promotes a hegemonic ideal whereby others are considered *less than*. The effects of multiple oppressed identities are cumulative, and it is important to generate a feminist solidarity around the intersectionality of oppression. Feminism places ageing 'within a context of inequalities – sexism, racism, anti-Semitism, heterosexism, capitalism, beautyism, etc' (Reinharz, 1997, p. 76). A feminist lens can further our understanding of social constructions that act to 'other' certain groups and promote a narrow idea of acceptability (Hooyman et al., 2002). Feminist gerontology seeks to understand women within their context and through an ecological lens that accounts for social, political and economic factors (Hooyman et al., 2002). Feminist gerontology highlights the lifelong pattern of differential treatment and silencing of women and provides a comprehensive lens for understanding the social hierarchy of power and privilege that favours men, youth, whiteness, heteronormativity and middle-class values. 'Women's lives [are] intertwined' (Reinharz, 1997, p. 83) and, as such, women should be acknowledged across the life span.

This substantive area of theory and research is large, but we briefly consider several aspects of identity that intersect with ageing. Race is important to consider in terms of both gender and ageing. Women of colour are often overlooked in terms of how their experiences of ageing impact on them and even how their experiences then in turn are socially constructed. The reality for many women of colour is that their disadvantaged social position becomes even more pronounced in older age. The lifelong experience of barriers to education, employment, housing and health care leads to a shorter average life expectancy; however, this one intersection between race and class does not represent all women of colour and their ageing experience. In fact, their experiences are under-represented in contemporary feminist scholarship as most work in this area is written by and from the perspective of white, middle-class women (Cruikshank, 2009). Further research is needed to elucidate the ageing experience of women of colour across class.

'Like women of colour, lesbians are … unlikely to be seen as norms for ageing' (Cruikshank, 2009, p. 121). Research often makes the assumption of heterosexuality and limits the exploration of the challenges that can be faced by older women who are lesbians (Cruikshank, 2009). Coming out, for the first time or the thousandth time, can be a significant obstacle for older women. The heterosexual assumption and over-sexualisation of female relationships along with ageist stereotypes that paint older adulthood as asexual makes this a difficult social terrain to negotiate. Similarly, issues of care and recognition of relationships may not be available. That is, nursing facilities typically only accommodate a married, heterosexual couple, and policies as well as staff may be homophobic in nature. This illustrates the intersection of gender, age and sexual orientation that gives precedence to age over other identities.

Socioeconomic status is another important factor to consider in the context of ageing given that it impacts all other facets of oppressed identities. For example, older women are typically less well off then older men, and older women of colour are usually worse off than white women. All aspects of social life are influenced by social class. Housing, access to health care and exposure to discrimination are just the tip of the iceberg when considering the impact of lower socioeconomic status on older women. The interrelationship between race/ethnicity and poverty and women and poverty illustrates the cumulative effects of multiple vulnerabilities to oppression. Nonetheless, economic determinism is not always taken into account because it does not fit the middle-class worldview of many gerontologists (Cruikshank, 2009).

Feminist gerontology and social work practice

Ageing issues shape social work in myriad ways, and feminist gerontology impacts all spheres of practice: micro, mezzo and macro. First, one should recognise the increased need for gerontological social workers given that most western nations are experiencing an ageing of the population. In fact, approximately 20 per cent of the population in the USA, UK and Australia will be 65 years and older by mid-century. Furthermore, women live longer than men, and thus it is likely that social workers will work with older women. However, research indicates that social work students are resistant to working with older people. In one study, only 5.6 per cent of more than 1,000 international social work students indicated that geron- tology was their preferred area of practice (Chonody & Wang, 2014). Thus, gerontological work is likely to be influenced by cultural norms and attitudes, and addressing this within the profession will be key to generat- ing new feminist gerontologists in the future.

Ageist beliefs are deeply ingrained within the culture and normative in nature. They are communicated in a multitude of ways and are seen more like facts than stereotypes. The idea of a 'senior moment' has been incorp- orated into everyday language, and birthday cards that describe the receiver as 'over the hill' or senile are common. Moreover, when someone inquires as to 'how many years young' someone is or refers to an older woman as a 'young lady' they are reinforcing the idea that old is bad (Cruikshank, 2009). These negative perceptions are perpetuated in western cultures, and older adults are perceived to be physically, cogni- tively and sexually inadequate (Zebrowitz & Montepare, 2000).

These types of ageist beliefs are important to feminist social work prac- tice because they represent a cultural narrative that can be challenged. Feminist gerontology acknowledges the diversity of the ageing experience for women and incorporates the personal narrative as the point of refer- ence for the 'truth' of that experience (Cruikshank, 2009). Just as fem- inism would argue against the universal notion of 'women', feminist gerontology does not support an all-encompassing notion of 'old women' (Cruikshank, 2009). Thus, perspectives on ageing women are shaped by positions of privilege that dictate a virtually unachievable ideal of the ageing woman: youthful and with adequate income, she is without disabil- ity or illness; she is active and attractive and socially engaged. Confronting this ideal may be one component of a feminist social work practice with older women. Ageing is a gendered issue and social workers will need to be able to contextualise the impact that this will have on their client popu- lations as well as how it affects social policy.

Micro practice

Social workers working from a feminist gerontological perspective should employ an empowerment approach (Teater, 2014) and 'strive to empower older women through assisting them in developing new roles, in identify- ing their abilities and strengths, and in utilizing their knowledge' (Garner, 1999, p. 7). In terms of micro practice, this includes individual work with women to reject negative images and views of older women (Hooyman et al., 2002). Consciousness raising can help older women to identify and acknowledge the cultural and social messages that negatively impact on self-perception and self-esteem. An exploration of the evidence that disputes such messages along with a problem-solving approach to combat the thoughts, feelings and behaviours that arise when faced with such messages can be part of social work practice. Through this process, the social worker helps older women to identify their abilities, strengths and knowledge, which could 'facilitate the processes of older women learning to care about themselves as valuable human beings and to become empowered' (Garner, 1999, p. 7). Thus, working at the micro level, social workers can help older women change the discourse about ageing by educating clients about biased norms that act to erode self-esteem and equipping them with tools to overcome these pressures.

As older women are more likely to access social services, social workers can advocate for women to receive the services they need and work with women to self-advocate for services. Social workers should be knowledgeable about welfare benefits and eligibility requirements in order to enhance the economic security of older women.

Finally, as social relationships are important for older women, social workers should assess the extent to which women may be experiencing social isolation and loneliness, and suggest resources and supports to enhance social relationships. For example, a social worker could find resources to fund a computer for an older woman to use Skype to contact friends or relatives who live a distance away, or a social worker could suggest local community activities, such as singing or coffee groups, for the older woman to attend. Employing an empowerment approach requires the social worker to collaborate with the older woman to assess what types of social activities would be of interest and suitable to her needs.

Mezzo practice

Consciousness raising can be further translated into mezzo-focused practice by facilitating groups with older women where they identify and challenge messages and biases and formulate alternative, more positive responses to ageing. The group could provide a supportive environment where women can share experiences and problem-solving skills and give and receive support with the aim of enhancing self-perception and fulfilment (Garner, 1999). Through individual and collective work, consciousness raising could compel women to manifest 'acts of resistance' – that is, to 'wear their bodies proudly' (Holstein, 2006, p. 328). Agency and resistance are key elements of a feminist social work practice, and thus they are essential to practice with older women. Encouraging woman to question the performance of age may free her from self-imposed constraints dictated by culture that propel the individual to feel that she *should* be 'this way' because of her age. In addition, working with older women in groups could involve group interventions such as assertiveness training, self-help groups, support groups, survivors groups and consensus-building groups (Garner, 1999).

Mezzo practice should also consider the extent to which older women give or require care. After perhaps caring for others throughout her life, older women may find themselves in a position of needing some care. Options for this care often fall to either adult children or nursing facilities, but peer care may offer an alternative (Cruikshank, 2009), particularly as it could foster social relationships and connections. Peer care allows women to work together to meet their particular needs while possibly avoiding the pitfalls of power dynamics that can occur when an adult child or a nursing home attendant is providing the caregiving. However, it requires a large enough group of women who are healthy to share responsibilities amongst the group for those who may be temporarily or permanently suffering from illness, disability or decline.

Mezzo practice not only involves working with groups of older women, but also involves social workers challenging cultural and societal norms, messages and biases through multi-professional working. Social workers working with older women often work with other professionals, such as nurses, doctors, care assistants and occupational and physical therapists who may disempower, discriminate and oppress older women through their language and actions, particularly those that are supported by the social and economic systems of a patriarchal social system. A social worker can educate and work with other professionals to challenge discriminatory and oppressive behaviours and promote empowerment through the use of feminist skills (Garner, 1999). Feminist gerontologists may help other practitioners gain an increased understanding of how ageist practices (Garner, 1999) – even the seemingly banal – can erode the self-esteem of older women. For example, calling an older woman 'honey' or 'sweetie' communicates the message that she is a child or childlike. While this language may actually originate from a place of empathy, older women want to be spoken to as adults, not children.

Macro practice

Empowerment is also key to creating social change that supports women as they age. Social workers working from a feminist gerontological perspective will also aim to challenge cultural and societal norms, messages and biases at the macro level, particularly through advocacy and political action. For example, the 'Representing Self-Representing Ageing' project funded by the Economic and Social Research Council (ESRC) aims to implement the Second World Assembly on Ageing's strategy to challenge stereotyped images of ageing and older women (see Hogan & Warren, 2012).

Social workers will need to advocate for older women within the political arena, but equally encourage older women to advocate for themselves collectively (Garner, 1999). Social workers can individually or collectively challenge cultural and social messages that discriminate and oppress older women as well as the patriarchal social systems that limit social and economic opportunities. Social workers can be political in terms of voting for politicians who acknowledge gender inequalities and advocate for woman's social and economic rights and support programmes that address the effects of gender inequality for older women. Social workers can also join social work interest groups that lobby politicians to pass legislation and develop policies that promote gender equality.

Additionally, social workers can encourage women to participate in academic research that aims to explore the ways in which older women perceive themselves through the ageing process, which can provide evidence to challenge cultural and societal norms, messages, biases, policies and practices and can further influence best practice approaches to working with older women (Freixas, Luque & Reina, 2012; Hogan & Warren, 2012; Liechty, 2012).

Finally, considering intersectionality in feminist gerontological social work practice requires social workers to acknowledge that 'older women' are not a homogeneous group, but rather race, class, sexuality and other factors can further define and divide older women. Therefore, when working at the micro, mezzo and macro levels, social workers will need to acknowledge and consider how the impact of ageism and ageing is impacting upon women, but equally how this is exacerbated by others 'isms'. For example, low-income women and women of colour are more likely to provide unpaid work in the home, which is not as valued as paid labour, and lesbian women and women of colour may have experienced homophobia and racism throughout their lives (Hooyman et al., 2002). The variation in older women's history and life experiences will further tailor the social work interventions.

Conclusion

There are a variety of feminist frameworks, such as radical, Marxist, liberal, global, postmodern and womanism (Teater, 2014), and each can be adapted and applied to gerontology and to social work practice with ageing women. This chapter has focused on feminist gerontology, which 'points to the value in analysing ageing from women's life experiences, not just because they are women, but because this analysis reveals the power dynamics that contour the ageing experience' (Hooyman et al., 2002, p. 5). Applying feminist gerontology to social work practice calls for action and interventions on the three levels of social work practice. Individual work at the micro level requires an empowerment-based approach that enables the woman to feel valued and worthy and provides access to services that enhances the woman's needs. Group work at the mezzo level can provide a sense of solidarity among older women and a place of mutual support that facilitates empowerment as well as caretaking. Equally important is work at the macro level, which involves challenging the structural and cultural norms that perpetuate the struggles of ageing for women. All three areas of social work practice require tailored interventions based on the intersections of age, race, class and sexuality. The aim of this chapter is for women to feel fulfilled during the ageing process.

Further reading

Calasanti, T.M. & Slevin, K.F. (2006) *Age Matters: Realigning Feminist Thinking.* Routledge, New York.

Cruikshank, M. (2009) *Learning to be Old: Gender, Culture, and Aging,* 2nd edn. Rowman & Littlefield, Plymouth, UK.

Garner, J.D. (ed.) (1999) *Fundamentals of Feminist Gerontology.* Hawthorne, New York.

References

Acker, J. (1988) Class, gender and the relation of distribution. *Signs,* 13, pp. 473–493.

Arber, S. & Ginn, J. (2005) Gender dimensions of age shift. In M.L. Johnson (ed.), *The Cambridge Handbook of Age and Ageing.* Cambridge University Press, Cambridge, pp. 527–537.

Calasanti, T. (2005) Ageism, gravity, and gender: experiences of aging bodies. *Generations,* Fall, pp. 8–12.

Calasanti, T., Slevin, K.F. & King, N. (2006) Ageism and feminism: from 'et cetera' to center. *NWSA Journal,* 18, pp. 13–30.

Calasanti, T.M. & Slevin, K.F. (2006) Introduction: age matters. In T.M. Calasanti & K.F. Slevin (eds), *Age Matters: Realigning Feminist Thinking.* Routledge, New York, pp. 1–18.

Chonody, J.M. & Teater, B. (forthcoming) Why do I dread looking old? A test of social identity theory, terror management theory, and the double standard of aging. *Journal of Women and Aging.*

Chonody, J.M. & Wang, D. (2014) Predicting social work students' interest in gerontology: results from an international sample. *Journal of Gerontological Social Work,* 57(8), pp. 773–789.

Cruikshank, M. (2009) *Learning to be Old: Gender, Culture, and Aging,* 2nd edn. Rowman & Littlefield, Plymouth, UK.

Davidson, K. (2001) Late life widowhood, selfishness and new partnership choices: a gendered perspective. *Ageing and Society,* 21(3), pp. 279–317.

De Jong Gierveld, J. (2003) Social networks and social well-being of older men and women living alone. In S. Arber, K. Davidson & J. Ginn (eds), *Gender and Ageing: Changing Roles and Relationships.* Open University Press, Maidenhead, UK, pp. 95–110.

Estes, C.L. (2005) Women, ageing and inequality: a feminist perspective. In M.L. Johnson (ed.), *The Cambridge Handbook of Age and Ageing.* Cambridge University Press, Cambridge, pp. 552–559.

Freixas, A., Luque, B. & Reina, A. (2012) Critical feminist gerontology: in the back room of research. *Journal of Women and Aging,* 24(1), pp. 44–58.

Garner, J.D. (1999) Feminism and feminist gerontology. *Journal of Women and Aging,* 11, pp. 3–12.

Hogan, S. & Warren, L. (2012) Dealing with complexity in research processes and findings: how do older women negotiate and challenge images of aging? *Journal of Women and Aging*, 24(4), pp. 329–350.

Holstein, M.B. (2006) On being an aging woman. In T.M. Calasanti & K.F. Slevin (eds), *Age Matters: Realigning Feminist Thinking*. Routledge, New York, pp. 313–334.

Hooyman, N., Browne, C.V., Ray, R. & Richardson, V. (2002) Feminist gerontology and the life course. *Gerontology and Geriatrics Education*, 22, pp. 3–26.

Liechty, T. (2012) 'Yes, I worry about my weight … but for the most part I'm content with my body': older women's body dissatisfaction alongside contentment. *Journal of Women and Aging*, 24(1), pp. 70–88.

Moody, H.R. (1988) Toward a critical gerontology: the contribution of the humanities to theories of aging. In J.E. Birren & V.L. Bengtson (eds), *Emergent Theories of Aging*. Springer, New York, pp. 19–40.

Nelson, T.D. (2011) Ageism: the strange case of prejudice against the older you. In R.L. Wiener & S.L. Willborn (eds), *Disability and Aging Discrimination*. Springer, New York, pp. 37–47.

Reinharz, S. (1997) Friends or foes: gerontological and feminist theory. In M. Pearsall (ed.), *The Other Within Us: Feminist Explorations of Women and Aging*. Westview Press, Boulder, CO, pp. 73–94.

Sontag, S. (1997) The double standard of aging. In M. Pearsall (ed.), *The Other Within Us: Feminist Explorations of Women and Aging*. Westview Press, Boulder, CO, pp. 19–24.

Teater, B. (2014) *An Introduction to Applying Social Work Theories and Methods*, 2nd edn. Open University Press, Maidenhead, UK.

Umberson, D. & Montez, J.K. (2011) Social relationships and health: a flashpoint for health policy. *Journal of Health and Social Behavior*, 51, pp. S54–S66.

Zebrowitz, L.A. & Montepare, J.M. (2000) Too young, too old: stigmatizing adolescents and elders. In T.F. Heatherson, R.E. Kleck, M.R. Hebl & J.G. Hull (eds), *The Social Psychology of Stigma*. Guilford Press, New York, pp. 334–373.

19 Feminism and disability

Barbara Fawcett

Introductions

Just as there are many forms of feminism, there are different ways of both conceptualising and constructing disability. Since the onset of second wave feminism in the 1970s, feminism has become more nuanced and different strands – called variously liberal feminism, radical feminism, socialist feminism, black feminism, standpoint feminism, ecofeminism and postmodern feminism – have been developed. However a core element of all feminisms has been an analysis of the operation of power, including the social construction of power relationships as well as the accompanying power imbalances. The various feminisms, particularly those that have mounted a strong political challenge, can be seen to have influenced the disability rights campaigns based around the social model of disability and also to have shared the challenges associated with acknowledgements of difference and diversity. In this way, both can be regarded as having contributed in a variety of ways to social work practice. In this chapter, I will explore the points of convergence between 'disability' and the various feminisms and examine the contribution that feminist forms of analysis can make to constructive critique with regard to the social model of disability. As part of this process, I will appraise assumptions of homogeneity and difference, consider the place of experience in challenging oppression and review controversies surrounding discussions of impairment and the body. I will then examine what social work has learned and also can learn from feminist analysis applied to the social model of disability. This encompasses a critical appraisal of matters surrounding care, control, risk and vulnerability.

Disability and feminism: points of convergence

I argue that there can be seen to be many points of convergence between the various feminisms and the social model of disability. Just as second wave feminists challenged gender-neutral views embedded in taken-for-granted ways of relating and behaving, proponents of the social model of disability have sought to unpick the centrality of able-bodied perspectives. Both have concentrated on deconstructing everyday notions about what it means to be a woman or a disabled person. As Shakespeare pointed out in 1994, in culture, in the media and in everyday social interaction, disabled women and men, in a similar way to women generally, have had to contend with ongoing processes of objectification. This has both limited and constrained and also constructed binaries out of the positions that women and disabled people can hold. For women this has traditionally veered from mother/saint to whore/sinner, and for disabled people from pitiful but brave cripple, to deformed outcast.

The various feminisms, by directing attention towards embedded prejudices, inequalities and the creation of binary positions, have opened up debate and critically explored dominant social and cultural processes of categorisation and 'othering'. As Oliver (1996) has pointed out, this has resulted in disabled women and men being responded to in a variety of negative ways, including being ignored, dismissed and feared. Once a heterogeneous group is viewed in a negative and homogenising fashion, all kinds of 'othering' processes come into play, and practices that are unthinkable for those not seen as part of the devalued group become justifiable.

Feminist critiques of processes of 'othering' can be seen to have played a significant role in the development of the social model of disability and its rejection of medicalised classification and categorisation systems. Proponents of the social model initially highlighted the key problem that someone could be regarded as a 'paraplegic', rather than as a person with similar hopes, aspirations and dreams to everyone else. They therefore redefined 'disability' to refer to how those with impairments were, and indeed continue to be, disabled by social, political and economic barriers and by overt and covert forms of prejudice and discrimination. As a result, they rejected a medicalised emphasis on responding to a condition, coming to terms with a condition and living with a condition and equated 'disability' with externally driven oppressive and discriminatory forces. Similarly, they critiqued medically or individually oriented responses to 'disability', such as those associated with forms of grief therapy and rehabilitation. This led to these practices being seen as counterproductive and as deficit oriented and pathologising. Such practices were also seen to privilege able-bodiedment or approximations of it and to present this as the only way to be.

Critiques of constructions of the body and the often-marketed message that there is an ideal body are embedded within all forms of feminism. Again, there can be seen to be a clear point of convergence with the social model of disability understandings. Both the many feminisms and the social model of disability have sought to challenge representations of 'perfect' bodies and have contributed many insights into the effect that this form of standardisation has had. However, the question of impairment remains a much debated topic within the disability movement and again there can be seen to be parallels with discussions that have taken place within the more politically oriented forms of feminism about the place of individual experience within an encompassing group identity. This is an important area and it is one that I will return to later in this chapter.

Disability and feminism: the development of critique

Within the various strands of feminism, feminist analyses have continually challenged and reformulated accepted understandings and practices. However, I argue that it is perhaps postmodern feminism which has brought to the fore the most pronounced deconstructive critique, and that this has added further layers of meaning. Clearly there are feminists who are wary of postmodern associations and Di Stefano famously drew attention to the fact that feminism without some kind of clear standpoint can be reduced to being 'an other among others' (1990: 77). This concern about postmodern analyses has been shared by proponents of the social model of disability, although there are also those who have considered such contributions positively (for example, Corker & Shakespeare, 2002; Wilson & Beresford, 2002). However, I maintain that postmodern feminist forms of analysis can draw attention to pressure points both within feminism generally and also within the social model of disability.

As with all of the feminisms there are many versions of postmodern feminism but, for the purposes of this chapter, I direct attention towards those that foreground the operation of power and knowledge and also consider concepts of difference. As I have highlighted (Fawcett, 2000), this form of analysis can facilitate the exploration of areas associated with assumptions of homogeneity, the place of experience in challenging oppression and considerations linked to impairment and the body. I will now look at these aspects in greater detail.

Assumptions of homogeneity and difference

As I discussed earlier in this chapter, it is often assumed that all disabled people comprise one very similar or homogenised group. This is best illustrated by the application of 'the' to disabled people, reducing a diverse grouping of women and men from different backgrounds and cultures and with different experiences to a group uniformly referred to as 'the disabled'. However, it is also possible to detect signs of this homogenising tendency within some forms of feminism and also the social model of disability. An example can be when feminism appears to encompass and speak for *all* women and when the social model of disability appears to speak for *all* disabled people. Clearly, any politically motivated movement has to present what appears to be a unified position in order to achieve and maintain credibility. There is the fear that diversification or fragmentation will result in disunity and in the dissolution of the core political platform. However, assertions of unity also prompt questions about whether feminism or the social model of disability can speak for those from different socioeconomic backgrounds, environments and sexual as well as cultural locations.

It is also notable that in the early days of the disability movement a consideration of gender and gendered issues was largely absent. This changed due to the input of disabled women activists such as Wendell (1996), Morris (1993) and French (1993), who drew from the feminist slogan 'the personal is political' to challenge ungendered assumptions. However, as with considerations of impairment, tensions emerged between those who viewed gendered perspectives as promoting greater theorisation within the disability movement and those who feared that a more nuanced discussion would fragment the clear political message.

In relation to disability, I maintain that there are analyses drawn from the various feminisms which can widen the debate about the incorporation of difference within what are also political campaigns. An example is Flax's (1992) analysis, which utilises postmodern feminist understandings. She focuses on citizenship and on de-coupling this from modernist, structuralist and universalistic underpinnings. By doing this she retains the connection with justice which she views as a process. She argues that, by concentrating on elements such as reciprocity, recognition, reconciliation and justice, differences can be positively valued yet also seen as variable and changing over time. Accordingly, matters associated with homogeneity and difference are reconciled in different contexts and emphasis is placed both on negotiation and also on the timing of political rallying points. This formulation connects citizenship with justice in a way that gives interconnected social subjects the responsibility for constructing and upholding it, and for making changes in an inclusive and consensus-oriented manner. Undoubtedly, discussions about difference and diversity within movements with a pronounced political message will always pose a challenge, but the example given above illustrates that there are productive ways of reconciling positions.

The place of experience in challenging oppression

Some forms of feminism have actively promoted consciousness raising on the basis of individual experiences, and the slogan 'the personal is political' retains a meaningful resonance. Clearly personal experiences are a powerful means of drawing attention to discrimination and formulating challenges to oppressive structures and ways of operating. However, as evidenced by the debates within radical and standpoint forms of feminism in particular, they also lead to contestation about whose experience is most significant or most valid. To paraphrase Adams' famous quotation from 1989, it can result in more time being spent in demonstrating oppression and having this acknowledged than dismantling it. It can also, sometimes by default, foreground victimhood rather than confront it.

Within the disability movement, there has also been a tendency to list oppressions. Begum (1992), to make a significant point, talked of the triple oppression of being a black, disabled woman. This drew attention to the ways in which forms of discrimination can be multiple. However, it can also confirm a negative identity and reduce complex experiences to a series of labels. More recently, attention has been directed towards inter-sectionality and how gender, 'race' and disablism are multidimensional and can connect and interconnect in a variety of ways (for example, Erev-elles & Minear, 2010; elle, 2014). The importance of theorising from experience and making links between a variety of experiences has also been emphasised. Drawing from postmodern feminism, I contend that conceptualising identities as fluid, as being linked to context and as multi-faceted, can add to this discussion (Fawcett, 2000). Clearly it is important both to name and to confront discrimination and oppression in their various manifestations, and experiences that are personal, shared and also theorised play a part in this. However, in terms of experience, as Maynard stressed, 'It is not always necessary to include women who are white, black, working class, lesbian or disabled ... to be able to say something about racism, classism, heterosexism and disablism' (1994, p. 24).

Impairment and the body

Discussions about 'the body' tend to incorporate both the actual physical, biological body as well as conceptualisations of abstract bodies. The first of these draws attention to individual impairments which, as I highlighted earlier, has proved contentious within the disability movement. However authors such as Beckett (2006) and Crow (1996), amongst others, have emphasised that we all have impairments and that we ought to focus on commonalities rather than potentially divisive and often externally con-strued differences. Crow (1996), in particular, argues for the self-interpretation of impairment within a more inclusively framed social model of disability where shared autobiographies, which include the experience and history of impairments, become part of the liberating process. Wendell (1996) talks of 'embodied difference' and again this is a concept that can be used to highlight that we all have 'embodied differ-ences', but this can also be regarded as constituting our shared similarity.

With regard to conceptualisations of abstract bodies, Foucault saw the body as 'the inscribed surface of events' (Rabinow, 1991, p. 83) and concen-trated on the body as a site of power. Foucault did not differentiate between the bodily experiences of men and women, but his work on docile bodies, where individuals self-discipline themselves in accordance with the opera-tion of dominant discourses, has been seen to have relevance for feminism (for example Bartky, 1988; Bordo, 1993) and also disability (Fawcett, 2000).

The notion of genealogy has played a part in this discussion. Foucault formulated the concept of genealogy as a deconstructive tool. According to Foucault, the task of genealogy is to 'expose a body totally imprinted by history and the process of history's destruction of the body' (in Rabinow, 1991, p. 83). Foucault (in Drefus and Rabinow, 1983) asserted that where there is power there is also resistance, and this draws attention to how a positioned body can reposition and also challenge. The key example here is how 'disability' has been reframed by proponents of the social model of disability to refer to individuals with a variety of corporeal impairments being disabled by social, political and economic constraints. Similarly, as with the movement 'mad pride', it draws attention to how pejorative labels can be revalued and ascribed a new meaning.

Deleuze and Guattari (1988) formulated an abstract conception of the body and introduced the notion of a 'body without organs' (BwO). Their work is complex, but a key point to emphasise is that they did not differentiate in a generalised manner between 'able' and 'disabled' bodies. Rather than placing emphasis on what the BwO is and the way in which it is composed, they concentrated on the body in terms of its actions, effects, functions and productive capacities. I argue that these ideas, picked up and used in social work practice in the disability field, can be used not only to represent discursive inscriptions, but also to inscribe and create a commonality of the body which is free from categorical divisiveness. At a theoretical level, but also with an accompanying practical element, this can challenge representations of 'ideal' bodies and the prioritisation of able-bodiedness.

Social work, feminism and disability

When turning attention to what social work can learn from feminist understandings, the discussion above highlights the centrality of feminism to social work in the arena of disability. However, there are also specific aspects which can be particularly emphasised. These include the ways in which feminism's concentration on relationships and power paves the way for an interrogation of areas associated with concepts of 'care', 'risk' and 'vulnerability'.

Relationships and power

As has been seen in this chapter and indeed throughout this book, power and knowledge frameworks and the ways in which these influence interaction and relationships are at the core of feminist analyses. In terms of social work practice, this draws attention to the importance of social workers not making decisions on the basis of 'taken-for-granted' assumptions. It also highlights the need for all knowledge claims to be questioned, no matter how powerfully presented or embedded in current procedures or ways of operating they appear to be. This brings to the fore the importance of acknowledging that meanings have to be shared and negotiated in all sets of circumstances. It can never be assumed, for example, that all those involved in any situation or interaction view what is going on in the same manner. Similarly, the ways in which some understandings, processes and outcomes can be privileged over others requires ongoing recognition and attention.

In the field of disability, as elsewhere, analyses drawn from the various feminisms promote social work practice that explores and critically reflects on what the issues are seen to be, who is affected and in what ways, what are the constraints of the social worker's role in a particular set of circumstances and how justified or binding these constraints actually are. Additionally, feminist forms of analysis direct attention towards what actions are required and by whom (or indeed whether action should be an option), what the expectations of the outcome are (and again by whom) and the extent to which these can be achieved. Social workers currently occupy a world dominated by assessment procedures, checklists and protocols, and social work practice often appears prescribed. However, feminist analyses emphasise the importance of social workers continually asking questions, exploring meanings and reviewing the implications for all those involved in the interactions taking place.

Critical reflection is widely used in social work and is an operational example of social workers maintaining a constructively critical yet productive approach. This form of analysis can be seen both to have drawn from and also to have parallels with feminist analyses and critiques. A number of writers have produced forms of guidance to promote critical reflection (for example Fook, 2002, 2009; Thompson & Thompson, 2008) and these have been built upon by Fawcett, Weber and Wilson (2012). Critical reflection that draws on feminist analyses can include the following questions:

- What is the range of assumptions operating?
- What are the strengths as well as the problems associated with these different assumptions?
- What do we (used inclusively to refer to all those involved) want to do or not do?
- How are we going to operationalise this?
- How are we going to evaluate the outcomes?
- How do we learn from this process?
- What could we have done differently?
- How might we transfer this learning to other contexts?

(based on Fawcett, Weber & Wilson, 2012, p. 147)

Applied to the field of disability, these questions avoid a deficit orientation and ensure that actions are negotiated and agreed. This avoids a 'one-size-fits-all' approach and concentrates attention on 'what works' for an individual in their situation. Social workers are under considerable pressure and often have high workloads. However, incorporating feminist analyses into a framework like this one can militate against a slide into a reductionist way of operating that can prove counterproductive for all concerned.

'Care', 'risk' and 'vulnerability'

In this chapter, I take forward the argument that the social model of disability takes from feminist practices the importance of social workers forming partnerships with disabled women and men and moving away from 'us' and 'them' or 'expert'/patient or service user dichotomies. I have highlighted that this recognises that all parties bring a variety of experiences, positions and agendas to any discussion and that relational power imbalances need to be both recognised and responded to. Accordingly, with regard to disability and social work, the social model of disability places emphasis on social workers foregrounding the importance of autonomy rather than paying attention to levels of dependence and independence. A disabled woman, for example, may not want to spend hours getting dressed or preparing food in order to demonstrate her independence. She may rather want to spend more time socialising or being involved in areas that interest her. This brings into the frame the arena of 'care' and its embedded corollary 'control'. Disabled women and men for a long time have been involved in expanding the meanings associated with 'care' and challenging organisational definitions that frequently equate 'care' with being 'looked after'. The social model of disability reformulates understandings of 'care' to emphasise the importance of reciprocity, of caring about, about roles not being fixed but fluid, and the ways in which, in a variety of situations, we all wear different hats (Morris, 1993; Beckett, 2006).

'Care' in organisational contexts can all too easily start to equate to control and, as for example the Francis Report (2013) into the abuses at the Mid Staffordshire Hospital in the United Kingdom (in common with many other reports) points out, forms of control can easily start to spill over into abuse. This happens when there is a clear divide between staff and patients or residents and when standardised practices slide into gradually incorporating routinised abuses, such as not responding or responding appropriately to requests for personal assistance to go to the toilet, or to have a drink or a meal. These in turn, particularly when scrutinising bodies do not focus on the quality of relationships but on areas more amenable to a simple tick-box approach, can all too quickly escalate into direct forms of physical abuse such as slapping, rough treatment or withholding food or direct assistance. The disability movement calls for personal assistants to be directly responsible and accountable to the disabled person they are working with in order to ensure that their role is to assist the disabled woman or man to do whatever they want to do. As Oliver (1996) and Oliver, Sapey and Thomas (2012) emphasise, this incorporates the mandatory foregrounding of full citizenship rights with associated educational, social, political and economic opportunities.

Any discussion of rights quickly leads on to considerations about assessments of 'risk' in social work. Increasingly social workers are being pressured into defining 'risk' in a negative manner, with policy and procedures focusing on ways to prevent risk and to safeguard 'vulnerable' individuals. This raises a number of issues in relation to disability. Being categorised as 'disabled' in the medicalised sense can lead to an individual also being perceived as 'vulnerable'. Safeguarding 'vulnerable' people is a key aspect of social work practice, but, as with 'care' and 'control', this can relatively easily slide into a restriction of autonomy, especially if an individual's capacity to make decisions for themselves is called into question. Many countries have legislation in place that deal with issues of capacity. However, it is possible to argue that even the most recent and well intentioned can militate against the exercise of autonomy by those positioned as 'vulnerable'. The Mental Capacity Act 2005 in England, for example, sets out clear principles for assessing capacity. However, it can also be seen to incorporate in-built challenges. In order to illustrate how these can affect a disabled person, it is useful to turn a feminist lens on the criteria.

The Mental Capacity Act 2005 (MCA) in England (like others, such as that in force in NSW, Australia) makes it clear that the initial presumption has to be that a person has capacity. The MCA also states that people have the right to make unwise decisions and that a person who makes a decision that is regarded by others as unwise should not automatically be viewed as lacking the capacity to make a decision (MCA s 1(4)). It is also emphasised in the legislation that people should receive support to enable them to make their own decisions and that capacity should be determined on a decision-by-decision basis (MIND, 2012).

Section 3 of the Act specifies that a decision about lack of capacity must relate to an individual's inability to understand information relevant to the decision, retain the information for long enough to be able to make a decision, weigh up information as part of the decision-making process and communicate the decision by formal or informal means of communication. The accompanying code of practice to the Act also specifies that an individual should not be assumed to lack capacity as a result of their age, appearance, a mental health diagnosis or any other impairment or mental condition.

Under the legislation, assessments about capacity and the concomitant making of a decision on behalf of a person can be undertaken by a variety of individuals. These include relatives, friends, informal carers, professional carers, doctors, social workers and medical personnel. Once a decision about lack of capacity is taken, the person making this decision, or another, is then charged with operating in the individual's best interest and making a decision on that person's behalf. Decisions made for an individual should restrict their freedom as little as possible.

As MIND (2012) point out, although the MCA does not provide a definition of 'best interest', section 4 provides a non-exhaustive checklist that should be considered by a person acting or making a decision on behalf of a person assessed as lacking capacity. This checklist includes: the consideration of relevant circumstances, whether the individual could make the decision in the future; supporting the participation of the individual concerned as fully as possible; and taking into account the individual's expressed wishes and feelings, beliefs and values as well as those of significant others.

Applying feminist analysis to this area makes it possible to disentangle positive aspects from those which are unclear and problematic. On one level, the legislation and accompanying guidance to the Mental Capacity Act 2005 appears comprehensive. However, on another, the range of people who can assess for incapacity and make a decision on an individual's behalf indicates that there will be variation about what constitutes 'best interest'. Accordingly, despite the proviso that an individual can make an unwise decision, whether an individual has the capacity to make a decision that to the assessor appears to be against their best interest is likely to remain a contentious issue. Similarly, the extent to which the capacity to make a decision will be assessed on a decision-by-decision basis and whether key decisions are revisited following further and perhaps different assessments of capacity constitute exceedingly grey areas.

Overall then, being regarded as disabled in the medicalised sense (where emphasis is placed on the nature of the impairment) can easily lead to an individual being regarded as vulnerable. They are then 'vulnerable' to having their capacity questioned if they want to make a decision that a family member or professional does not believe to be in their best interest. This can relate to sex, to getting drunk, to travelling, to undertaking a course or complex project and so on. It is also not unusual for organisations to promote safeguarding procedures that are routinely risk adverse and as a result prioritise the interests of the organisation rather than the individual.

All of these aspects highlight the important role of the social worker. It is the social worker who is in a prime position to mediate and ensure that, whether operating as an assessor or as an adviser, the Mental Capacity Act 2005 and the accompanying code of practice are fully adhered to and that prevailing assumptions are fully scrutinised. This brings us back to the importance of feminist analyses, and to the need to review continually the ways in which power/knowledge frameworks are operating in any given situation.

Concluding remarks

There are many ways of practising social work and many forms of feminism. In relation to both, I have argued that it is crucial to include fully all those involved in decision-making processes, to operate reflexively and to consider what is influencing interaction and the making of decisions and what is being left out. The social model of disability has drawn from feminist perspectives in order to challenge and change disabling constructions. In this chapter I have explored 'disability' by utilising the lenses that the various forms of feminism have to offer. I have drawn attention to the opportunities and also the challenges posed by these perspectives and have appraised how feminist forms of analysis have influenced and can influence social work responses. This, I contend, locates feminist understandings and analysis at the centre of social work practice in the field of disability. It also emphasises the centrality of feminist analyses of gender and power to the whole arena of social work practice.

Further reading

Beckett, A.E. (2006) *Citizenship and Vulnerability: Disability and Issues of Social and Political Engagement.* Palgrave Macmillan, Basingstoke, UK.

Fawcett, B., Weber, Z. & Wilson, S. (2012) International Perspectives on Mental Health: Critical Issues Across the Lifespan. Palgrave Macmillan, Basingstoke, UK.

Oliver, M., Sapey, B. & Thomas, P. (2012) *Social Work with Disabled People*, 4th edn. Palgrave Macmillan, Basingstoke, UK.

References

Adams, M.L. (1989) There's no place like home: on the place of identity in feminist politics. *Feminist Review*, 31, pp. 23–33.

Bartky, S.L. (1988) Foucault, femininity and the modernization of patriarchal power. In I. Diamond & L. Quinby (eds), *Feminism and Foucault: Reflections on Resistance.* Northeastern University Press, Boston, MA, pp. 61–86.

Beckett, A.E. (2006) *Citizenship and Vulnerability: Disability and Issues of Social and Political Engagement.* Palgrave Macmillan, Basingstoke, UK.

Begum, N. (1992) Disabled women and the feminist agenda, *Feminist Review*, 40–42, pp. 70–84.

Bordo, S. (1993) Feminism, Foucault and the politics of the body. In C. Ramazanoğlu (ed.), *Up Against Foucault: Explorations of Some Tensions Between Foucault and Feminism.* Routledge, London, pp. 179–202.

Corker, M. & Shakespeare, S. (eds) (2002) *Disability/Postmodernity: Embodying Political Theory.* Continuum, London.

Crow, L. (1996) Including all of our lives: renewing the social model of disability. In C. Barnes & G. Mercer (eds), *Exploring the Divide: Illness and Disability.* Disability Press, Leeds, UK, pp. 55–73.

Deleuze, G. & Guattari, F. (1988) *A Thousand Plateaus.* Athlone, London.

Di Stefano, C. (1990) Dilemmas of difference: feminism, modernity, and postmodernism. In L.J. Nicholson (ed.), *Feminism/Postmodernism.* Routledge, London, pp. 63–82.

Drefus, H.L. & Rabinow, P. (eds) (1983) *Michel Foucault: Beyond Structuralism and Hermeneutics.* University of Chicago Press, Chicago, IL.

elle (2014) Eleanor Lisney: intersectionality and disability. *Sisters of Frida,* 7 March. www.sisofrida.org/2014/03/07/intersectionality-and-disability/   (accessed   4 August 2014).

Erevelles, N. & Minear, A. (2010) Unspeakable offences: untangling race and disability in discourses of intersection. *Journal of Literary and Cultural Disability Studies,* 14(2), pp. 127–145.

Fawcett, B. (2000) *Feminist Perspectives on Disability.* Prentice Hall, Harlow, UK.

Fawcett, B., Weber, Z. & Wilson, S. (2012) *International Perspectives on Mental Health: Critical Issues across the Lifespan.* Palgrave Macmillan, Basingstoke, UK.

Flax, J. (1992) Beyond equality: gender, justice and difference. In L. Bock & S. James (eds), *Beyond Equality and Difference.* Routledge, London, pp. 193–205.

Fook, J. (2002) *Social Work: Critical Theory and Practice.* Sage, London.

Fook, J. (2009) Critical reflection: overview and latest ideas. Paper presented at AASSWE Workshop, Melbourne.

Foucault, M. (1981) Question of method: an interview with Michel Foucault. *Ideology and Consciousness,* 8, pp. 1–14.

Francis, R. (2013) *Report of the Mid Staffordshire NHS Foundation Trust Public Inquiry.* The Stationery Office, London.

French, S. (1993) Disability, impairment or something in between? In J. Swain, V. Finkelstein, S. French & M. Oliver (eds), *Disabling Barriers: Enabling Environments.* Sage, London, pp. 17–25.

Maynard, M. (1994) Methods, practice and epistemology: the debate about feminism and research. In M. Maynard & J. Purvis (eds), *Researching Women's Lives from a Feminist Perspective.* Taylor & Francis, London, pp. 10–26.

MIND (2012) *The Mental Capacity Act 2005.* MIND, London. www.mind.org.uk/ information-support/legal-rights/mental-capacity-act-2005/ (accessed 28 July 2014).

Morris, J. (1993) *Pride Against Prejudice.* Women's Press, London.

Oliver, M. (1996) *Understanding Disability: From Theory to Practice.* Macmillan, Basingstoke, UK.

Oliver, M., Sapey, B. & Thomas, P. (2012) *Social Work with Disabled People,* 4th edn. Palgrave Macmillan, Basingstoke, UK.

Rabinow, P. (ed.) (1991) *The Foucault Reader.* Penguin, Harmondsworth, UK.

Shakespeare, T. (1994) Cultural representations of disabled people: dustbins for disavowal? *Disability and Society,* 9(3), pp. 283–299.

Thompson, N. & Thompson, S. (2008) *The Critically Reflective Practitioner.* Palgrave Macmillan, Basingstoke, UK.

Wendell, S. (1996) *The Rejected Body: Feminist Philosophical Reflections on Disability.* Routledge, London.

Wilson, A. & Beresford, P. (2002) Madness, distress and postmodernity: putting the record straight. In T. Shakespeare & M. Corker (eds), *Disability/Postmodernity: Embodying Disability Theory.* London, Continuum, pp. 145–158.

20 Engaging men in feminist social work

Theory, politics and practice

Bob Pease

Introduction

I first engaged with feminism in the 1970s in response to being challenged by women about my privilege as a man. My partner would come home from women's consciousness-raising meetings and challenge my limited participation in housework and my over-commitment to paid work at the expense of our relationship. I had to work out what these challenges would mean not only for my personal relationship, but also for my chosen career of social work and my political activism on issues of social justice.

I first took gender seriously in intellectual work in a Master's thesis on radical social workers in the mid-1980s (Pease, 1987, 1990). By then, feminism had played an important role in shaping my personal, professional and political concerns. Close personal relationships with feminist women, cooperative working relationships with feminist co-workers and my experience in an anti-sexist men's consciousness-raising group provided the direct impetus for bringing a gender consciousness into my practice in social work.

Thus, my engagement with feminism ran parallel with my study, practice and teaching in social work. I was fortunate to come to my second academic position in social work in a school that espoused a radical philosophy of social work that was influenced by critical theory and feminism. I was also fortunate in being mentored by a senior feminist social work academic who suggested that I take responsibility for addressing the negative responses of many male students to feminist content in the curriculum.

As a result, I developed and taught a course on men, masculinities and social work which was first offered in 1985. Although the elective course was originally intended primarily for male social work students, it became popular with female students who wanted strategies for dealing with men in their personal lives as well as in their professional roles. The course provided an opportunity for me to bring a feminist-informed scholarship on men and masculinities into the social work curriculum to address such issues as theorising masculinity, men's sexuality, men and intimacy, fatherhood and men in families, homophobia and men's friendships, men and work, men's health, men and ageing, men's violence, men's movement politics, and men and gender equality (Pease, 1997).

In the early 1990s I was also involved in attempts to construct a pro-feminist activism. I had previously been involved in men's consciousness-raising groups in the 1970s and 1980s. However, it was not until 1991 when I co-founded Men Against Sexual Assault (MASA) that I moved into concerted activism against men's violence against women. Even in those early days, my sense was that work done by men with men against men's violence should be accountable to critical reference groups of women who worked in women's services (Pease, 1995).

This engagement with activist work on men's violence against women took me into theorising and research with men about the pathways by which some men become pro-feminist and how to analyse men's power and resistance to change (Pease, 2000). It is often difficult for men to acknowledge the oppression of women because they are implicated in it. Gender is differentiated from many of the other social divisions because it is experienced in the context of intimate relationships at home (Ridgeway & Correll, 2004). It is likely that men have participated in the subordination of the wives, mothers, sisters and daughters who are a part of their life. Many men are reluctant to acknowledge that male privilege exists because they fear they will have to face guilt and shame for their part in maintaining their privileges (Johnson, 1997).

In Connell's (2000) view, the primary motivating factor for men to support gender equality will come from their 'relational interests' winning out over their egotistic interests. It is men's relationships with partners, daughters, mothers and sisters and so on that will provide the basis upon which men will come to support change.

Developing a pro-feminist sensibility among men in social work

Men *can* change in the direction of feminism. They have choices as to whether they accept patriarchy or work collectively against it. Before men can organise collectively, though, they must transform their subjectivities and practices.

Although we cannot individually or as a group escape our material position in patriarchy, I believe that we can change our ideological and discursive position. A standpoint relates both to structural location as well as to the discursive construction of subjectivity, allowing us to distinguish between a 'traditional men's standpoint' and a 'pro-feminist men's standpoint'.

A traditional men's standpoint is based on the privileges and powers men have, and excludes the perspective of women. A pro-feminist men's standpoint involves being critical of men's position in society and how it contributes to the inequality of women, and developing an ethical and moral commitment to addressing that inequality and discrimination because of the harm it causes (May, 1998).[1] It is possible then for men to change their subjectivities and practices to constitute a pro-feminist men's standpoint. Men have to change their vantage point if they want to see the world from a different position and this requires them actively to engage in pro-feminist struggles in both the private and public arenas.

As I have noted elsewhere (Pease, 2009), pro-feminism involves a sense of responsibility for men's own and other men's sexism, and a commitment to work with women to end men's violence (Douglas, 1993). It acknowledges that men benefit from the oppression of women, drawing men's attention to the privileges men receive as men and the harmful effects these privileges have on women (Thorne-Finch, 1992). Pro-feminist men also recognise that sexism has an impact on men as well as women. To oppress others, it is necessary to suppress oneself.

Social work practice with men, however, should focus on ways of working towards gender equality rather than focusing solely on the issues facing men and consequently it is important to locate practice with men in the context of feminist theories. Feminist theory began with a critique of masculinity and men's practices, and the study of men by men needs to incorporate these insights and the questions they raised about men (Hanmer, 1990). The 'bottom line' is acknowledging the debt that is owed to feminist activism and theory and articulating the power inequalities in one's personal and political life (Luck & Jackson, 1995).

Most feminists agree that 'a critical understanding of dominant group members is needed' (Hyde & Bricker-Jenkins, 1995, p. 314). Comprehending how dominant group members understand and interpret the world is seen as an important element on the road to women's liberation. So analyses of men's experiences and practices in patriarchy are essential to the project of transforming gender relations. Feminist-informed critical studies on men can therefore contribute to our understanding of how men gain, maintain and use power to subordinate women (Hanmer, 1990). It can expose and demystify men's culture from the inside out.

Towards pro-feminist practice with men in social work

Masculinity and the place of men in social work has until recently been a neglected area in social work writing. Although there is a mass of literature in social work that has much to say about men and masculinities, this is usually done in an implicit and untheorised way.

Feminists in social work have drawn attention to the prevalence of sexist attitudes and practices in social welfare, and during the last 30 years feminist social workers have developed interventions and policies aimed at overcoming sexism. Feminist practice with women has thus made a significant contribution to critical social work practice. However, feminist social work has not had a lot to say about working with men either. The key feminist social work texts make only passing references to men and there is only one feminist text that looks systematically at feminist practice with men (Cavanagh & Cree, 1996).

However, it is increasingly recognised that addressing sexism necessitates an understanding of men as well as women. All social workers will have contact with men. Furthermore, the majority of the concerns that women bring to social workers are connected to their relationships with men.

Over 25 years ago, Tolman et al. (1986) articulated 11 principles for a pro-feminist commitment among men in social work: develop a historical, contextual understanding of women's experience; be responsible for themselves and other men; redefine masculinity; accept women's scrutiny without making them responsible; support the efforts of women without interfering; struggle against racism and classism; overcome homophobia and heterosexism; work against violence in all its forms; do not set up a false dichotomy between oneself and other men; act at individual, interpersonal and organisational levels; and attend to process and product. They noted at the time that very few men had been proactive in promoting feminist values such as these in social work and that men had contributed very little to ending sexism (Tolman et al., 1986). Dominelli (1999) made a similar observation 13 years later. Writing in 2014, little has changed.[2] Nevertheless, men in social work have an important part to play in challenging sexism.

If men are to play an anti-oppressive role in relation to gender in social work, they will need to embrace a commitment to pro-feminist practice. In the context of wider anti-oppressive theory and practice, social work education thus needs to develop specific knowledge and skills to inform a pro-feminist commitment by men in social work. If men gain unearned benefits from their presence in social work, they have a responsibility to challenge the basis of those entitlements (Pringle, 2001).

Masculinity and the issues facing men

Lichtenberg (1999) argues that men will change when they consider the costs of masculinity for themselves. I have argued previously, however, that the focus on the problems facing men has placed too much emphasis on the costs for men associated with patriarchal relations and given insufficient attention to the costs to women and children of men's practices (Pease, 2000). In this regard, Cowburn and Pengelly (1999, p. 198) make the distinction between 'men with problems' and 'men as problems'. The latter include rape and sexual assault, violence against women in the home, sexual harassment and sexual misconduct as a group norm.

Although men are privileged, it does not mean that men do not experience pain in their lives. Men can be both privileged and miserable at the same time. Kaufman (1994) argues that men's lives involve both power and pain and that much of men's pain arises from men's power and privilege to constitute what he calls 'the contradictory experiences of men's power'. Thus the patriarchal dividend is not totally successful in advantaging men because men experience emotional and physical costs associated with their dominant position (Whitehead, 2002).

When the costs of masculinity are documented in popular books about men, however, they are rarely framed in terms of the unintended consequences of men's advantages. Populist writers of books about men talk about a 'crisis in masculinity' as men find their traditional privileges and symbolic power being eroded (Horrocks, 1994). Whitehead (2002) argues that 'the male crisis discourse' distorts the connections between hegemonic masculinity and men's health. The idea of masculinity in crisis may itself be a strategy enacted by men to reinforce men's power. Connell (2000) also makes the point that most of the costs associated with patriarchy for men are not necessarily experienced by the men who gain most of the benefits. Many current men's health policies and programmes, for example, fail to recognise the social and economic context of men's lives and the impact of class and race divisions on their health (Pease, 2009).

To develop a feminist framework for practice with men, we have to conceptualise the issues facing men adequately. It is important to understand men's experiences within the context of the patriarchal structures in society and their relationship to class, race and gender regimes. Men and women who work with men in social work should have an analysis of the social construction of masculinities and they need to understand how the forces that construct dominant masculinities embed men and women in relations of dominance and subordination that limit the potential for them to be in partnership with each other. If men do not grasp the basic notion of gender as a social construction, then feminist critiques of patriarchy, dominant masculinity and abusive male behaviours are going to be felt by men at a deeply personal level.

Hence, approaches to working with men will be shaped by how we understand masculinity and men's lives. Whether masculinity is framed primarily from a biological, psychological or sociological perspective will impact on the ways of understanding the issues facing men. It will certainly influence whether the focus is more on men's pain or men's privilege (Featherstone, Rivett & Scourfield, 2007). Work with men has also been differentiated in terms of whether it has been supportive of feminism and gender equality, or non-feminist (or even anti-feminist) and oriented towards reproducing traditional gender roles and inequalities.

There is currently an enormous volume of literature on men and masculinities. Theoretical approaches have ranged from socio-biological, psychoanalytical, Jungian and sex role theories through to materialist and discursive approaches. My aim is not to provide an overview of the different theories, as I have done that elsewhere (Pease, 2002). My focus here is specifically to theorise men's gender privileges and situated dominance in relation to women as a basis for pro-feminist practice with men.

Feminist-informed perspectives on men and masculinities emphasise that gender and masculinity are socially constructed throughout life. Following Connell (2000), I believe that it is most useful to understand men and masculinities as involving six key dimensions: (1) multiple masculinities that arise from different cultures, different historical periods and different social divisions between men; (2) different positions reflected in these multiple masculinities in relation to power with some forms of masculinity being hegemonic and dominant, while other masculinities are marginalised and subordinated; (3) institutionalised masculinities embedded in organisational structures and in the wider culture as well as being located within individual men; (4) embodied masculinities that are represented physically in how men engage with the world; (5) masculinities produced through the actions of individual men; (6) fluid masculinities that change in relation to the reconstructive efforts of progressive men and in response to changes in the wider society. Within this theoretical context, Connell (1995) identifies four forms of masculinity: hegemonic, complicit, marginalised and subordinate.

Hegemonic masculinity is the culturally dominant form of masculinity that is manifested in a range of different settings. Such masculinity is idealised and promoted as a desirable attainment for boys and young men to strive towards. It is presented as heterosexual, aggressive, authoritative and courageous (Connell, 2000). Although the majority of men do not adhere to hegemonic masculinity, it nevertheless represents the most valued form of masculinity and all men are positioned in relation to it (Connell & Messerschmidt, 2005).

The majority of men engage in what Connell (1995) refers to as complicit masculinity. Complicit masculinities refer to those men who do not meet the normative standard of hegemonic masculinity but nevertheless benefit from it in various ways. The concept of complicit masculinity is useful in understanding how men who do not regard themselves as oppressors nevertheless act in ways that reproduce men's dominance and male privilege. While the majority of men may not engage in excessive forms of hegemonic masculinity, they nevertheless do not challenge patriarchy and male privilege that supports this form of dominance (Mills, 1998) because they adhere to the dominant discourse.

Marginalised and subordinate masculinities are useful in understanding the relationship between gender and other dimensions of stratification such as class, race and sexuality. Connell (2000) uses these concepts to illustrate how the diversity of masculinities is marked by hierarchy and exclusion. This hierarchy of masculinities means that men do not benefit equally from male privilege.

Historical and contemporary debates within pro-feminism

Pro-feminism is not a homogeneous movement, any more than feminism is. Different approaches from within pro-feminism have shaped different practices with men. Each of these different approaches reflect different understandings of feminism.

The early debates were between liberal pro-feminist and radical pro-feminist men. Nearly 25 years ago, Clatterbaugh (1990) noted the differences between focusing on perceived symmetries between women and men in terms of limitations of male and female sex roles in liberal pro-feminism and the focus on male privilege and power in radical pro-feminism.

Liberal feminism is largely focused on campaigns for gender balance within the government and corporate sectors. This approach regards men as having a positive contribution to make to addressing gender inequality (Holmgren & Hearn, 2009). Radical and socialist feminists argue, however, that this approach fails to consider the extent of men's dominance and are concerned that gender balance approaches often mean that women are pressured to become like men to attain positions of power. For them, a radical transformation of patriarchy is required to address gender inequality (Holmgren & Hearn, 2009).

Blais and Dupuis-Deri (2011) argue that contemporary developments in liberal pro-feminism are not at all concerned with women's oppression but rather are focused primarily on the issues facing men. This form of pro-feminism is shaped by individualism and still informed by sex role theories. They argue that this form of pro-feminism is anti-feminist in its politics and practices.

Pro-feminist strategies that focus on macro-structural issues are informed by radical feminist and socialist feminist theories, both of which were part of second-wave feminism. In these views, men's subjectivities and practices are interconnected to macro-level power structures. These approaches are less concerned with men's identities and the problems they face associated with these identities, and more concerned with changes in the structural dimensions of gender inequality (Ashe, 2011).

Beasley (2005) locates pro-feminism's largely sociological orientation to social theories in the 1980s and 1990s. She argues that pro-feminist masculinity studies is predominantly modernist in its approach to gender inequality and maintains that it has largely ignored or dismissed the postmodern and post-structural turn in feminist theories. While she does not argue explicitly that these 'older' theoretical frameworks are necessarily less useful for pro-feminism, it is inferred that pro-feminism has fallen behind the newer theoretical developments within feminism.

Post-structural feminist perspectives are critical of the centralised model of power underpinning the concept of patriarchy, and emphasise the multiplicity of power in localised contexts (Ashe, 2011). Third-wave feminism, as it is sometimes referred to, focuses on gender primarily as a form of self-presentation and lifestyle choices. Some forms of third-wave feminism suggest that feminism is no long necessary as a social movement for women's empowerment and gender equality (Bailey, 2012). I argue here that third-wave feminism does not provide a solid foundation for pro-feminist practice with men in social work.

Diversifying men and masculinities

We are now entering a new stage in which variations among men are seen as central to the understanding of men's lives. Thus, we cannot speak of masculinity as a singular term but rather should explore masculinities. Men are as socially diverse as women and this diversity entails differences between men in relation to class, ethnicity, age, sexuality, bodily facility, religion, world views, parental/marital status, occupation and propensity for violence.

Differences are also found across cultures and through historical time. The discourse about 'masculinity' is constructed out of 5 per cent of the world's population of men, in one region of the world, at one moment in history. We know from ethnographic work in different cultures that non-western masculinities can be very different from the western norm (Connell, 2000).

Because men are not homogeneous, they do not benefit equally from the operation of the structures of gender domination. Issues of race, sexuality, class, disability and age significantly affect the extent to which men benefit from patriarchy. Thus some men in social work will experience marginalisation on the basis of their class origins, sexuality, level of able-bodiedness and ethnicity or race (Pease, 2000). These other social divisions will complicate men's gender dominance in social work.

An intersectional analysis makes it clear that almost everyone experiences both privilege and subordination. Multiple forms of social difference shape both unities among and differences between men. Such an analysis provides a framework for designing interventions with men that take into account their different positionings in relation to privilege and oppression.

Messner (1997) argues that pro-feminist men should place multi-racial feminism with its respect for difference at the centre of their strategies. There is an ongoing debate within pro-feminism, however, about the focus on difference and diversity in men's lives and what this means for analysing men's structural power and dominance as men. There is concern among many feminist women and pro-feminist men that focusing on multiple masculinities shifts attention away from the power differences between women and men.

Schwalbe (2014) critiques the concept of multiple masculinities for obscuring men's privileged positioning within structurally based gender inequality. He argues that this leads to a de-radicalisation of gender theory. For him, masculinity has become separated from men's domination of women. The approach to pro-feminist social work practice advocated here maintains an emphasis on men's institutionalised privilege and power.

Working with men at multiple levels in social work

Pringle (1995) identifies four levels in which male social workers should engage in anti-oppressive practice: one's own behaviour, individual work, group work and structural change at the community and societal levels.[3] Notwithstanding the developments within pro-feminism in the last 20 years, this is still a useful framework to unravel the various dimensions of pro-feminist social work practice with men.

Working on one's own social location and behaviour

The starting point for men's pro-feminist practice with men must thus involve a critical reflection upon the privileges associated with men's own position in the gender order and the gendered division of labour within social work.

While social work is often regarded as a 'women's profession' due to its female majority workforce, predominantly female clientele and its association with caring, many of the values associated with hegemonic masculinity such as emotional distance, rationality and technical expertise are also characteristic of social work (Pringle, 1995; Christie, 1998). In fact, Orme (2009) argues that social work practice is predominantly a rational-technical project that reflects dominant forms of masculinity.

Women's majority status in social work leads to social work being referred to as a female-dominated profession (Simpson, 2004). McPhail (2004) challenges the representation of social work as a female-dominated profession because, although women constitute the majority of members, they do not have control of the profession. McPhail argues that framing social work as a female-dominated profession hides sexism and male prejudice within social work. In her view, it is more accurate to refer to social work as a 'male-dominated female majority profession'.

Men are shown to be over-represented in both management and higher status jobs in the social services. Studies of social workers demonstrate that women are less likely than men to be undertaking managerial roles in the human services and that women in these roles earn less money than men in comparable positions (Anastas, 2007; Bent-Goodley & Sarnoff, 2008; Sakamoto et al., 2008). These inequalities are reflected in various forms of horizontal and vertical occupational segregation in social work. Notwithstanding the influence of feminist ideas on social work, I argue here that the social work profession still retains patriarchal gendered practices and that these gendered practices can be understood as representing an unequal gender regime.

Christie (2001) has stressed the importance of male social workers critically reflecting upon and challenging their gendered privilege and the gendered nature of their work. Pringle similarly argues that male social workers 'have a particular responsibility to engage in challenging those oppressive structures of power from which they may benefit directly' (2001, p. 45). This requires male social workers to monitor and challenge their own behaviour. It also means that male social workers need to recognise the contradictions and dilemmas arising from their position.

Individual work with men

Men often want things to change but they do not want to relinquish their power. A pro-feminist approach encourages men to rethink their power. It involves what Cree calls 'critical engagement': how to 'build open connection with men while at the same time not being seen to condone their behaviour or attitudes' (2001, p. 161).

Many of the beliefs men hold are the cause of the troubles in their lives. Thus, the starting point for work with men is to assess their beliefs. What beliefs does the man hold about masculinity? What are the sources of these beliefs? What are the potential harmful effects of these beliefs? (Allen & Gordon, 1990). Men's socialisation leads to individual beliefs that can promote abusive behaviours (Russell, 1995). Men need to be helped to acknowledge their tendencies to act oppressively and they should be assisted to devise strategies to avoid those situations and change their behaviour. They should also be encouraged to develop wider repertoires of behaviour and models of masculinity not associated with violence, control and objectification (Pringle, 1995).

Feminist social work with women has been guided by the recognition that women's individual struggles are located in oppressive social arrangements (Goodman et al., 2004). Likewise, pro-feminist social work with men must locate men within the context of patriarchy and the divisions of class, race, sexuality, age and other forms of social inequality, while at the same time exploring ways in which patriarchal belief systems become embedded in men's psyches (Pease, 2009).

Social work with men that does not acknowledge the existence of gender power inequalities is likely to reproduce men's dominance over their female partners. The failure to view men's relationships with women in the context of a wider relational and structural context will end up endorsing men's sexism and coercive control over women's lives (Dolan-Del Vecchio, 1998). If social work with men is to encourage greater empathy and respect for women it will need to address gender-based inequalities in their relationships with women.

Group work with men

Anti-patriarchal consciousness-raising group work with men can clarify the social dimensions of and historical shifts in masculinities (Pease, 2003). Such consciousness raising in men's groups can provide a link between personal experiences and the wider social context of men's lives. Men can come to understand their own sexist behaviour and develop emotional support for other men to encourage their anti-sexism.

Pro-feminist group work emphasises the importance of working in groups with men who oppress and disempower others, where men's prejudices and oppressive behaviours can be challenged (Pringle, 1995). As Hearn (2001) comments, pro-feminist group work models educate men about the oppressiveness of their beliefs and behaviours and involve them in analysing their use of power and control tactics to enable them to move towards more equal relationships with women.

I have been running workshops for men for some years aimed at engaging men's emotions in challenging their privilege. I aim to foster social empathy in men by encouraging their understanding of the consequences of men's structural power and privilege for women. A practice that I have used here is facilitating Patriarchy Awareness Workshops based on the Racism Awareness model. These workshops use presentations, small-group discussions and simulation exercises to explore such issues as analyses of patriarchal culture, men's experience of power and domination, alternatives to patriarchal power, the impact of men's domination on women, social and personal blocks to men's ability to listen to women, and visions and potential for men to change. The workshop provides an opportunity for men to move beyond their feelings of powerlessness in relation to gender issues and to identify ways of taking pro-feminist men's politics beyond the arena of personal change to incorporate collectivist and public political action (Pease, 2012).

Creating change at community and societal levels

Feminist and pro-feminist writers in social work emphasise that personal change does not go far enough and advocate the importance of connecting personal change with cultural and structural change (Cree, 2001; Pease, 2004–2005). Work with men should be one aspect of a broader strategy for changing unequal power relations between women and men.

For example, men need to become more actively involved as partners with women in social movements against violence towards women. However, as the involvement of men in men's violence prevention has become more widely supported, I have become concerned that the tensions, dilemmas and dangers of such involvement have not been adequately addressed These dangers include: reducing funding for women's services and programmes, weakening the feminist orientation, silencing women, taking over the campaign, colluding with violent men, gaining more praise and failing to earn women's trust (Pease, 2008).

When developing alliances between women and men, particular conditions need to be met and specific principles need to be adopted to address the potential problems associated with such partnerships (Pease, 2008). The theoretical premises underpinning men's involvement in violence prevention need to be based upon feminist theory and the critical scholarship on men and masculinities. We have to ensure that, in involving men in men's violence prevention, we do not replicate the same structures and processes that reproduce the violence we are challenging.

Conclusion

If we fail to examine the social construction of masculinities in social work, we will be unable to acknowledge the ways in which masculinities impact upon women's lives. To the extent that issues of men and masculinity are discussed in social work, the focus tends to be on the costs of sexism for men and how such costs may encourage men to be more responsive to feminism (Christie, 1998; Lloyd & Degenhardt, 1996).

It is important that social work with men locates men's lives within an understanding of patriarchal gender relations and that such work is committed to transforming those gender relations. While men's gendered belief systems are only a part of the processes that perpetuate gendered inequality, they are amenable to intervention at the individual level and hence challenging men's abusive beliefs makes an important contribution to respectful and egalitarian practices (Featherstone et al., 2007).

If we are to engage more men in pro-feminist social work, we need to open up a debate within the profession and within social work education about the gendered nature of caring work. The social work profession and social work education need to interrogate the gendered assumptions about nurturing, caring, intimacy and love which are embedded within social work. Ascribing caring to women and femininity reproduces patriarchal discourses by devaluing women's practices in social work and legitimating men's avoidance of caring (Camilleri & Jones, 2001). The challenge for the profession is to encourage men and women in social work to understand how affective inequalities in the doing and receiving of care and love reproduce inequalities in economic, political and social relations (Lynch et al., 2009). Thus, fostering caregiving masculinities (Hanlon, 2009) is an essential part of promoting gender equality in the profession and the wider society.

There are progressive and important roles for men in social work in promoting a more egalitarian profession. However, we need to be clear about what constitutes 'good practice' for men and be aware of the dangers and problems, as well as the possibilities, associated with increasing men's presence in social work.

Clearly, some men in social work do not subscribe to dominant forms of masculinity. Social work as a profession needs more men who are critical of hegemonic masculinity and who are aware of the gendered injustices associated with male privilege and unearned entitlements. However, I argue that, if men in social work are not actively promoting pro-feminist practices, they will reproduce an unequal gender regime within the profession.

Notes

1 I use the language of 'pro-feminism' to articulate men's support for a feminist perspective. I believe that men should not call themselves feminists both because feminism is grounded in women's experiences of patriarchy and because I believe that there are dangers in men appropriating women's work. I recognise, however, that some men committed to feminism may not necessarily share this distinction.
2 While the debates within critical masculinity studies and pro-feminism have developed significantly over the last 20 years, these developments have had very little impact on extending pro-feminism among men in social work.
3 In this section of the chapter, my focus is on male social workers who work with men. While there are similarities between how men and women might address male privilege in working with men, female workers also face different issues which I have not addressed here (see for example, Cavanagh & Cree, 1996; Walker, 2001).

Further reading

Cavanagh, K. & Cree, V. (eds) (1996) *Working with Men: Feminism and Social Work.* Routledge, London.
Christie, A. (ed.) (2001) *Men and Social Work: Theories and Practice.* Palgrave, London.
Featherstone, B., Rivett, M. & Scourfield, J. (2007) *Working with Men in Health and Social Care.* Sage, London.
Pease, B. & Camilleri, P. (eds) (2001) *Working with Men in the Human Services.* Allen & Unwin, Sydney.
Scourfield, J. (2003) *Gender and Child Protection.* Palgrave, Basingstoke, UK.

References

Allen, J. & Gordon, S. (1990) Creating a framework for change. In R. Meth & R. Pasick (eds), *Men in Therapy: The Challenge of Change.* Guilford Press, New York, pp. 131–151.
Anastas, J. (2007) Theorizing (in)equity for women in social work. *AFFILIA: The Journal of Women and Social Work*, 22(3), pp. 235–239.
Ashe, F. (2011) *The New Politics of Masculinity: Men, Power and Resistance.* Routledge, New York.
Bailey, J. (2012) *What Happens when Men get Involved in Feminism? Contemporary Mixed Gender Activism in England.* PhD thesis, University of Sheffield, Sheffield.
Beasley, C. (2005) *Gender and Sexuality: Critical Theories, Critical Thinkers.* Sage, London.

Bent-Goodley, T. & Sarnoff, S. (2008) The role and status of women in social work education: past and future considerations. *Journal of Social Work Education*, 44(1), pp. 1–8.

Blais, M. & Dupuis-Deri, F. (2011) The masks of anti-feminism: 'masculinity in crisis', 'masculinism' and 'liberal profemism'. *European Women's Voice*, Autumn, pp. 13–17.

Camilleri, P. & Jones, P. (2001) Doing women's work? Men, masculinity and caring. In B. Pease & P. Camilleri (eds), *Working with Men in the Human Services*. Allen & Unwin, Sydney, pp. 25–33.

Cavanagh, K. & Cree, V. (eds) (1996) *Working with Men: Feminism and Social Work*. Routledge, London.

Christie, A. (1998) Is social work a 'non-traditional' occupation for men? *British Journal of Social Work*, 28, pp. 491–510.

Christie, A. (2001) Gendered discourses of welfare, men and social work. In A. Christie (ed.), *Men and Social Work: Theories and Practice*. Palgrave, London, pp. 7–34.

Clatterbaugh, K. (1990) *Contemporary Perspectives on Masculinity: Men, Women and Politics in Modern Society*. Westview Press, Boulder, CO.

Connell, R. (1995) *Masculinities*. Allen & Unwin, Sydney.

Connell, R. (2000) *The Men and the Boys*. Allen & Unwin, Sydney.

Connell, R. & Messerschmidt, J. (2005) Hegemonic masculinity: rethinking the concept. *Gender and Society*, 19(6), pp. 829–859.

Cowburn, M. & Pengally, H. (1999) Values and processes in groupwork with men. In J. Wild (ed.) *Working with Men for Change*. UCL Press, London, pp. 197–206.

Cree, V. (2001) Men and masculinities in social work education. In A. Christie (ed.), *Men and Social Work: Theories and Practices*. Palgrave, London, pp. 147–163.

Dolan-Del Vecchio, K. (1998) Dismantling white male privilege within family therapy. In M. McGoldrick (ed.), *Re-Visioning Family Therapy: Race, Culture, and Gender in Clinical Practice*. Guilford Press, New York, pp. 159–175.

Dominelli, L. (1999) Working with men from a feminist perspective. In J. Wild (ed.), *Working With Men for Change*. UCL Press, London, pp. 17–38.

Douglas, P. (1993) Men equals violence: a profeminist perspective on dismantling the masculine equation. Paper presented at the Second National Conference on Violence, Australian Institute of Criminology, Canberra, 15–18 June.

Featherstone, B., Rivett, M. & Scourfield, J. (2007) *Working with Men in Health and Social Care*. Sage, London.

Goodman, L., Liang, B., Helms, J., Latta, R., Sparks, E. & Weintraub, S. (2004) Training counseling psychologists as social justice agents: feminist and multicultural principles in action. *Counseling Psychologist*, 32, pp. 793–837.

Hanlon, N. (2009) Caregiving masculinities: an exploratory analysis. In K. Lynch, J. Baker & M. Lyons (eds), *Affective Equality: Love, Care and Injustice*. Macmillan, Basingstoke, UK, pp. 180–198.

Hanmer, J. (1990) Men, power and the exploitation of women. In J. Hearn & D. Morgan (eds), *Men, Masculinities and Social Theory*. Unwin Hyman, London, pp. 21–42.

Hearn, J. (2001) Men, social work and men's violence towards women. In A. Christie (ed.), *Men and Social Work: Theories and Practice*. Palgrave, London, pp. 63–86.

Holmgren, L. & Hearn, J. (2009) Framing 'men in feminism': theoretical locations, local contexts and practical passings in men's gender-conscious positionings on gender equality and feminism. *Journal of Gender Studies*, 18(4), pp. 403–418.

Horrocks, R. (1994) *Masculinity in Crisis.* St Martin's Press, London.

Hyde, C. & Bricker-Jenkins, M. (1995) Women's studies or gender studies: a feminist discussion. *Journal of Social Work Education,* 31(3), pp. 310–321.

Johnson, A. (1997) *The Gender Knot: Unravelling the Patriarchal Legacy.* Temple University Press, Philadelphia, PA.

Kaufman, M. (1994) *Cracking the Armour: Power, Pain and the Lives of Men.* Viking, Toronto.

Lichtenberg, P. (1999) Men: overview. In R.L. Edwards & J.G. Hopps (eds), *Encyclopedia of Social Work,* 19th edn. National Association of Social Workers, Washington, DC, pp. 1691–1697.

Lloyd, S. & Degenhardt, D. (1996) Challenges in working with male social work students. In K. Cavanagh & V. Cree (eds), *Working with Men: Feminism and Social Work.* Routledge, London, pp. 45–64.

Luck, M. & Jackson, D. (1995) The exploration of men and masculinities from an anti-sexist perspective. *International Association of the Study of Men Newsletter,* 3(2), p. 5.

Lynch, K., Baker, J., Cantillon, S. & Walsh, J. (2009) Which equalities matter? The place of affective equality in egalitarian thinking. In K. Lynch, J. Baker & M. Lyons (eds), *Affective Equality: Love, Care and Injustice.* Palgrave Macmillan, Basingstoke, UK, pp. 12–34.

McPhail, B. (2004) Setting the record straight: social work is not a female-dominated profession. *Social Work,* 49(2), pp. 323–326.

May, L. (1998) A progressive male standpoint. In T. Digby (ed.), *Men Doing Feminism.* Routledge, New York, pp. 337–354.

Messner, M. (1997) *Politics of Masculinities: Men in Movements.* Sage, Thousand Oaks, CA.

Mills, M. (1998) *Challenging Violence in Schools: Disruptive Moments in the Educational Politics of Masculinity.* PhD thesis, University of Queensland, Brisbane.

Orme, J. (2009) Feminist social work. In M. Gray & S. Webb (eds), *Social Work: Theories and Methods.* Sage, London, pp. 87–98.

Pease, B. (1987) *Towards a Socialist Praxis in Social Work.* Master of Behavioural Science Thesis, La Trobe University, Melbourne.

Pease, B. (1990) Towards collaborative research on socialist theory and practice in social work. In J. Petruchenia & R. Thorpe (eds), *Social Change and Social Welfare Practice.* Hale & Iremonger, Sydney, pp. 86–100.

Pease, B. (1995) MASA: men against sexual assault. In W. Weeks & J. Wilson (eds), *Issues Facing Australian Families,* 2nd edn. Longman Cheshire, Melbourne, pp. 258–266.

Pease, B. (1997) Teaching anti-patriarchal men's studies in social work. *Issues in Social Work Education,* 17(1), pp. 3–17.

Pease, B. (2000) *Recreating Men: Postmodern Masculinity Politics.* Sage, London.

Pease, B. (2002) *Men and Gender Relations.* Tertiary Press, Melbourne.

Pease, B. (2003) Critical reflections on profeminist practice in men's groups. In M. Cohen & A. Mullender (eds), *Gender and Social Groupwork.* Routledge, London, pp. 53–65.

Pease, B. (2004–2005) Rethinking profeminist men's behaviour change programs. *Women Against Violence,* 16, pp. 32–40.

Pease, B. (2008) *Engaging Men in Violence Prevention: Exploring the Tensions, Dilemmas and Possibilities,* Issues Paper 17. Australian Domestic and Family Violence Clearinghouse, University of NSW, Sydney.

Pease, B. (2009) Challenges and directions for profeminist practice with men. In J. Allan, L. Briskman & B. Pease (eds), *Critical Social Work: Theories and Practices for a Socially Just World*, 2nd edn. Allen & Unwin, Sydney, pp. 160–174.

Pease, B. (2012) The politics of gendered emotions: disrupting men's emotional investments in privilege. *Australian Journal of Social Issues*, 47(1), pp. 125–140.

Pringle, K. (1995) *Men, Masculinities and Social Welfare*. UCL Press, London.

Pringle, K. (2001) Men in social work: the double edge. In A. Christie (ed.), *Men and Social Work: Theories and Practice*. Palgrave, London, pp. 35–48.

Ridgeway, C. & Correll, S. (2004) Unpacking the gender system: a theoretical perspective on gender beliefs and social relations. *Gender and Society*, 18(4), pp. 510–531.

Russell, M. (1995) *Confronting Abusive Beliefs: Group Treatment for Abusive Men*. Sage, Thousand Oaks, CA.

Sakamoto, I., McPhail, B., Anastas, J. & Colarossi, L. (2008) Status of women in social work education. *Journal of Social Work Education*, 44(1), pp. 37–62.

Schwalbe, M. (2014) *Manhood Acts: Gender and the Practices of Domination*. Paradigm Publishers, Boulder, CO.

Simpson, R. (2004) Masculinity at work: the experiences of men in female dominated occupations. *Work, Employment and Society*, 18(2), pp. 349–368.

Thorne-Finch, R. (1992) *Ending the Silence: The Origins and Treatment of Male Violence Against Women*. University of Toronto Press, Toronto.

Tolman, R., Mowry, D., Jones, L. & Brekke, J. (1986) Developing a profeminist commitment among men in social work. In N. van Den Bergh & L. Cooper (eds), *Feminist Visions for Social Work*. National Association of Social Workers, New York, pp. 61–79.

Walker, L. (2001) A feminist perspective on men in emotional pain. In G. Brooks & G. Good (eds), *The New Handbook of Psychotherapy and Counseling with Men*. Jossey-Bass, San Francisco, CA, pp. 683–695.

Whitehead, S. (2002) *Men and Masculinities: Key Themes and New Directions*, Polity Press, Cambridge, UK.

Conclusion

Sarah Wendt and Nicole Moulding

In this concluding chapter, we draw together key ideas about contemporary feminist social work that have emerged throughout the book, and highlight the different ways in which feminism remains central, even indispensable, to social work knowledge, ethics and practice. We outline these ideas not as universal statements of what feminist social work is or should be, but as principles that seem common to feminist social work across diverse theoretical traditions and practice contexts. We also consider what feminist social work into the twenty-first century might look like, identifying some of the main challenges we face as in a rapidly changing global context.

To briefly recap, the book has explored the centrality of feminism to social work at two main levels: conceptually and in terms of day-to-day practice. Thus, the first part of the book involved critical feminist discussion of the core theoretical concepts and practice modalities that comprise social work. Social work theory, ethics, research, leadership, community development, policy, organisations and globalisation were therefore considered but with the question of gender at the forefront. The book then showcased the many and varied feminist projects within social work, including feminist-informed approaches to working with Indigenous communities, refugees, older women, women living with disabilities and feminist approaches to mental health, homelessness, sexualities, domestic violence, rape and sexual assault and child wellbeing. Throughout the different chapters, authors have offered up a range of feminist theoretical frameworks for viewing the world, and demonstrated how these influence their approaches to practice. Some authors have explicitly subscribed to a particular set of ideas within feminist scholarship, including Carole Zufferey's use of intersectional feminism in exploring women's homelessness; Annie Pullen Sansfaçon's engagement with standpoint theory to explore ethics, Barbara Fawcett's post-structural feminist approach to women and disability; Margaret Rowntree's engagement with materialist feminism to explore sexualities in social work; and Fiona Buchanan's use of radical feminism to examine working with children. Other authors have traversed a range of different feminist theories in order to elaborate the particular social problem in question. For example, Deirdre Tedmanson and Christine Fejo-King drew on postcolonial theory and standpoint feminism in their exploration of Indigenous issues; Laurie Cook Heffron, Susanna Snyder, Karin Wachter, Maura Nsonwu and Noël Busch-Armendariz draw from postcolonial, Chicana, anti-oppression and black feminist scholarship; while Nicole Moulding applied the concept of situated intersubjectivity to navigate the discursive and material dimensions of women's mental health experiences. In some ways, then, it could be argued that the book reflects the coming together of modernist and postmodernist feminist traditions that is occurring more broadly in feminist scholarship and perhaps to a lesser extent across the social sciences more generally at this point in time. Finally, some authors do not name a specific feminist theoretical approach but a feminist lens is nonetheless adopted that reflects this diversity of feminist thought over the past four decades. Most importantly, this combined effort in feminist scholarship is illustrative of how feminism is flourishing in contemporary social work across diverse areas of knowledge and practice. Thus, while there is no one single accepted version of feminism, the authors in this book have shown that feminism nonetheless provides an important critical lens for social workers in engaging with their practice worlds. This engagement enables acknowledgement of the gender relations framing women's and men's lives, and analysis, theorisation and thoughtful, feminist-informed responses to the social problems encountered in day-to-day practice. The chapters in this book therefore represent a celebration of the sophisticated development of diverse feminisms within social work over the past 40 years.

Within the richness, complexity and diversity of feminist social work that is captured in this book there are nevertheless some key ideas that have emerged which are important to acknowledge because they speak to the challenges facing contemporary social work at this historical juncture. This is not an attempt to try and pin down any one feminism for social work but instead to highlight some 'key (anchoring) principles and practices' of feminism that are visible in social work today (Lazzari, Colarossi & Collins, 2009, p. 351). It is these principles and practices that enable the visibility and growth of feminism within social work, offering an anchoring point for further conversation and recognition into the future.

1   Feminism promotes social justice

As Mel Gray and Lake Schubert point out in their chapter, feminism promotes a social justice agenda because it seeks change and empowerment. With all of its diversity, at its heart, feminism is primarily about the attainment of a more just society through critical thinking, empowerment and social change. As such, gender inequality is named and discussed throughout all of the chapters. For example, Margaret Alston, Lena Dominelli, Lesley Laing, Sue King and Deidre Tedmanson opened up conversations about women's equality and wellbeing in terms of policy, community and global development. The critical lens used by these authors provided valuable insights into relations of power and gender inequalities. They showed how the 'masculine' is often constructed as the norm in social, economic and environmental initiatives and politics. At the same time, they emphasised the exclusion of women in policy, global development and service delivery. Feminism therefore enables a questioning of power and knowledge, and foreshadows the need for collective action that aims to support women in the shaping of their own futures.

2 Feminism promotes reflexivity and reflective practice

The different authors have shown that it is common practice for feminist social workers to acknowledge positions of power and privilege related to race, class and other social positionings in addition to gender in their theorising, research and practice. For example, Laurie Cook Heffron, Susanna Snyder, Karin Wachter, Maura Nsonwu and Noël Busch-Armendariz acknowledge the risk of speaking 'for' rather than 'with' refugee women because of positions of power and privilege related to race, class and formal education. Deirdre Tedmanson and Christine Fejo-King exposed and explored subtle performances of everyday racism. In both of these cases, the authors explored claims of knowing and highlighted the importance of reflexivity for feminism and social work so that alternative ways of being and knowing are recognised. Bob Pease demonstrated his own growth and insights about working in feminist-informed ways as a male social worker. More generally, Lia Bryant opened up a conversation about the production of knowledge in social work while Sarah Wendt argued that the self-critical stance and diverse nature of feminism, and its acknowledgement and tolerance of contradiction, represents an embrace of reflexivity that is vital for the future of social work knowledge and practice.

3 Feminisms are about relationships and inclusive styles of engagement

Feminisms ground their perspectives in the experiences of women and hence feminist social workers aim to be highly engaged and inclusive in their scholarship and practice. All authors consider relationships in their chapters in different ways. For example, Annie Pullen Sansfaçon provided a rich description of relationships and inclusive engagement in her chapter on ethics. She draws on her own experiences and advocacy work related to human rights of trans children and young people. Sarah Wendt draws on her years of relationship building in the domestic violence field and quotes women's stories from her own research to form her arguments about the gendered nature of domestic violence. Carole Zufferey engages with intersectional feminism to broaden feminist activism in the areas of homelessness and build more inclusive engagements with different groups of women experiencing homelessness.

4 Feminism involves critical and contextual analysis of power

As Swigonski and Raheim (2011) point out, analysing power is a key idea within feminism but it is also central to social work. All chapters in the book feature critical discussions about power. There were reflections about one's own power as a feminist social worker, and the power dynamics in social work more generally. There was also exploration of the ways gender frames women's experiences, engaging with both modernist and postmodernist notions of power. Thus, attention was drawn to how gender power relations frame women's lived experiences of violence and abuse, poverty, inequality and discrimination, but attention was also devoted to the connections between power and knowledge, and the effects of dominant gender discourses and their implications for women's understandings and experiences. Power was also theorised at a number of different levels including structural and institutional, interpersonal and interrelational, and at the level of the individual. The nature of power, sources of power, access to power and how power is exercised, were therefore questioned, and debated throughout. For example, within the mental health arena, Nicole Moulding argued that feminist-informed approaches enable a more situated perspective that locates women's distress in the contradictory gender discourses and power relations that frame their lives, thereby avoiding victim blaming and offering greater scope for both individual and social change. Fiona Buchanan opened up conversations about how particular approaches in social work, such as attachment theory, do not consider gendered roles and unequal power relations within families, including the disempowering impact of gendered expectations on mothering. Barbara Fawcett argued that feminism enables a challenging of taken-for-granted assumptions and a questioning of knowledge claims in the field of disability.

5 Feminism values intersectional and fluid identities

Melanie Shepard and Lake Dziengel point out that feminism is well positioned to provide a paradigm for examining and deconstructing gender in social work. Through engagement with intersectional theory, feminism has committed to a more inclusive approach to other social positionings such as those of race, class and sexual orientation. For example, Fiona Buchanan and Lynn Jamieson argue that in situations of rape and sexual assault, the lens of intersectional feminism makes more visible women's experiences across diverse ages, abilities, cultures, socio-economic classes and sex-gender identities, such as lesbian and trans-sexual women. Jill Chonody and Barbra Teater examine age, gender, power and the intersection of oppression throughout the life span, arguing that this allows a better understanding of social relationships, care giving, work, income and retirement, health care, social and personal issues, and abuse as they are experienced across different groups of women. Through engagement with post-structuralism and the influence of postmodernism, feminism has also demonstrated that gender is a social construct that is fluid and diverse. Gender is theorised as not something people have but rather something they do (Swigonski & Raheim, 2011). For example, Margaret Rowntree engaged with feminist philosopher Rosi Braidotti and her materialist theory of becoming, applying this to sexualities in social work. In contrast, Nicole Moulding showed how contradictions between generic selfhood and feminine identities can be reinforced by gendered violence and abuse, and implicated in women's emotional distress.

6 Feminism acknowledges the relationship between the personal and political

The slogan of the personal is political is longstanding in feminism, emanating as it does from the second wave. However, this book has shown how relevant this position remains across diverse contemporary feminisms. In every feminist tradition, the valuing of personal experience and the positioning of it in the political realm remains a powerful means of drawing attention to discrimination and formulating challenges to oppressive structures, discourses and practices. Within this value base is a respect and affirmation of women's agency and the importance of local contexts. Feminist social workers have successfully led diverse research and practice projects through respecting the lived everyday experiences of women's lives in an effort to name multiple challenges and enable change.

This is a critically important time for feminist social work on a number of fronts. Challenges include responding to the effects of rapid globalisation and growing socioeconomic inequalities within and between countries in the context of the continued rationalisations of government spending. Gender is at the forefront of these concerns because women are over-represented among those living in poverty, while the gender pay gap in some countries, including Australia, has widened over the past two decades. Gendered violence and abuse continue at high rates in all countries across the globe, forcing many women and their children into poverty and placing their lives, as well as their physical and mental wellbeing, at significant risk. Women's reproductive rights are continually under siege, reminding us that the gains won by the feminist movement can never be taken for granted. However, young women appear to be re-engaging with feminist ideas after a period of retreat, with the internet a new and significant force in contemporary feminist thought, organisation and action.

The digital realm is a medium that social work is yet to engage fully with, offering enormous potential for the development of new forms of practice and social action into the future. In view of these challenges and changes, it is more important than ever that feminist social workers continue to bring a gender perspective to all levels of practice, from one-to-one and group work, to community work, policy development and social action, drawing on the wealth of feminist scholarship and activism that has been built over time and which continues to strengthen and flourish into this century.

References

Lazzari, M.M., Colarossi, L. & Collins, K.S. (2009) Feminists in social work: where have all the leaders gone? *AFFILIA: The Journal of Women and Social Work*, 24(4), pp. 348–359.

Swigonski, M. & Raheim, S. (2011) Feminist contributions to understanding women's lives and the social environment. *AFFILIA: The Journal of Women and Social Work*, 26(1), pp. 10–21.

Index

Page numbers in *italics* denote tables.

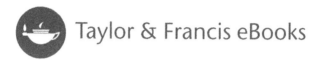

Taylor & Francis eBooks

Helping you to choose the right eBooks for your Library

Add Routledge titles to your library's digital collection today. Taylor and Francis ebooks contains over 50,000 titles in the Humanities, Social Sciences, Behavioural Sciences, Built Environment and Law.

Choose from a range of subject packages or create your own!

Benefits for you

- » Free MARC records
- » COUNTER-compliant usage statistics
- » Flexible purchase and pricing options
- » All titles DRM-free.

 REQUEST YOUR FREE INSTITUTIONAL TRIAL TODAY

Free Trials Available
We offer free trials to qualifying academic, corporate and government customers.

Benefits for your user

- » Off-site, anytime access via Athens or referring URL
- » Print or copy pages or chapters
- » Full content search
- » Bookmark, highlight and annotate text
- » Access to thousands of pages of quality research at the click of a button.

eCollections – Choose from over 30 subject eCollections, including:

Archaeology	Language Learning
Architecture	Law
Asian Studies	Literature
Business & Management	Media & Communication
Classical Studies	Middle East Studies
Construction	Music
Creative & Media Arts	Philosophy
Criminology & Criminal Justice	Planning
Economics	Politics
Education	Psychology & Mental Health
Energy	Religion
Engineering	Security
English Language & Linguistics	Social Work
Environment & Sustainability	Sociology
Geography	Sport
Health Studies	Theatre & Performance
History	Tourism, Hospitality & Events

For more information, pricing enquiries or to order a free trial, please contact your local sales team:
www.tandfebooks.com/page/sales

Routledge
Taylor & Francis Group

The home of
Routledge books

www.tandfebooks.com